The Menopause Industry

"This is the story that asks the question: Would menopausal women have become a growing market share if there were not 80% profits to be made in synthetic estrogens? Every woman approaching age 40 should read Sandra Coney's clear-eyed, carefully documented account of the dangerous duping of midlife women by the medical pharmaceutical complex. Otherwise, she may be at increased risk for breast cancer, endometrial cancer, and other serious illness associated with hormone replacement therapy (HRT).

Coney debunks the stereotypes of menopausal women as diseased by examining how different cultures approach this part of the life cycle, by sharing excerpts of her many interviews with menopausal women, and by comparing menopausal symptoms with midlife experiences of men. She quotes from pharmaceutical advertising, showing how hormone replacement therapy has been promoted to physicians, reinforcing their paternalistic attitude toward their female patients who 'see only the inevitability of old age awaiting' them.

Sandra Coney has given women an invaluable gift in *The Menopause Industry:* the facts they need to make informed decisions about their own health.

— Nancy Evans, President, Breast Cancer Action

"This book offers a unique view of menopause. Unlike Germaine Greer's *The Change,* which addresses the broad social issues, and Eileen Hechas and Denise Foley's *Unequal Treatment* which discusses the general medical neglect of women, Coney focuses on the way physicians and pharmaceutical manufacturers have changed menopause from a natural life transition into a disease requiring treatment. By labeling midlife women as estrogen-deficient, they can intervene to prevent the consequences, necessitating medical visits, tests, and hormone therapy . . . . Illustrations from drug advertisements support her thesis. A fascinating book; highly recommended for all collections."

— *Library Journal*

"Women's value has historically been tied to their ability to reproduce. Menopause, marking the end of a woman's childbearing years, is therefore more stigmatized than male midlife. Coney believes that doctors and drug manufacturers have exploited this social prejudice, and middle-aged women's attendant insecurities, by exaggerating both the menopausal 'symptoms' (hot flashes, depression, etc.) and the curative powers of estrogen and by underselling the dangers of hormone treatments . . . . Coney's depictions of the sexism surrounding the hormone craze are well supported; she provides examples of ads with misogynist slogans, such as 'Menrium treats the menopausal symptoms that bother him the most,' and doctors' descriptions of the physical unattractiveness of the postmenopausal female body . . . . [A]dds a valuable perspective to a highly charged debate."

— *Kirkus Reviews*

About the Author

Sandra Coney has been involved with women's issues for many years, particularly in the area of women's health. She has been a consumer representative on the expert group advising the New Zealand Minister of Health on a national cervical screening program and has been a member of the Working Party on Osteoporosis Prevention. She was a founding member of the feminist magazine *Broadsheet* and was one of its editors for 14 years. She lives in Auckland, New Zealand.

Other books by Sandra Coney:

Standing in the Sunshine: Centenary of Women's Suffrage in New Zealand 1893–1993 (1993)

Hysterectomy (1990)

Out of the Frying Pan (1990)

The Unfortunate Experiment (1988)

Every Girl: A Social History of Women and YWCA in Auckland (1986)

Ordering Information

Trade bookstores and wholesalers in the U.S. and Canada, please contact

Publishers Group West
4065 Hollis, Box 8843
Emeryville CA 94608
Telephone 1-800-788-3123 or (510) 658-3453
Fax (510) 658-1834

Special sales

Hunter House books are available at special discounts when purchased in bulk for sales promotions, premiums, or fundraising.
For details, please contact
Special Sales Department
Hunter House Inc.
P.O. Box 2914
Alameda CA 94501–0914
Telephone (510) 865-5282
Fax (510) 865-4295

College textbooks/course adoption orders

Please contact Hunter House at the address and phone number above.

Orders by individuals or organizations

Hunter House books are available through most bookstores or can be ordered directly from the publisher by calling toll-free
1-800-266-5592

THE
MENOPAUSE
INDUSTRY

How the Medical Establishment
Exploits Women

Sandra Coney

Library of Congress Cataloging-in-Publication Data

Coney, Sandra
The menopause industry: how the medical establishment exploits
women / Sandra Coney
p. cm.
Includes bibliographical references and index.
ISBN 0-89793-161-0 : $24.95. — ISBN 0-89793-160-2 (soft cover) : $14.95
1. Menopause—Popular works. 2. Middle aged women–Medical care–
Social aspects. 3. Women—Health and hygiene—Sociological aspects.
4. Menopause—Hormone therapy. I. Title.
RG186.C628   1994
618.1'75—dc20   94-11673

Manufactured in the United States of America

9   8   7   6   5   4   3   2   First U.S. edition

Project Credits

Project Editor: Lisa Lee   Production Manager: Paul J. Frindt
Cover design: Jil Weil Graphic Design   Book design: *Qalagraphia*
Cover photography: Julian C. R. Okwu   Model: Jeanne Brondino
Copy Editor: Janja Lalich   Research: Kate McKinley
Proofreading: Susan Burckhard   Production Assistance: María Jesús Aguiló
Sales & Marketing: Corrine M. Sahli   Publicity & Promotion: Darcy Cohan
Customer Support: Sharon R.A. Olson, Sam Brewer
Order Fulfillment: A & A Quality Shipping Services
Publisher: Kiran S. Rana
Typeset in Adobe Garamond by 847 Communications, Alameda CA
Printed and bound by Data Reproductions, Rochester Hills, MI

Contents

Important Note

The material in this book is intended to provide an overview of the medical and social issues surrounding menopause. Every effort has been made to provide accurate and dependable information.

Professionals in the field may have differing opinions and research is always taking place. Therefore, the author, publisher, and editors cannot be held responsible for any error, omission, or outdated material.

The author and publisher disclaim any liability, loss, injury, or damage incurred as a consequence, directly or indirectly, of the use and application of any of the contents of this volume.

If you have any questions or concerns about the information in this book, or your health care or treatment, please consult licensed health-care professionals.

Acknowledgments

There are a number of people who were helpful during the writing of this book. First, my thanks to the many women who responded to my request for their thoughts about menopause and aging, and also to the women whom I interviewed. Their experiences and ideas both confirmed that I was on the right track and gave me new insights into the shape this book should take. Judi Strid and Ruth Henderson helped with administrative details when I was at my most desperate about meeting my deadline.

A number of other people helped with advice on scientific matters. I would like to thank them, although it should be noted that they were not asked to endorse the contents so should not be taken to have done so. The ideas and interpretations in the book are mine alone. I received valuable advice from Associate Professor Ian Reid of the Department of Medicine at Auckland School of Medicine; Dr. Ruth Bonita of the University Geriatric Unit at Auckland School of Medicine; Dr. Helen Roberts, Medical Director of Auckland Family Planning Association; Dr. John Aiken of Tauranga; Professor Robert Beaglehole of the Department of Community Health at the Auckland School of Medicine; Betsy Marshall of the Auckland Division of the Cancer Society; and three doctors who did not wish to be named.

I would also like to thank Peter Hosking for, as always, his support and also for distracting me from my task from time to time.

My thanks to Renee for giving permission to quote from her *Broadsheet* article on menopause (Chapter 5) and Fiona Kidman and Richards Literary Agency for permission to print the poem "Doing It Badly" (Chapter 5).

Lastly, I would like to thank Barbara Seaman for her foreword and Paula Doress-Worters for her preface to this edition. I appreciate their generous words and their support.

Sandra Coney
Auckland, New Zealand

Foreword

by Barbara Seaman

"The right to choose is meaningless without the right to know."
Cindy Pearson, National Women's Health Network

"All we know for sure is that the term menopause was coined in 1821, picked up by those in the medical establishment who hoped to profit from it, and that before then women noticed only that they were growing older."
Carol Heilbrun, Author

"Menopause Manor . . . is a house or household, fully furnished with the necessities of life. In abandoning it, women have narrowed their domain and impoverished their souls. There are things the Old Woman can do, say, and think that the Woman cannot do, say, or think."
Ursula LeGuin, Author

"If you don't really need a drug, any risk is unacceptable."
Dr. Philip Corfman, FDA

This book, a hot "underground" property for the past three years, has a publishing history that is both dramatic and puzzling. It is a testimony to the importance of this information as well as to how "vested interests" can sway an industry.

The Menopause Industry was brought to my attention in 1991 by Dr. Sheldon Cherry, a gynecologist who is the author of two well-respected books on menopause. His daughter discovered Coney's book on a trip to Australia and brought it home to New York. Cherry urged me to read it, assuring me that the author's viewpoint was similar to mine. He informed me that *The Menopause Industry* was originally published by Penguin New Zealand and assumed, as I did, that Penguin USA would soon make it available here.

Were we wrong! I made numerous calls to Penguin's New York offices, and then back to Cherry. Penguin USA had never heard of this book, nor of Ms. Coney. Had I gotten the title wrong or misspelled the author's name? It was hopeless. They had no intention of publishing it, nor would they import it from their New Zealand affiliate—not even if I took five copies, which I offered to do. An employee in the Penguin publicity department did stay on the case for me, and shared my bemusement.

By 1992 it was obvious that menopause books were becoming a genre in themselves. Some achieved bestsellerdom, and many publishers were scrambling to add menopause books to their lists. Why was Penguin unwilling to bring *The Menopause Industry* to the USA, when sophisticated health professionals and patient advocates here were already giving it enthusiastic word-of-mouth advance reviews?

I tried to borrow Cherry's copy but was unsuccessful. (He might well have feared that if he didn't get it back, he would *never* be able to replace it.) I spread a wider net. It seemed everyone in the women's health movement had heard about the book, had seen reviews or excerpts, or possessed some photocopied chapters, but still lacked a copy of her own. I wrote to friends in Australia and was informed it had sold out there. I kept asking.

After substantial time, Rose Sorger of Healthsharing Women in Melbourne triumphantly obtained and mailed me a copy. Obviously, by now I harbored high expectations—but even so I was dazzled. *The Menopause Industry* is a superb book, truly a great work of investigative health reporting, and I do not use the word "great" lightly! I did feel obligated to lend my copy out (but only to the most reliable people, and with stern warnings attached). I talked the book up to every editor I ran into, some of whom made the counter-proposal that I update my own 1977 book, *Women and the Crisis in Sex Hormones* instead. I told these editors that I was flattered, but there would be no point to it. *The Menopause Industry* was the 1990s book that I wish I had written myself, but I didn't; Coney did.

Some time later, in February 1994, Sandra Coney filled in more of this intriguing publishing history. She explained to Lisa Lee, her editor on this edition:

"When it came to *The Menopause Industry*... I cannot know why Penguin Australia chose to take only 100 books, when *The Unfortunate Experiment* [Coney's earlier work] had sold thousands there, except that they had Germaine Greer's book *The Change* coming out in a couple of months after mine and chose to put their effort into that.

"Consequently, although news of my book spread through the women's health network in Australia, women couldn't get the book.

I kept on being told that women couldn't get it. By the time Penguin in Australia ordered more books, Penguin in New Zealand couldn't supply it because they had sold out and didn't reprint. When I went to Australia I had to take a box of books with me!"

So, that answered one question for me. Rose Sorger had rescued my own prized copy from the box the author carried to Australia by hand. It also answered another question. The book was scarce in Australia because of an accident in timing—the Penguin affiliate there perceived Coney's book to be in competition with Greer's, which it is not. (I would say rather that the two books complement each other and between them go far to help "debrief" the midlife reader who today is constantly brainwashed—in the magazines and papers, on TV, in some books, and in many doctor's offices—against viewing herself as a naturally healthy woman in her prime.)

But what about Penguin in the United States, where Greer is published by Knopf? Their position remains a mystery, but never mind, for at last *The Menopause Industry* is available here.

The Truth About Estrogen Replacement Therapy

In fact, the timing of this Hunter House edition may be ideal. More readers may be ready for this book than would have been in 1991, since a backlash against exaggerated claims for estrogen is now developing. For example, in November 1993 a blue ribbon panel of scientists from the Institute of Medicine roundly chastised the National Institutes of Health for concealing the real risks of estrogen in the consent forms that the agency designed for the Women's Health Initiative, a research project on hormones that will ultimately enroll 160,000 women. Under duress, the consent forms were revised in a more truthful direction, apt to discourage many prospective volunteers.

Around the same time, a chilling essay in the British journal, *Lancet,* suggested that we are awash in a "sea of estrogens," which might help explain the rise in male prostate cancer paralleling the rise in female breast cancer. (Men, too, have had immeasurable exposure to estrogens by eating commercially raised, DES-tainted beef and poultry for 35 years, and being exposed to pesticides and chemicals mimicking estrogens that are ubiquitous in our environment.)

As to the specifics of the menopause industry, Premarin is the #1 bestselling prescription drug in the United States, and with ups

and downs has remained in the top 50 since 1966. Not coinciden-
tally, in January of 1966 Dr. Robert Wilson, a handsome, avuncular
Brooklyn physician, published his bestselling tract, *Feminine Forever.*
(Only one other pharmaceutical has stayed in the top 50 as long as
Premarin—Dilantin, an anticonvulsant.)

Do not be fooled, however, into believing that most women who
start on Premarin stay with it, for they do not. A fairly well-kept
secret is that fewer than 30% of women who fill a first prescription
for Premarin are taking it at the end of a year. Most of the population
on Premarin rotates; they do not remain on it for the long haul.

Why should this be so? The first reason, oddly, is that a doctor
can make it very hard to refuse that first prescription. A certain (vo-
cal) minority of doctors are quite evangelical, pushy, unpleasant, and
even threatening to patients who don't want hormone therapy. "Don't
call me when you get your first heart attack," one doctor chided my
friend Daisy. Daisy felt she would either have to swallow her medicine or change doctors, so she walked. But Daisy is better informed
and more independent than many patients. As a medical writer she
knows that the FDA never approved Premarin for the prevention of
heart disease, and that as a woman with a uterus she would have to
take Premarin in conjunction with progestin, which would probably
have wiped out any possible, but unproven benefits of estrogen to
the heart. She also knows that Premarin increases her risk of getting
breast cancer. And above all, Daisy knew she didn't need it: she had
no hot flashes. She had no night sweats. She felt just fine. For every
woman like my friend, who refused hormone therapy, I must know
two or three others who let their doctors coerce them into giving it
a trial, who "tough it out" for a few cycles or longer, then drop off.

The second type of women who take Premarin do so for what I
consider a sensible reason: they truly suffer from temporary menopausal complaints. They take Premarin to carry them through the
rough spots, then soon taper off, perhaps adding Vitamin E, primrose
oil, or certain herbs to modulate their period of adjustment.*

Lastly, there are women who ask for Premarin and expect to love

---

* To obtain ongoing, continuously updated information on alternatives
  to hormones, consider subscribing to *A Friend Indeed for Women in the
  Prime of Life,* a monthly newsletter published in Canada by Janine
  O'Leary Cobb. For information and a sample copy: Box 1710,
  Champlain NY 12919-1710. Also read *Menopause Without Medicine*
  by Linda Ojeda, Ph.D. For information see the back of the book.

it, but are disappointed. The progestin that many now take with it is definitely not a feelgood preparation. If often causes irritability, depression, unpredictable bleeding, and on and on. Premarin alone makes some women feel euphoric, but even so, in time they may get conditions and symptoms requiring them to stop. These include, but are by no means limited to uterine cancer, rapid growth of fibroids, endometriosis, blood pressure and gallbladder disturbances, breast cancer and other breast disorders, extreme water retention and bloating, nausea, migraine, and blood clots.

Since Premarin has been available since the 1940s and a top-fifty seller since 1966, one would expect to find a plenitude of older women celebrating their 20th or 25th anniversaries on it, but this is not the case. Yes, such veteran users do exist, but in nowhere near the numbers the manufacturers would have us believe. In any circle of women, one death of an estrogen user from hormone-dependent breast cancer or uterine cancer leads most of her friends to swiftly reevaluate. (So successful have hormone promoters been in trivializing uterine cancer that most women perceive it as "mild" or "easily curable." In fact, the death rate from this cancer is 17%.)

Since 1975, when it was conclusively established that the increase in uterine cancer among Premarin users is four- to eight-fold or higher, standard practice has been to add progestin to the prescription for all women who have not had a hysterectomy. But in the words of Sheldon Cherry, "Progesterone is the wild card, an unknown." Most of the studies that indicate a beneficial effect of estrogens on blood lipids were performed on women taking estrogen alone. Unfortunately, it appears that when it comes to cardiovascular disease, any benefits of estrogen are opposed by the addition of progestin. Indeed, an article in the New England Journal of Medicine published April 14, 1994 states that "continuous estrogen-progestogen therapy seems to have deleterious effects on serum HDL cholesterol levels." Thus, even if it should one day be proven beyond any doubt that estrogen (alone!) is good for your heart, the hormone formulation that most doctors prescribe today may well be bad for it.

The Power of Vested Interests

During the 1980s I made a serious misjudgment. As the author who had first proposed the idea of patient labeling on prescription drugs

(*Doctors' Case Against the Pill,* 1969; *Free and Female,* 1972), I was approached by several key persons at government agencies, consumer organizations, and the pharmaceutical industry and asked if I would oppose the marketing of prescription drugs directly to the public *provided warnings, precautions, and contraindications were included with these advertisements.* I said this advertising was okay with me, since I trusted consumers not to part lightly with their money for powerful potions they didn't need. I even hoped that such ads might help spread understanding that, in general, "the more the pharmaceutical action, the more the reaction."

I was wrong. The ensuing magazine ads do include prescribing information, but in print so tiny that a magnifying glass is required to read it. The TV ads contain no cautionary information at all. As a result, according to a 1993 poll conducted by Scott-Levin Associates, a healthcare marketing firm in Pennsylvania, 78 percent of doctors said that patients had brought up symptoms they had seen mentioned in ads. Four years earlier, in 1989, that figure was only 30 percent. We are letting ourselves be increasingly persuaded that our normal discomforts of living are "diseases" requiring elaborate tests and heavy treatments. The model for this method of manipulation is Premarin's longstanding, highly-effective promotion of menopause as an "estrogen-deficiency disease."

We are also targeted on a slightly more subtle level. Pharmaceutical companies widely support promotional campaigns that do not directly mention brand names—and don't need to. The manufacturer of Prozac, Eli Lilly, underwrites the National Mental Health Associations's multimedia advertising campaign to "increase public awareness" about depression. The manufacturer of Premarin, Wyeth-Ayerst, sponsors osteoporosis screening and pays doctors to appear on talk shows. The doctors push estrogen treatments but eschew the name "Premarin," and they certainly do not mention who they represent. (The hosts of these shows are also to be faulted for so rarely bringing this out.)

When acquiescing to the intrusion of the prescription drug industry into mass media, I failed to foresee that I would help to silence my own voice. Now the pharmaceutical industry has power to exercise unofficial censorship, and to (largely) keep its critics out of the magazines and off the air.

In the 60s, 70s, and 80s most discussions of menopause permitted several points of view. At one extreme were the evangelistic proponents such as Robert Wilson, who maintained that every woman should take estrogen and once said to me, "They say we should do nothing to retard menopause. Just think of that. Isn't that dreadful? The estrogen regimen should start at age nine—nine to ninety. It's necessary to begin then and to check your estrogen level all through life, so that it never leaves you. Don't allow it to."

In the center were those who believed estrogen might be beneficial for many or most women, but that some conditions precluded it: cancer, blood clots, high blood pressure, and perhaps fibroids or gallbladder disease.

Lastly, in the conservative corner, were believers that hormones should be prescribed only for the relief of significant symptoms and, with rare exceptions, should be reserved for relatively short-term use of less than two years. The holders of these views are generally rendered uneasy at the prospect of long-term usage of any powerful or carcinogenic drug by healthy people. Some of these conservatives observed that estrogen therapy signaled a daring, potentially dangerous departure in "prevention," an example of what Dr. Adriane Fugh-Berman of the National Women's Health Network dubbed "disease substitution," i.e., trading off possibly lower risks of one disease for higher risks of another."

Feminists were further offended at the image of mature women conveyed in such constructs as "estrogen deficiency disease" or "outliving our ovaries," but fear of hormone toxicity was hardly limited to feminists. One need only scan the current edition of an esteemed reference work, *Goodman and Gilman's Pharmacological Basis of Therapeutics,* to discern that (thus far) estrogen's benefits to the heart and bones remain unproven or unimpressive, while its role in cancer promotion is thoroughly established. *Goodman and Gilman* conclude, "The routine, prophylactic use of estrogen is difficult to justify.... When used, estrogens should be administered in the lowest effective dose for the shortest possible time .... " These last two sentences express the essence of the conservative view. The long-term preventive benefits of hormonal treatments remain unproven; the short-term use, for symptoms, should be handled cautiously.

As a result of the vested interest pharmaceutical advertising supports, the conservative view on hormone therapy is no longer admitted on talk shows and is rarely seen in magazines that seek advertising. Instead of acknowledging the spectrum of positions, only extreme and middle-of-the-road proponents of estrogen therapy are acknowledged. That long-term hormone treatment is still controversial, still experimental, still considered dangerous by more than a few authorities is concealed from general viewers and readers. In the 90s, I have given interviews to scores of magazine writers, only to have my comments removed from the final copy. In the 90s I have been called by and booked on all three network morning programs, only to be canceled out with some lame excuse.

I share the conservative, estrogen-suspicious position with Sandra Coney and many other women.

Much of the information contained in *The Menopause Industry* has effectively been censored in recent years, and thus the publication of this exemplary book is a genuine milestone.

To fairly judge a work of health reporting or popular science there are several questions we must ask:

First, is it free of any 'conflict of interest' or is it overtly or covertly trying to sell you something?

Second, is it thoroughly researched, objective, and accurate?

Third, is it readable?

Fourth, is it sensible, profound, wise, and does it *illuminate?*

When looked at with these questions, *The Menopause Industry* seems to me to be almost perfect, a powerful and a pleasing read from an author whose gifts go beyond research and political analysis. Coney is a marvelous writer, and for that reason I believe you will take pleasure in *The Menopause Industry,* even as it rattles your confidence in modern medical practice.

Barbara Seaman is the founder of the women's health movement in the U.S. and a cofounder of the National Women's Health Network. Her first book, The Doctor's Case Against the Pill *(1969), exposed the serious health risks of oral contraceptives which were being ignored by physicians and the FDA. The book resulted in Senate hearings, patient package inserts, and an awareness among women of "informed consent."*

She has also authored Free and Female *(1972),* Women and the Crisis in Sex Hormones *(1977)—possibly the most quoted book on women's health—and* Lovely Me: The Life of Jacqueline Susann *(1987), and is a contributing editor to* Ms. *magazine. The U.S. Library of Congress called her the author who "raised sexism in health care as a worldwide issue." Her current commitments include work on designing appropriate medical responses to domestic violence, and caring for her two granddaughters while her daughter teaches at CUNY.*

Preface

by Paula B. Doress-Worters

Sandra Coney has amassed in *The Menopause Industry* a wealth of empowering information and analysis. She not only makes the research on menopausal hormone treatment accessible to the lay reader, but creates a most valuable tool for all women to demystify the medical approach to menopause.

Hormone therapy has been called a product in search of a market. Most research on menopause is designed to demonstrate the desirability of medicalized interventions. Although the use of hormones to help women cope with common signs of menopause, such as hot flashes, has been known since 1937, hormone treatment was popularized for a mass market in the 1960s. It was promoted not simply as a palliative for the discomforts of menopause but also as a panacea for "psychological problems" supposedly related to the change of life. Such claims were unproven but were treated as common knowledge. These assertions promoted a stereotyped view of postmenopausal older women as asexual, neurotic, and unattractive. As a result, exogenous estrogen was approved for prescription use without adequate testing and soon became one of the five top-selling prescription drugs.

In the mid-1970s, several studies tied the use of estrogen to an increased rate of uterine cancer, and sales plummeted. To bolster their sagging sales, drug companies began to promote hormone treatment as a way to prevent chronic diseases of aging such as osteoporosis and heart disease. So, women who had no or few discomforts due to menopause were now marketing targets for hormone treatment.

The women's health movement in the United States has been vocally critical of promotions that imply that *all* women need to be worried about osteoporosis and heart disease, rather than those who are likely to be at risk. We have also continually demanded more stringent standards before the use of unproven treatments on healthy populations.

Sandra Coney's analysis from halfway around the world reinforces the criticisms made by American feminists and brings a new perspective to these issues. Yet Coney is evenhanded in her critique, admonishing those feminists who minimize some of the difficulties women face at midlife. As Coney points out, this image may not jibe with the experience of most middle-aged and older women who face loss of status as they age. The way women are treated at midlife may exacerbate the stressfulness of menopausal discomforts and undermine our ability to experience a natural menopause and a dignified old age.

As women we learn very early in life to consult obstetrician-gynecologists (ob-gyns) about normal life events such as menstruation, sexuality, and reproduction. By the time we arrive at the midlife transition of menopause, it may seem natural to consult an ob-gyn and look to medical solutions to avoid changes and occasional minor discomforts. Yet, the majority of women manage this transition without medical intervention, and according to one of the few community-based American studies involving large numbers of women, the majority regard the cessation of menses with neutrality or relief.

We women know that too many physicians give out hormones indiscriminately to women at midlife, despite the fact that the risks and benefits of such treatment are still controversial. Physicians would do better to carefully evaluate who is likely to benefit from hormone treatment and who is not.

We also know that women who take hormones are subject to increased medical visits and are at increased risk of medical procedures and surgeries. Thus the individual woman who buys into this regimen is made increasingly dependent on the medical care system. Ironically, medical practitioners, who are taught that all of a midlife woman's problems stem from menopause, overtreat what is really a normal life transition while frequently undertreating and misdiagnosing chronic diseases in this same population. From a social policy standpoint, medical care is used more to support the hormone regimen than to serve real medical needs.

Coney's argument highlights the pitfalls of focusing on disease at midlife rather than assuming that the years from 40 to 60 are a period of health and well-being. We are made to feel that if we are not vigilant about preserving our health and if we fail to utilize the medical approach to do so, our bones will crumble and our minds and bodies deteriorate. In essence, we are asked to question nature and trust the doctors and the pharmaceutical companies.

As more women enter the middle years, we face a choice. Will we be perennial patients organizing our lives around pills and medical procedures? Will we be passive consumers of every treatment, unguent, and snake oil that promises eternal youth? Or, will we work together as a powerful constituency actively seeking empowering information to help us shape the kind of lives we want after 50? The choice is ours.

The depth of knowledge and thoughtful analysis presented in these pages can empower us. The questioning of newly "orthodox" wisdom can provide us with tools and resources for evaluating facile advice, whether from popular articles or from our health care providers. Every woman at or approaching midlife must read this book.

Paula B. Doress-Worters is the founder of the Boston Women's Health Book Collective. She is also the coauthor of The New Our Bodies, Ourselves *(1992) and* The New Ourselves, Growing Older *(1994).*

Introduction

If the world were kinder to women, this book need never have been written. The relationship between midlife women and the health system is distorted by negative stereotypes of aging women which are exploited by vested interests for their own ends. The midlife woman is oblivious to the deeply sexist ideology underlying the options that are placed before her. Naively she may think these are offered simply for her own benefit. She is not cognizant of the others whose benefit may also be served by her decisions. She is unaware too that the options themselves may be incompletely tested, that there may be considerable controversy about them in the medical literature and that doctors differ in their views.

What she is told—how much and how—is mediated by her doctor. He or she acts as a gatekeeper for medical knowledge, applying a kind of censorship system in deciding which information to hold back and which to pass on. In many cases, the information the doctor possesses has already been prepackaged by commercial interests, in the process losing a certain amount of objective truth. The end result is a woman poorly placed to decide for herself.

The Menopause Industry seeks first of all to explain the politics of medicine's interest in the midlife woman, and second, to give information. In bypassing the gatekeepers, it short-circuits the system by which women customarily obtain medical information.

Much of this book is based on research papers published in medical journals that are kept in medical school libraries. This work is not readily accessible to women but holds the key to the truth about medicine. Doctors are much more frank in the literature they produce for each other than they are to their patients. The medical literature can alert us to the risks, uncertainties, and controversies surrounding various interventions, as well as to the benefits. Women need to know the former as a balance against the latter.

In a way, this book is simply a matter of giving back to women what is rightfully theirs. The papers in medical journals are based on the experiences of women; medical knowledge has been learned on women's bodies. The medical system ordinarily considers that it "owns" this knowledge, which properly belongs to women. What I have done in *The Menopause Industry* is to reclaim that knowledge, and then interpret it from the standpoint of one of the "studied" rather than the "studiers."

The medical viewpoint is commonly biased by the ideology of medicine, which proceeds from the injunction to diagnose and treat. This is all very well when the object of interest is a sick person who has sought help; it is less appropriate when applied to populations of well people who have not asked to be treated. I have approached medical knowledge about midlife women as one of the objects of interest—a well woman at midlife—who thinks that people should be left alone to get on with their lives as much as possible. The justification for interfering in well people's lives must be firmly established before it is acted upon.

Although this is a book with a point of view, I have tried not to manipulate the information to suit my "case." My intention was to be evenhanded, so that women can decide for themselves. I was already aware of some areas of doubt. Often, however, I was surprised to find that benefits I had understood to be firmly established were not so clear-cut in the literature at all.

I am not "against" any of the interventions explored in this book. All have their place. I do believe, however, that at least some of them have been promoted to women in a widespread way before the risks and drawbacks have been fully resolved. Women are not told this. They think they are being offered something beneficial and safe when often the true situation is far more equivocal.

This book proceeds from the premise that women at midlife, which I define as around 40 to 60 years of age, should expect to be well and enjoy life, not to live life in a state of apprehension waiting for decrepitude or disease to strike. A minority of women *will* experience ill health or problems related to menopause in this age group, but the majority will not. There is something essentially irrational about persuading the majority that their wellness is conditional and that they can only ensure their good health by becoming preoccupied with disease.

A Guide to Reading
The Menopause Industry

Hormones

The two main hormones discussed in this book are the female hormones *estrogen* and *progesterone*. The principal estrogen of the postmenopause is *estrone*. Artificially produced progesterone given as a drug is called *progestogen* or *progestagen*.

Hormone replacement therapy (HRT) can consist of estrogen given alone or estrogen and progestogen combined. In much of the medical and lay literature, writers are not specific about which form they are talking about. It is important to be precise because the risks and benefits differ for the two kinds of therapy. In this book, the term hormone replacement therapy or HRT will only be used when it does not matter which form of therapy is being discussed. When it is important to differentiate, the terms *estrogen* or *unopposed therapy* will be applied to estrogen used alone, and the terms *estrogen/progestogen therapy*, *opposed therapy*, or *combined therapy* used when both hormones are discussed.

Research

This book contains considerable information taken from the results of research, and different study designs will be mentioned.

Research is *prospective* when it follows people over a period of time to see what happens to them. The form of prospective research believed to give the most reliable results is the *randomized controlled trial*. This takes a group of people and randomly allocates them into two subgroups. One group is then investigated or treated in some way, while the other group—the control group—is not investigated or treated. At the end of the study, the outcomes for the two groups are compared. A randomized controlled trial is *experimental* because it tries to change something about the first group of people through behavior or treatment.

It is not always possible to conduct randomized controlled trials to answer a research question, especially when huge groups of people would be needed to obtain reliable results or when they would need to be followed up for decades. For instance, a randomized controlled trial looking at whether HRT prevented hip fracture in women would need to follow the subjects for about 30 years—from the age at which HRT is started (usually in one's fifties) to the age at which hip fractures occur (usually the eighties). Similarly, a randomized controlled trial that wished to look at whether there was an increase in endometrial cancer in users of HRT would need to involve tens of thousands of women to detect any increase in the disease because it is an uncommon condition.

Three other types of studies are used to try to answer research questions. These are called *observational* studies because they do not intervene in the people's treatment in any way. The three types of studies, described below, are case control, cohort, and cross-sectional.

(1) The *case control study* takes people—cases—who have a particular disease or intervention and compares them to other people—controls—who do not have the disease or intervention. The study aims to discover what is different between the two types of people. For instance, if studying hip fracture, the cases would be people with hip fracture, while the controls would be people of the same age, sex, and race who had not had fractures. The research question the study might be trying to answer could be whether the people who had fewer fractures had taken postmenopausal hormones, or whether they had bigger body mass, were more active, had higher calcium intake, or smoked less.

(2) Another type of study is a *cohort study* which takes a group of healthy people and follows them forward in time. The people are divided into subgroups according to whether or not they have been exposed to a potential cause of or protection from disease. For example, a cohort of postmenopausal women might later be divided into two groups according to whether or not they were taking hormones to see if there were more or fewer breast cancer cases among the hormone users compared to nonusers after a period of time.

(3) A *cross-sectional* study measures the prevalence of a condition or disease at one point in time. For instance, to ascertain the proportion of women experiencing hot flashes, a group of women might be questioned to see how many had flashes, the severity of the flashes, and the menopausal status of the women.

Lastly, I interviewed many women and quote them throughout the book. In addition to numbers and statistics, these very real experiences of women provide the personal dimension that studies and statistics often lack.

While writing this book, I asked women to comment on their experiences. This poem from Jenny Tuck summed up for me in a few lines what my book was about. I did wonder at this point why I was bothering with thousands of words when she had captured it in a few!

This is me,
I'm fifty-three,
Jenn—y.

I'm not in the paid workforce, but I have been,
Off and on,
Moved around the country with my husband's job,
And made some wonderful women friends;
I'm on good terms with my four children,
And my nine grandchildren,
My husband, brothers, sisters, my Mum and Dad;
I'm slowly doing a social science degree and
All the Women's Studies papers I can get my hands on;
The rest of the time I play bridge and garden,
Those very white-middle-class hobbies.

I haven't had a period for a year and I'm still waiting
For the lightning bolt of menopause
To strike me;
But, no hot flashes
    no palpitations
    no depression
    no bloating
    no prickly sensations under my skin;
I can't be normal, I've always known it,
My mother told me,
My husband tells me,
And my children like to remind me;
I'm only feeling better, more positive.

I reckon that bleeding business really gets you down,
And what Margaret Mead
Called Post Menopausal Zest
Is nothing
More than a rest from having to make up that bloody
    blood
Every month.

Part One

Women at Midlife

Chapter 1

The Medicalization of Midlife

> In the detection of sickness, medicine does two things: it
> "discovers" new disorders, and it ascribes these disorders to
> concrete individuals. To discover a new category of disease is
> the pride of the medical scientist. To ascribe the pathology
> to some Tom, Dick, or Harry is the first task of the
> physician acting as a member of a consulting profession.
> Trained to "do something" and express his concern, he feels
> active, useful, and effective when he can diagnose disease.
> —Ivan Illich, *Limits to Medicine*

In the 1990s it is Sally, Helen, and Lynne, aged in their forties and
fifties, who are most at risk of being bestowed with a disease by their
physicians. Modern medicine, having long regarded her with a modicum of pity, even contempt, has "discovered" the midlife woman. She
is now a sought-after commodity. Entire health services and massive
research programs are focused on her—whether she likes it or not.

In previous years medicine treated the midlife woman as a kind
of a stateless refugee, denying her citizenship in the land of the sick.
When they visited doctors, midlife women were very likely to be
called hypochondriacs, their complaints put down to anxiety,
neuroticism, or the trauma of "the change." For a quarter-century of
her life, any complaint she reported, physical or mental, could be laid
at the door of menopause, that apparently grueling transition from
the desirable state of nubile youth to redundant old age. There were
no important disease labels to place on the midlife woman, no im-

pressive tests and treatments that could be conjured up for her benefit. Accordingly, doctors were uninterested in the midlife woman—
she was simply a nuisance, an unavoidable embarrassment in their
waiting rooms.

No more. The midlife woman is a prime target for the new pre-
vention-oriented general practice. Faced with a midlife woman, the
general practitioner can now feel active, useful, and effective. He does
not cringe when he sees this woman in the waiting room, he invites
her to come in. Research careers are being built around her: there are
doctors and medical entrepreneurs who wish to measure her bones,
her breasts, the cells on her cervix, and her hormone levels. People
build machines to scan, photograph, x-ray, and magnify the most
intimate parts of her body. The pharmaceutical companies have a veri-
table chocolate box of pills, patches, pessaries, and implants for the
midlife woman. She can swallow them, have them sewn into her flesh,
or even insert them in her vagina—from where the magic hormones
will course through her body transforming everything they touch.

The midlife woman now has her very own disease—estrogen
deficiency syndrome—specific to her sex and time of life. Medicine
has determined that in her normal state, the midlife woman is sick.
The idea of normal aging has been collapsed into a definition of
pathology. The menopause is no longer simply the end of periods or
a life stage, rather it has been construed as an illness that no woman
can escape. She will suffer from this from the moment her ovaries
start to falter until she dies—a period of at least half her lifetime. In
the eyes of the medical industry, this has raised her status enormously.
She is now diagnosable and treatable, in vast numbers. Women are
living longer. One third of all women will live well into their eighties.
The potential this provides for various interested parties is limitless.

And what of the object of all this interest—the midlife woman?
What is she to make of it all?

Modern medicine creates dilemmas for midlife women. As much
as they might feel healthy and fit in their natural state, there is always
a niggling doubt, a sneaking suspicion that some vile, sinister disease
process is all the while surreptitiously invading some body part, rendering bones in danger of imminent collapse, breasts about to erupt
with mountainous lumps. And will their vaginas wither up, as the
doctors say, cracking and desiccating like an old seed pod left too
long on the tree? Will the body inexorably sag and droop in a land-
slide of flesh, no longer able to withstand the force of gravity?

Fear has been planted in the psyche of the midlife woman. If she ignores the siren call of the medical industry, offering her longer life and the prolongation of her youth, will she pay for it somehow in the end? As she creeps around, bowed by her burdensome dowager's hump, or winces in pain on the marriage bed, will she regret her belief in herself and the normal resilience of her sex?

On the other hand, if she takes the proffered potions and pills, is she risking some other kind of retribution? Will her normal body tissues rebel and mutate, growing freakish and sick? If she takes the tests, will she only win her clean bill of health through baptism with the surgeon's knife?

My Mission Statement

The "menopause industry" in the title of this book refers to medicine's discovery of the midlife woman and looks at this industry in all its manifestations and the vested interests it serves. It is called an industry because it is managed, marketed, and makes profits. For the midlife woman it is a paradox, for it contains both potential benefit and potential harm. The trick is to gain the first, while avoiding the second. This book is offered as a tool for women to use in accomplishing that task.

Before we embark on our odyssey through the world of the midlife woman and medicine's relationship with her, it must be stressed that the subject of all this attention is *well* women. Not women who are sick, not women with disease states, but normal well women. These women may be growing older, but they have busy active lives, friendships and relationships, good times and bad times. More than at any other time of their lives, they are actors in the world.

Not every well woman is being targeted: middle-class Caucasian women are the particular object of interest. There is a logic to this for some of the health issues that will be discussed. Polynesian women, for instance, are not at risk of osteoporosis: they are protected by their race. But there are other causes for the focus on white middle-class women. These women are health conscious. They are good at attending to medical services and checkups and they wish to preserve their health because they have responsibilities—to children, aging parents, and employers.

The fact that they also have money enhances their attractiveness to the health industry. Women have more disposable income at midlife than at any other life stage. They can afford to pay for the various services being offered to them, whereas younger and older women and non-Caucasian women might not.

Middle-class Caucasian women place high value on health and their physical attractiveness. They regard these as assets, important to their social status and their sexual marketability. They may be feeling a little anxious about these assets as they enter their forties. They know that at this age serious illnesses can occur for women and, as far as beauty is concerned, in the world's eyes their worth is inexorably declining. Susan Sontag talks about "the double standard of aging" that women encounter: men's status and attractiveness is enhanced by growing older whereas women's is diminished.

> The great advantage men have is that our culture allows two standards of male beauty: the *boy* and the *man* . . . . A man does not grieve when he loses the smooth, unlined, hairless skin of a boy. For he has exchanged one form of attractiveness for another: the darker skin of a man's face, roughened by daily shaving, showing the marks of emotion and the normal lines of age.
>
> There is no equivalent of this second standard for women. The single standard of beauty for women dictates that they must go on having clear skin. Every wrinkle, every line, every gray hair, is a defeat. No wonder that no boy minds becoming a man, while even the passage from girlhood to early womanhood is experienced by many women as their downfall, for all women are trained to want to continue looking like girls.(1)*

Sontag also points out that the money and power that can come at middle age add to men's value and make them more desirable. What they do rather than how they look determines their status. On the other hand, similar success for women can lessen their attractiveness.

Far from challenging such sexist stereotypes of aging and women, medicine accommodates and even exploits them. Women are susceptible to messages that tap into these fears, promising freedom

---

* Numbers in parentheses are bibliographic references, which are listed by chapter in the References section beginning on page 331.

from ill health or the perpetuation of youthful femininity. Women, medicine tells us, will "look better" and "feel better" on hormones, as if these are legitimate indications for medical treatment. Medicine depoliticizes the situation of the midlife woman by reducing her socially-caused anxieties and complaints to "symptoms" of bodily processes that can be solved by medication. The social prejudices and stereotypes midlife women experience fuel their dependence on the health system and facilitate medical control.

Commercialism distorts the medical environment that offers these interventions to midlife women. For instance, it is common for women as young as 35 to have a baseline mammography, despite a lack of evidence that it is of any use at this age. In fact, while most women are urged to have regular mammographies starting at age 45, there is no proof of benefit from regular screening until about 50.

In the private sector, health education is employed manipulatively. To use the example of mammography again: women are not informed of the risks of false negatives, which can wrongly assure a woman she is safe, or of false positives, which can result in needless biopsies. Patient information within the private health sector often amounts to nothing more than a marketing exercise, a way of selling the service and inducing patient compliance.(2) It is notable that private mammography clinics tend to be sited in affluent areas within easy reach of middle-class Caucasian women, rather than in poorer socioeconomic areas.

The medical interventions discussed in this book are not inherently harmful. They do have benefits, but they also have risks. Women tend to be oversold the former and barely told about the latter. Although much lip service is paid to the concept of informed consent, women are not given the prerequisites necessary to achieving it.

At times, it may seem that the picture painted in this book is unduly negative. There is an explanation for this. Most readers will already have been exposed to hyped-up claims for the benefits of the various topics discussed, couched in unrealistic terms of "miracles" and "cures." Conversely, they will probably know little about the drawbacks. This book is an attempt to redress that imbalance.

As well as this, a different balance of risks and benefits has to apply when we are discussing interventions for well people. The person with a serious illness will be prepared to take risks for the chance of a cure; for the well person, the risks have to be measured, not against the gloomy prospect of continuing illness, but against their present good health. An intervention must offer a clear advantage before the risk can be contemplated. If the benefit is minimal or only remotely possible, while the risk is grave, it would seem irrational to recommend it.

This understanding has led to a cautious approach in this book. Where adverse effects have been suggested by research, these have been fully explored. A "guilty until proven innocent" stance has been adopted, rather than the approach taken by the medical profession, which tends to be the other way around.

Such interventions as prophylactic use of hormone replacement therapy, mammographic screening for under-50-year-olds, and bone density testing have been introduced without adequate information about their safety and/or effectiveness. The research results are not yet in. In the case of HRT, the problems being grappled with by researchers are ones that have emerged from actual use of the drugs by women. The research was not done when it should have been—before the product was widely marketed.

Nevertheless, despite the lack of proof of safety or usefulness, these interventions are already on their way to becoming an accepted part of the health scene. This establishes a legitimacy for them that they have actually yet to earn. Once again, women are duped by the apparent "normality" of these interventions to believe that they must have been proved safe. Women can be oblivious to the actual controversies that rage within medical circles, the contradictory research findings, and the biases of the various parties involved. Science does not like sharing its unresolved problems with the public.

This book lays bare and explores those unresolved problems. This is not necessarily a reassuring process. More doubts may be thrown up than easy certainties. The technologies discussed are complex and difficult. While it is possible to simplify the issues further than attempted here, it is difficult to do so and still tell the truth.

The Illusion of "Choice"

Modern medicine claims that it provides the midlife woman not with dilemmas but with "choices." Women can choose whether to undergo tests, they can choose whether to take part in screening, they can choose whether to take the proffered drugs.

"Choice" is a bland term implying one can make simple decisions between easily understood options as well as have ready access to objective information on which to base the decisions. It suggests that the options offered to women are entirely beneficial and that the consumer is powerfully placed to select or reject from an attractive range of products. Sociologist Victoria Grace warns that this model in which the market claims to empower the consumer is deceptive and false.(3) She says that although consumers appear to have choices, the market has actually constructed their needs. Women may be able to make individual "choices," but the range of those choices will be predetermined and outside their control.

Midlife women have actually had no say in the services being provided for them. The "choices" available to them have been largely selected by commercial interests who have products and services to sell. There is another curious factor here that should alert us to the fact that all is not straightforward. The industry that has grown up around the provision of "choices" to midlife women is primarily controlled by men. The scientists building careers by researching menopausal women are men, and those who proselytize about the value of the various interventions tend to be male. Women have not been asked what their priorities are—no one has consulted them. Instead, women have simply been told that it is for their own good.

Women's ability to have any kind of free "choice" is compromised by the complexity of the issues they are faced with and the confusion in the scientific knowledge about them. Information about the interventions must be mediated to them through their doctors, increasing their dependency on the medical system. Alternatively, women rely on bowdlerized versions of medical wisdom published in the mass media.

Victoria Grace talks about premodeling or control of people's choices. This is vividly demonstrated by the way women have been trained through the mass media and advertising industries to see osteoporosis as a major threat in their lives, a threat that can be lifted by the taking of hormones or calcium supplements. They have been primed to generate a demand. When women ask for what the menopause industry has to offer, they do so because they have been told to want it and they have been told they need it—not because they ever had a "choice."

The "choice" argument is an attempt to personalize what is essentially political. Menopause is now a commodity that can be exploited for commercial gain. There is much more at stake for women here than individual choice. The menopause industry is about the colonization of a sex, the redefining of a normal life stage as a medical event. It is difficult for women to make choices freely when they have been subjected to a demoralizing propaganda campaign aimed at brainwashing them into accepting that they are "estrogen deficient," in other words, defective in their normal state. Modern medicine does not make women more powerful and in control of their lives. It disempowers them, sending them on an endless quest for the Holy Grail of youth and perfect health.

Medicalization Gone Mad

This book explores the interface between well midlife women and preventive medicine, that branch of medicine that intervenes in people's lives to prevent disease from occurring, as opposed to waiting to treat it after it has appeared. Preventive medicine aims to keep well people well, as opposed to concentrating on healing the sick. On the surface, this would appear to be a simple task, calling for less technology and minimal involvement in people's lives. In practice, this is not so at all, at least as far as the midlife woman is concerned. Under the old reactive medical model, she could avoid contact with the medical system unless she had some symptoms of disease. Now, she is exhorted to regularly have checkups to confirm that she is well.

This has the effect of intensifying her involvement in the health system. Doctors have the power not only to bestow disease labels on people, but also they control the technologies of diagnosis and treatment. In the case of midlife women, the boundaries of what is considered normal have disappeared, so that all menopausal women are seen to be in need of diagnosis and treatment. This process which has accorded doctors increased jurisdiction over normal people's lives is called medicalization.

Preventive medical programs medicalize people's lives as they inexorably "make patients out of well people."(4) In *Medicine Out of Control* Richard Taylor describes this process as "the patientization of the population": "The implication is that we are all under a cloud of possible illness (of which we are unaware) until we have been proven by objective means to be healthy." With this model, health becomes "a state of successive negative tests for hidden disease."(5)

A whole battery of investigations and tests has been devised for midlife women, not because they are sick but perversely "to tell well women that they are well" and "to reassure women they do not have cancer."(6)

It is no longer possible for an individual to simply regard herself as a healthy woman in the prime of life. This can only be stated with authority if medicine has confirmed it by "screening" various parts of her body. She should submit to "monitoring" by periodic testing. For her breasts, there should be a "baseline mammogram," against which any changes in her tissues will be measured. She will develop a surrogate identity or alter ego—femina medica—in which she is defined by a series of computer printouts and x-ray films. Her body becomes a machine that must be given its "warrant of fitness" to be deemed in proper running order. The woman who eschews protecting herself in this way is seen as inexplicably reckless and careless of herself. When women enter the medical environment for one purpose, they also risk further unasked-for interventions, as the story starting on page 27 so clearly illustrates.

There are parallels here with the process by which pregnancy and childbirth have become medicalized. No woman can believe her pregnancy is normal, her unborn child healthy, and the birth happening without scans of the womb, tests of the fetal fluid, and electronic monitoring of her labor. As with midlife women, the price to be paid for this intense technological surveillance of normal events is loss of control and erosion of confidence, a process eloquently described by Ivan Illich:

> Diagnosis always intensifies stress, defines incapacity, imposes inactivity, and focuses apprehension on non-recovery, on uncertainty, and on one's dependence upon future medical findings, all of which amounts to a loss of autonomy for self-definition. It also isolates a person in a special role, separates him from the normal and healthy, and requires submission to the authority of specialized personnel. Once a society organizes for a preventive disease-hunt, it gives epidemic proportions to diagnosis. This ultimate triumph of therapeutic culture turns the independence of the average healthy person into an intolerable form of deviance.(7)

To save the few, preventive programs must be aimed at the many. No one should escape the net. For instance, in one "successful" breast

Getting Caught Up in the System

The first mistake I made was to let myself be persuaded to have hormone replacement therapy (HRT). I went through menopause at about 40, so according to the experts I am a prime target for the dreaded osteoporosis. I have to say, however, it was not my GP who suggested the HRT, but a friend, who is a GP's wife. I was never really convinced about the hormones. The more I read about their possible effects, the more I wondered what I was doing taking them. My lack of commitment meant that I was always forgetting to take the pills. In the end I gave them up altogether.

After I had been taking the HRT (off and on) for a year, my GP suggested it would be a good thing to get a "baseline mammography" against which any subsequent changes in my breasts could be measured. The reading I was doing had made me even more skeptical about mammography than HRT, so I carried that referral around with me in my handbag until it was scruffy and grimy. In the end, I went ahead and had the mammography, as much out of curiosity about the procedure as anything. It was interesting to see how the machine worked and to look at the X-ray of my breasts. The radiographer said the radiologist would look at the X-rays and send a report to my GP. I left and promptly forgot all about it.

Some months later my GP phoned me in a state of anxiety. She said she had been trying to contact me for a long time and asked with a note of reproach in her voice why I had not been in touch to learn the result of my mammogram. I told her I knew she would phone if there was anything the matter. It turned out that the report did note an area of density in one of my breasts that the radiologist thought might possibly require further examination. I asked her to read me the report, which stated reassuringly that there were no indications of malignancy. The comment about the unexplained dense patch seemed to me to be implying that there was only the most outside chance that it might be hiding a tumor.

"Well, what do you want to do?" my doctor asked. "You could have another mammography."

I told her I have no faith in mammography as a diagnostic tool, and that on the basis of the report I was prepared to do nothing. She became rather more anxious at that stage and it was clear that she was not happy to let the matter rest. In the end we agreed that she should send the X-rays to a breast specialist and get his comments and that if he thought it was necessary I should go and see him.

Some days later she contacted me again. The specialist did want to see me, and he wanted me to have some more mammograms done, including some magnifications and a view at a different angle with greater compression. He also asked for an ultrasound scan. He would then give me a physical examination and discuss the results of all these tests with me.

Now, as I am a supporter of New Zealand's dwindling public health system, I do not have medical insurance. It was December, a time of year when it is difficult to find extra money for medical treatment. I pointed this out to my doctor, but she was unsympathetic. I therefore went ahead and made appointments to have the mammography one morning and to visit the specialist at his clinic directly afterward. I discussed the issue of cost with the specialist, but he too was unmoved.

"If you go to the public hospital," he told me, "you won't get an appointment until late January. Better come and see me this week, so you won't spend the whole of Christmas worrying about it."

It occurred to me to tell him that it was not me who was worrying but my GP, but I thought better of it.

I went to the x-ray clinic on a Friday morning, taking time off work to do so. My partner came with me for support. The radiographer who eventually took the mammogram was a straight-laced woman of the old school. When I had taken off my clothes and she saw my rather small breasts, she remarked accusingly, "With breasts as small as these it makes it terribly difficult to diagnose as well as photograph," and added, "You could have provided a bit more!" Clearly, if the X-ray did not turn out well, it was my fault, not that of her equipment or skill.

She took a number of views of the same breast to try to capture the elusive shadowy patch. I soon lost count. After about the sixth film I asked anxiously whether such a large number was really necessary, as I had no insurance and I would have to pay for them. This did not go down well. It was clearly not the kind of thing patients are meant to say in the middle of treatment. She told me rather tersely that she did not concern herself with money, and followed this up by remarking, "It's your life, not mine!"

I got the clear message that I was meant to be so worried about my survival that I should be everlastingly grateful for the wonderful service she was giving me and ready to mortgage my home to meet the cost.

The magnification meant a whole lot more x-rays. Perhaps feeling a little defensive after my earlier comment about cost, the radiographer volunteered the justification, "It's a life thing."

I went out to the specialist clutching a big envelope of X-rays. I insisted my partner stay with me as I wanted help in remembering what he said, and he was happy for that to happen. After examining the new X-rays and the ultrasound report, and giving my breasts a thorough examination, the specialist told me there did not seem to be anything there he could perform a biopsy on, but he thought he could just feel the patch that showed on the X-rays. He did not think it was anything to be concerned about, but just to be on the safe side, I should go in for another mammography in about six months' time. That would be one year after the first one.

The cost of the whole exercise came to just over $200— $112 for the X-ray and $95 for the specialist. Two hundred dollars just before Christmas is a lot to pay for reassurance, especially when you are not worried in the first place. I was convinced that the whole effort was a case of overtreatment. But I got hooked into a system that threatened me, both implicitly and explicitly, with the risk of death if I did not comply (and pay).

The question is, will I go for the mammogram in six months' time? At the moment, I am tempted to let it slip. I know I am at low risk for breast cancer. In terms of all the risk factors in my life and history, I am more likely to die of heart disease. But there is always that outside chance that they are right and I am wrong. If I let it go, and that shadow under my left arm becomes a cancer, I am not only going to look silly, I am going to look sick. And the straight-laced radiographer will be the first to tell me I have only myself to blame.

screening program, 1,850 women had to be screened with 75 false positive results to gain one extra survivor.(8) In 15 women who were found to have breast cancer the outcome was unchanged. The only benefit to the 1,760 other women was the reassurance of a negative test. This feature of screening programs—that the majority of the population must undergo an intervention for the benefit of a few, in this case one—has been called "the prevention paradox" and the "mass treatment trap."(9) To prevent harm to an unidentifiable minority of people, everyone must submit to tests or treatments that are themselves not without risks.

Illich talks about the difficulty of "equating statistical man with biologically unique men." One of the pitfalls of preventive strategies is the making of predictions for individuals based on population-based statistical averages. Such predictions are all-embracing. Thus a woman who is told she has a 1 in 15 chance of breast cancer before the age of 75 years will have no idea whether she will be amongst the fortunate 14 or be the one. She is then asked to make her "choice" on this statistical imponderable. Then, too, she may be told she is in a "high risk category" or a "low risk category." Once again, this will be a guess, but the implications of being labeled at "high risk" are unpleasant. It is not a label that is possible to outlive or cure. Instead, the recipient is marked for a lifetime—a living, breathing collection of risk factors waiting to fulfill the prediction. Consider the following: being a woman, being Caucasian, and being small are all deemed to be "risk factors" for osteoporosis, yet a substantial proportion of the population would fall within these categories.

Labeling is not a benign activity. Once labeled, "the person is required to enter the social role appropriate to the label—to undergo certain types of treatment, to modify his or her behavior in ways seen as therapeutic, perhaps to abandon all other social roles and enter an institution filled with similarly labeled persons (cancer ward, jail, mental hospital)."(10) To label a person is to deny his or her individuality, his or her social identity and right to self-definition.

Preventive medicine habitually talks in terms of risks, as if normal life is a very precarious business during which we are continually in danger of being struck down by dread disease. Addressing this issue, one writer said:

As a people, we have become obsessed with health.
There is something fundamentally, radically unhealthy about

this. We do not seem to be seeking more exuberance in living as much as staving off failure, putting off dying. We are losing confidence in the human form.

The new consensus is that we are badly designed, intrinsically fallible, vulnerable to a host of hostile influences inside and around us, and only precariously alive. We live in danger of falling apart at any moment, and are therefore always in need of surveillance and propping up. Without the professional attention of the health-care system, we would fall in our tracks.(11)

Emphasizing the possibility of illness focuses the mind on human mortality rather than resilience. The success of prevention programs is measured in terms of deaths forestalled. Healthy women are exhorted to use hormones, for instance, to prevent deaths from hip fractures and heart attacks, even though the risk of these is hypothetical and the risks of the treatment unknown. The medical evangelists promoting this strategy place an absolute value on the prolongation of life, no matter what the quality of the extra years so earned. Against the weighty matter of increased survival, women can only protest about "trivial" matters such as return of menstruation and weight gain.

In 1990 Geoffrey Rose, Professor of Epidemiology at the London School of Hygiene and Tropical Medicine, noted that decisions about preventive policies were "made by expert groups who usually do not have access to the recipients' opinions and values." He pointed to an increasing disjunction between the values of medical practice and the community: "If patients share in the decisions then the decisions will often be different because their values and ours are often different. Doctors regard health, and especially survival, as paramount and they tend to favor vigorous investigation and action. For patients, health is only one among a number of values and is often not the highest."(12)

Part of the problem lies in the failure of medicine to see women as whole people. Medicine is traditionally organized to see people in bits: as blood, skin, reproductive organs, hearts, and so on. The bits that break down get sent to the body shop to get fixed, but the soul of the person? There is no place in the medical curriculum for that. This mechanistic attitude has spilled over into preventive medicine, where programs focus on one body part to the exclusion of all else. The person interested in bones may recommend hormones to a woman to prevent bone loss, even though this treatment has not been cleared of a possible link to breast cancer. Somewhere else, a radiologist wants to look at the same woman's breasts to check for cancer. At the same time, we are told that mammograms are less effective in women using hormones. The contradictions are endless but invisible.

As already noted, when well women submit to medical investigation there can be a snowball effect, with the first intervention leading to more and more. This might be termed "secondary medicalization." Women on hormone replacement therapy, for instance, are often advised to have regular mammograms, endometrial biopsies, and other tests, while side effects of the therapy frequently lead not to withdrawal of it but to further medication. The medical response to shortcomings of the therapy is inevitably to propose more radical interventions. Take the example of women using postmenopausal hormones. If they have a uterus, they must take progestogen to prevent the development of endometrial cancer, but this can cause unpleasant premenstrual-like symptoms and might negate some of the beneficial effect of estrogen.

Several proposals have seriously been put forward to deal with this "problem." Without any mention of the risks and discomforts of IUDs, one doctor proposed that a progestogen-releasing IUD be inserted in postmenopausal estrogen users to confine the progestogen to the uterus rather than letting it enter other body systems as it does when it is swallowed.(13)

Another suggestion is to "ablate" (destroy or remove) the endometrium by laser—a procedure from which people have been known to die—before prescribing hormones.(14)

The doctor who started the first menopause clinic in London has proposed a "pelvic clean-out" before therapy is commenced, obviating the need for progestogen. In years to come

> women will elect to have a hysterectomy when their families are complete at forty or forty-five . . . . That operation will remove their ovaries, cervix and endometrium, the three major sites of gynecological cancer. They will then start taking Hormone Replacement Therapy and continue it indefinitely. It will be regarded as a very safe process—everything out and then HRT—very sensible.(15)

This is light-years away from the ethical injunction in the doctors' Hippocratic Oath: "First—do no harm."

The Machine Age

Preventive medicine depends on the existence of technology in the forms of tests and drugs. The growth of technology has facilitated the extension of "the medical gaze" over women's lives.(16)
　　Lesley Doyal argues that

> medical techniques themselves are not merely the logical conse-
> quence of "scientific progress," but rather the product of a par-
> ticular conjunction of social, economic and political forces.
> Hence we have to understand the existence of any particular
> practice or technology not simply in terms of its utility in helping
> the sick—indeed it may be of very little therapeutic value—but
> in terms of the activities of powerful groups in society whose
> various interests are furthered by the initial development and
> continued use of such technologies.(17)

In the case of the midlife woman, as we shall see throughout this book, the pharmaceutical industry has been a prime force in deter-mining which interventions are being promoted to women, as this industry has been instrumental in the development of the disease labels that justify the use of the interventions. The pharmaceutical industry has promoted the idea of menopause as a disease because it has the drugs to treat it. Similarly, raising the profile of osteoporosis and redefining it as a woman's disease has been the ambition of drug companies, accomplished with the willing cooperation of research scientists, the doctors who run menopause clinics, and family phy-sicians. It is a symbiotic relationship, for the existence of the tech-nology builds careers, thus enabling the expansion of the medical empire and in particular the menopause industry.
　　This interplay is invisible to women. The midlife woman who visits her doctor believes she is getting objective advice, the result of the doctor's scientific training and careful reading of the medical literature. She does not realize the doctor's information may in fact have come from a drug company video viewed at a "seminar" held at a holiday resort and paid for by the drug company. The journal articles the doctor reads may be only the selection handed out by the visiting drug retailer (along with the crystal wine glasses after the seminar), rather than the result of research conducted by the doctor himself.

There is no doubt that, properly used, all the interventions presented to midlife women have the potential to be beneficial. The woman whose life is being made hellish by hot flashes that come on the hour, every hour, day and night will be grateful for estrogen's calming powers. The woman whose preinvasive cervical lesion is seen through the keen eye of the colposcope will be grateful she has been spared from malignant disease. The woman whose tiny impalpable breast tumor is revealed by a telltale white spot on a mammogram will be glad that such early diagnosis has saved her breast and given her a better chance of survival.

At the same time, all these interventions have their negative side. They may cause discomfort, they may be imprecise, in which case there will be unnecessary investigations of women without disease, and they may also miss serious disease. Sometimes this is because of an inherent flaw in the technology, at other times it results from operator error. There is also the problem caused by improper application of the technology, such as the use of mammography to diagnose palpable breast lumps or the proliferation of storefront bone screening clinics in America.

There is a propensity to invest the machinery with magical powers, to believe that more technology must provide better medicine. Richard Taylor says:

> There is a tendency to assume that any human activity that involves these machines is superior to those which do not. Thus there is a general feeling by the public and doctors alike that diagnosis involving technological methods must be more accurate, and reveal conditions which are somehow more relevant than diagnoses using simpler techniques—if for no other reason than "science" itself is involved.(18)

This faith in the efficacy of technology devalues simpler human methods of medical treatment and self-care. For the doctor, the value of simple history taking (listening to the patient) and physical examination has been undermined by the existence of sophisticated tests. As a result, in mammographic screening programs it has been found that up to half the lumps detected by mammography could actually be felt. Midlife women contemplate hormones to save their bones, but do not consider simple preventive measures they can take, such as breast self examination. At the same time, they often persist in damaging personal habits, such as smoking.

Richard Taylor argues for control of technology, otherwise it can become "malignant" and dangerous to health. The rapid proliferation of technology threatens to outstrip the rational basis for its application. The existence of the technology seems to impel its use:

> Clinical actions are becoming as much determined by the *existence* of sophisticated gadgetry, as by any rational assessment of what more can be achieved by using these methods. What we have is science-fiction medicine, not medical science. We have an expanding technological empire which is rapidly developing its own intellectual and economic momentum. And at the control of "space-ship medicine" we find a group of technocrats whose ethos and actions more closely resemble the antics of Flash Gordon and his crew than actual human beings practicing the most applied of the biological sciences on their fellow travelers.(19)

How New Is the "New General Practice"?

The front line in preventive medicine is primary health care. On the surface of it, this appears to be a positive development, for it changes the role of community medicine from that of ambulance at the bottom of the cliff to one of preventing disease from ever occurring.

However, the placement of disease prevention within a medical setting gives rise to inherent problems in the way it is perceived and carried out. Medicine traditionally expects passivity from its clients and preventive medicine has taken over this approach. The human users of preventive services are described as the "target population" and the literature is littered with references to the problem of "noncompliance"—that is, people who do not show up for tests or fail to take their drugs. Thus prevention offered within a medical setting is more about what doctors can do to people than what people can do for themselves.

Doctors are normalized toward tests and drugs; these are the tools of their trade. It is frequently possible to make lifestyle changes to prevent particular diseases. For instance, women wishing to keep their bones strong could be advised to stop smoking, eat healthily, and be physically active. But because preventing osteoporosis has been claimed as a medical matter, the tendency is to rely on technology and drugs. It is much more consistent with the doctor's training to suggest a bone scan or hormones than to advise a woman to run around the block.

General practice is claiming preventive health care as its proper and exclusive business under the banner of the "new general practice." It is through preventive medicine that general practice has been able to claim status as trailblazer, at the cutting edge of modern medicine. Before this, general practitioners were the poor cousins of the medical profession: "The general practitioner was still a watered-down hospital doctor who had either fallen off the hospital career ladder through failure, poverty, or need for immediate income."(20)

The revival of general practice has been made possible through the exploitation of computer technology and the widespread adoption of the strategies of preventive medicine. The general practitioner no longer waits for patients to present themselves in his surgery with their diseases; he goes out looking for clients, he runs "clinics" rather than surgeries, he circulates newsletters and he maintains "surveillance" over his patients by means of his age-sex practice register and recall systems. Science was once the prerogative of the hospital doctor, the academic teacher, and the medical researcher; now the humble GP can bring science to the aid of his frontline care, immensely enhancing his status.

> The new general practices sought to use the microcomputer to unlock and utilize clinically the prevention potential locked up in conventional reactive general practice consultation; to move medical effort away from end organ salvage towards early diagnosis of risk; to shift from management of crises and response to illness that was led by demand towards proactive and anticipatory care and from management of disease in an individual patient to management of risk factors for populations and their members. This takes the bias towards prevention that is present in so much routine general practice on to a more systematic screening that is not always executed by doctors or initiated by patients but is based on the practice register. It applies above all to cardiovascular risk factors but also logically to any condition in which our present knowledge permits useful treatment before symptoms develop, including breast cancer, diabetes, depression, and cervical dysplasia.(21)

This description has strong similarities with a military or evangelical campaign! Susan Sontag has eloquently written about metaphors used to describe particular diseases in *Illness as Metaphor.*(22) Cancer, for instance, is always described in terms of warfare. Malignant cells are said to "invade" the body and must be "killed" by radiation and chemotherapy poisoning. People commonly refer to the "war" or "battle" or "fight" against cancer.

Many of the metaphors of preventive medicine are those usually associated with authoritarian states and dictatorships. Thus "populations" (rather than individuals) are "targeted" and "recruited" for "screening." They are then "kept under surveillance" and "monitored." People must take part for the collective good. The idea that the healthy population contains hidden disease parallels with the idea of the spy who passes himself off as one of the community but really aims to betray it. With mammography, we are told "breast cancer has virtually nowhere to hide."(23) Remember, says a New Zealand pamphlet for mammography, "what you don't know *can* hurt you."(24)

The aim of preventive medicine is to flush out the enemy within. This language betrays the underlying intention of primary healthcare-based screening, which is to *not* give people control over their own health, but to exercise control over them.

Ethics and Entrepreneurialism

The shift from the process of the sick patient seeking help from the doctor to the recruitment of large numbers of well people for potential treatment has taken place with very little discussion among the medical profession of the implications or the ethical questions involved.

Arguing for the need for policies on screening, Thomas McKeown, Professor of Social Medicine at the University of Birmingham, wrote that in screening

> there is a presumptive undertaking, not merely that abnormality will be identified if it is present, but that those affected will derive benefit from subsequent treatment and care. This commitment is at least implicit, and except for research on the protection of public health, no one should be expected to submit to the inconvenience of investigation or the anxieties of case finding

without the prospect of medical benefit. This obligation exists even when the patient asks to be screened or to have a health examination, for his request is based on the belief that the procedure is valuable, and if it is not, it is for medical people to make this known.(25)

Those comments were made in 1976, but the principle that a clear benefit must be able to be demonstrated from screening before people are invited to take part has not been applied in some present-day screening activities. It is possible to show benefits from cervical screening, although there are still drawbacks, as we shall see later; but it is far less possible to show a clear benefit from mammography, at least in some age groups. In discussing the British breast screening program, Rodgers commented: "In effect, we are asking women whether they want to find out that they have cancer earlier than they otherwise would. This action, without adequate counseling of women before the screen, to inform them of the implications and risks of screening, is ethically unjustifiable."(26)

One doctor warned that in preventive screening programs doctors needed to guard against the consequences of entrepreneurialism, especially in terms of the ethics of informed consent:

We have tended to take a marketing approach in telling the community what we think they should know, often with an element of subtle coercion using simplistic slogans . . . . Mass medicalized programs will bring more power and money to our profession and the whole health industry. In this new age of entrepreneurial practice, we should be careful not to descend to the ethic of commercial advertising with its accent on subjectivity, subtle deception and fashionable slogans.(27)

Women's need for disinterested advice, objective information, and control over their health care is glossed over when doctors resort to such marketing strategies. The information women are offered is crudely manipulated to ensure their cooperation rather than provided as an aid to informed decision making. What one writer has called "the commercialization of health" has distorted both the medical information and the climate in which it is imparted.(28)

The examination of the health issues facing midlife women is offered here as a tool to aid their decision making. It seeks to make them more powerful in their interaction with the medical system—first, by providing an examination of the medical topics, and second, by exposing the origins of the ideologies and interventions. Both the medical information and the political context are critical to understanding and then resisting the "menopause industry."

Chapter 2

The Fabulous Midlife Woman

So who is this creature, this midlife-woman who is the unwitting focus of so much medical scrutiny? She used to be called "middle-aged," a rather dreadful term carrying connotations of dull, unadventurous, and frumpish. Middle age was a kind of no-woman's land—a barren ground caught between the glorious past age of youth and the enemy, old age. The middle-aged woman had fulfilled the central purpose of her existence—to bear and raise children—and was then relegated to the sidelines of life to watch the world go by.

For women, middle age was the culmination of years of social conditioning to accept their place in the world. They were schooled not to expect self-fulfillment or social status. When the middle-aged woman, having completed the task society had demanded of her, discovered that no honor lay in her retirement, it was too late to do anything and she was well trained not to complain.

Until the mid-1970s women had few choices about how to lead their lives. After their education, they entered the workforce, but this was only a temporary condition. Traditionally, it was viewed as a stopgap until a woman's real career as "housewife" began. Most women resigned from their employment on marriage, either because it was socially unacceptable to do otherwise or because it was forced on them by the conditions of their employment. They bore two or three children and were almost exclusively responsible for their upbringing as well as for running the household. Their badge of office was their apron.

Within households, there was a strict division of roles along gender lines. Despite the fact that the role of motherhood was glorified, it was ignominious for men to have anything to do with it. Husbands believed they would be instantly rendered impotent if caught pushing a stroller. This sexual division of labor spilled over into the marketplace with work categorized as either "men's" or "women's." There were prohibitions on women entering some areas of employment or the training programs that led to them. Quota systems restricted the number of women entering fields such as medicine, and formal and informal barriers prohibited women from entering male-dominated trades. Women clustered in female employment ghettos, where their wages were poor and chances of advancement minimal.

Once a woman's children grew up she might find a part-time job as a source of "pin money." It was not permissible to be serious about paid work, to have ambitions or follow a career. The middle-aged woman might do good works but nothing that could interfere with her domestic duties—calling up these could absolve a woman of responsibility for virtually anything else. The future role to look forward to was becoming a grandmother.

It was a monolithic system. There was a set pattern and women were expected to follow it. The highest accolades were to be "a good woman," "a good mother," and "a good wife." These were shorthand for being a self-sacrificing, well-trained, uncomplaining, compliant, second-class citizen. Even women described themselves deprecatingly as "just a housewife."

A rigid code of behavior ensured that women carried out their proper role. When I was a young wife in the 1960s, I was told by a well-meaning older company wife that "the mark of being well-dressed is that after the party no one can remember what you wore." This advice symbolized for me precisely what I chafed against in the female role. My job was to be an asset to "him," which I could best achieve by being so bland that I stood out neither for my incongruence nor my individuality. It was just as unacceptable to be badly behaved as brilliant. All that was sought from me was that I be blank, like paper without writing or a garden waiting for the lettuces to emerge.

If women in the 1950s and 1960s experienced any personal distress—violent husbands, sexual dissatisfaction, unwanted pregnancy, frustrated ambition, or just plain boredom—it was kept invisible. Single girls went out of town for a while and returned with flat stomachs. A smile, however vacuous, could be put on the faces of troubled housewives with the simple expedient of drugs. As a last resort, there was always electroconvulsive therapy, guaranteed to render women trouble-free.

To divorce was a disgrace. A divorced woman was sinful, fast, and preyed upon other women's men. It was better to placate husbands than to leave them. There were no refuges, no benefits for solo mothers, and no right of access to the economic fruits of marriage.

Release from Domestic Thralldom

The sexual revolution of the 1960s and the women's liberation movement of the 1970s changed the way women lived forever. Women's lives in the 1990s are unrecognizable compared to those of women a generation ago. There has been a social revolution among women, and this has led to profound legislative and economic changes, as well as to a complete shift in self-definition. No area of women's lives has been untouched.

There is not room here to give anything more than the briefest summary of the changes women have wrought. There is still much work to do to improve the status of women, but enormous strides have been made. Virtually every legislative barrier to women's full participation in society has been removed. Divorce is easier to obtain, and women now have equal rights to the assets of a marriage, regardless of their contribution in financial terms. State benefits support solo women with children. Most of the formal barriers to equal employment have been removed, although this has not banished covert forms of discrimination.

Social attitudes have changed dramatically. Women expect to be fully participating members of society. It may still be a struggle in many areas, but any public report of sexism will be greeted with a howl of condemnation. Working mothers are accepted as the norm and are no longer berated for "dumping" their children in child care. Violence against women is still endemic, but the public attitude is one of sympathy for the victims rather than the former reaction that "she asked for it."

The midlife women of today have lived through this time of social change. Women who are in their forties in the 1990s were born in the 1940s and 1950s. The gender revolution of the 1960s and 1970 was part of their youth. The older cohort—women now in their fifties—was born in the 1930s, so their experience has been somewhat different. They were children in the tough depression years and young women during the war. After a taste of freedom and taking over men's jobs, they were caught up in the "back-to-the-home movement" of the 1950s, and extricating themselves from that life has been a struggle.

These midlife women are the generation that freed their sex. They did not inherit equality, they fought for it. It was their agitation—their blood, sweat, and tears—that led to all the reforms enjoyed by young women today. Many sacrificed their own personal advancement to work for the betterment of their sex. Ironically, these women in their forties and fifties have not been able personally to take the fullest advantage of the gains they made. It was the followings generations that reaped the rewards of those struggles. For midlife women were just a little too late, in much the same way as the women who fight for a local kindergarten have all their own children off to school by the time it is built.

Midlife women are caught on the cusp between the old world and the new. The shape of their lives had already been sketched by events that predated the social change. The decisions they made in their youth were limited by the prohibitions placed on their sex. They had left school, done arts at university, trained as nurses, become shorthand typists, given babies up for adoption, married, left the workforce, had children, and divorced. This restricted what they could then do, even if later, when the world changed, they seemed to be offered a cornucopia of choices. The turmoil many of these women went through in their thirties was about taking apart their lives and reconstructing them. As women gained more freedom, it was possible to have a second chance—at education, relationships, employment—but it was hard work and compromises had to be made.

The present generation of midlife women are a new breed. They cut their teeth on the feminist revolution of the seventies and eighties, and are unlikely to be content merely to follow the path their mothers took into middle age. Men at midlife have always been the movers and shakers; now women are finding their own power in their middle years. "Midlife" is uncharted territory. It is ripe for definition, to be made of whatever women wish. Today's midlife women—veterans of the "battle of the sexes"—are ideally placed to do it.

Facts and Figures about Midlife Women

Numerically, midlife women are a significant age group. There are almost 16 million American women aged 40–49 years and over 11 million aged 50–59. At 40 a woman has half her life ahead of her still, while the 50-year-old can expect to live another 30 years.(1)

In many ways their lives are greatly varied. Some have continued to lead quite traditional lives, either from preference or from lack of opportunity to do otherwise. Others are breaking new ground in many directions: in employment, public office, community activities, and living styles. The following statistical profile contributes to the picture of midlife women, but cannot depict the rich variety of their lives.

Workforce participation and income

The number of women in the civilian labor force has risen dramatically, from about 23,240,000 in 1960 to about 56,554,000 in 1990. This is not just due to the "baby boom" generation, since in 1960 only 35.5% of all women were employed, compared to 54.3% in 1990. Much of this rise, in fact, is due to new attitudes toward marriage and working. Whereas in 1960 women in their late teens and early twenties often worked, then left the workforce at marriage to become full-time homemakers, today more and more women are marrying later and keeping their jobs after marriage. Indeed, the number of married women with children under 6 years of age who are participating in the labor force has skyrocketed from a mere 18.6% in 1960 to 59.9% in 1990.

The double influx into the workplace in the 1970s of married women and baby boomers (sometimes the same woman) has caused an interesting shift in the age of the working woman. In 1960, 45.5% of the female workforce was in the 35–54-year-old age range; but in 1980, this same age group comprised only 34.4% of the workforce, and in 1990 the figure had risen back up to 41.3% as the baby boomers joined this group. However, the percent of the female workforce 45 years old or older has actually fallen from 39.4% in 1960, when younger married women with children were discouraged from working, to 28.2% in 1990. This is not surprising given that in nearly two-thirds of all married-couple families, the wife worked at least part-time in 1991.

While more women are working and a few have penetrated formerly male-dominated employment areas, more working women are still relegated to a restricted range of employment categories. Over half are in service, administrative support, clerical, and sales jobs—the only employment categories in which the number of women far exceeds the number of men.

This preponderance of women in the low-paying "pink collar" ghettos compounds the difference in pay that still exists between men and women. In 1992 the median weekly earnings of men in managerial and professional positions was $700 compared to $562 for women. Even in the female-dominated clerical jobs, women's median earnings were about 75% that of men in similar positions. This difference is most marked in the 45–64-year-old age range, when women's median income is less than half that of men. Women never really recover their income-earning potential after withdrawing from the workforce to have children.

As well as returning to the workforce, more midlife women are returning to college. While college enrollment rates have risen only slightly for women under 25, more or less in proportion with general population increases, the number of older women students has skyrocketed. Unfortunately, higher education does not give the same advantage to women as it does to men. In 1991 the average income of women with a bachelor's degree or more, working full-time, year-round was $33,144, as compared to the $50,747 a similarly qualified man could expect. The discrepancy is largest for those 55 and older, when women average $34,363 at 55–64 years old and $23,332 at 65 and older, while men average $59,164 and $56,164 for the same age groups.

Nor is wage the only indicator of the "glass ceiling." In jobs such as teaching and nursing where there are large numbers of highly qualified women, women still find it hard to gain the prestige of the higher echelons. For example, even though three-fourths of all public school elementary and secondary school teachers in 1990 were women, only one-third of the principals in those same institutions were women.

Although women's earnings alone are less than men's, especially in the middle years, the median household income is higher at that age than at any other. This reflects the fact that most midlife women are married to men at the peak of their earning ability.

Living arrangements

By far the majority of American households consists of a married couple, although single-parent households are much more likely to have a female head than a male. Only one third of all households are owned by women, and most of these are divorced or widowed women.

Only 5% of midlife women have never married, while 14% of women 35–44 years old have had a divorce or annulment. The number of widows rises through the midlife age groups, reaching 14.9% for women 55–64 years old. Although the number of unmarried couples has risen dramatically from 523,000 in 1970 to 3,308,000 in 1992, only about 475,000 include women 45 years or older.

Motherhood

There is also a noticeable trend toward late motherhood. In 1980 there were 6.3 first births per 1,000 U.S. women between 30 and 34 years old, compared to 10.7 in 1990. At the same time the rate of first births for women 15–29 years old has dropped from 48.6 to 40.9 per thousand women. This means that an increasing number of women are bringing up small children in their middle years.

Community work

Over 20% of all midlife women in America do volunteer work outside the home.

Health

Life expectancy for women is now 78.8 years, 7 years more than for men. There are differences according to race, with life expectancy for white women at 79.4 years, compared to 75.2 years for black and other minority women. In 1991 there were over 2 million women 85 years old or older.

The first-listed hospital diagnosis for women 45 to 64 years old is heart disease, followed by cancer. In 1991, 546,000 hysterectomies were performed, with an estimated 12 deaths in every 10,000.

Heart disease is the leading cause of death for women of all ages. Cancer is the next most important cause of death, the three main sites being the respiratory tract, the colon, and the breast. Between the ages of 45 and 64, the order of the principal cause of death is reversed. In this age group the most frequent cause of death is cancer, followed by heart disease.

Women's Views of Midlife

As we shall see in the following chapters, many of the components of the medical stereotype of menopausal women are drawn from decades-old studies and observations of women. They may not have been accurate even then; they are certainly a long way off the mark in the 1990s. It is still assumed that the domestic role is women's greatest source of self-esteem, and that women will therefore suffer a crisis when their mothering role diminishes. Apart from the advent of grandchildren, aging is viewed in an almost entirely negative light.

We have just seen that in fact women in this age group lead varied lives which are not focused solely on the home, but this kind of statistical profile cannot tell us about women's thoughts and feelings. So the questions remain: Are midlife women satisfied with the lives they lead? Do they find life rewarding in the middle years or has life become more difficult?

The Society for Research on Women in New Zealand conducted a survey of nearly 500 women aged between 35 and 60 years in 1986 that reinforces that idea. They were not a random sample in that participants chose to take part and some were patients of local practitioners or had been attending menopause clinics. These women tended to be better educated and in higher socioeconomic groups than midlife women in general. Because of these factors, it is not possible to say they represent a cross section of the population. Nevertheless, this survey does represent the only attempt made to find out about the experience of midlife women in New Zealand in recent years.(2)

The researchers commented that overall the picture that emerged "is a positive one and in no way endorses the stereotype of midlife women feeling depressed and aimless as a result of children leaving home and the loss of the motherhood role."

They found that 80–90% of the women had a quite positive or very positive attitude to their daily lives. As well, more than 80% felt positive about their physical appearance and health. Only 14% of the women were unhappy about what they were doing each day, and 80% were positive about the future.

Of the 445 women in the survey, 352 were living with their husbands, 36 were living with another person, and 58 were living alone. The level of dissatisfaction with their living arrangements in all these groups was around 10%.

With regard to sexual relationships, 64% were in an ongoing relationship and 20% were occasionally involved with another person.

One third of all the respondents reported some stress in their relationship with husband or partner, mentioning factors such as husband's unemployment, illness, long working hours, or financial stinginess. As women became older and their children grew up, it was clear they enjoyed their children more. In the 35–40 age group, two thirds of the women said their children caused some stress, whereas among 50–60-year-olds, two thirds said their children were not stressful at all. No woman expressed regret at her children leaving home.

While researching this book, through women's networks I invited comments from women on topics related to midlife and received replies from all over the country, from cities, provincial centers, and rural areas. I also conducted in-depth interviews of some women. These sources of information were unstructured and informal and there was no attempt to involve a cross section of women. Many of the women would identify as feminist and were more highly educated than the population at large. Nevertheless, they made valuable comments and helped in shaping the content of this book.

What stood out from these contacts was the range of attitudes women have to aging. Virtually none of the women was especially concerned about menopause, but all had some concerns about getting older, although these differed dramatically from person to person. A source of anxiety to one woman was of no importance to another.

Wrinkles and middle-aged spread

Some women seemed to go through a kind of grieving process about changes in their physical appearance: the inexorable arrival of lines, grey hairs, and changing body shape. They felt sad about the loss of their youthful attractiveness, knowing that they could never regain it. Others were unconcerned about such changes.

The women quoted below all had different attitudes to the physical signs of aging and the weight gain that seemed to be a common phenomenon among women at midlife:

I find aging quite difficult, although not as much now as in my thirties when I first began to notice it. Every now and then I see myself in the mirror in daylight and I'm shocked. I still think of myself as 25.

I look in the mirror and regret the face that I see there, long for the wrinkle-free, beautiful young me.

I think I've become more attractive as I've gotten older. I look more elegant and confident. I don't make mistakes with clothes anymore—I know what suits me. Exercise keeps my muscles firm, and as I know myself sexually very well by now, sex is a source of satisfaction and good feelings.

I find it sad that my hair is changing color and texture and drying out, also my skin, face, neck, etc.

It doesn't worry me that I'm going gray and getting wrinkles, what I've been doing with my body is the important thing. I look at my mother and think I'll look like that if I live to my seventies and I think she's not too bad. Because I am a lesbian, I have a positive view of women's bodies. I've had relationships with older and younger women—it's fitness I like. If I was still in a relationship with a man I would be conscious of my increase in weight and my physical appearance. The women I'm involved with don't see my blemishes, only my good qualities.

I seem to be steadily putting on weight. I asked the doctor if I was unhealthily overweight, and he said, well, you're at the upper limit for your height but there's no health reason to take it off. My husband likes me the weight I am. He likes me cuddly when I take off all my clothes. Women who are a little bit on the heavy side look better. The best thing is a husband who loves you the way you are. He thinks aging is natural and does not want me to be a designer object.

Seeing ourselves as others see us

Social attitudes and other people's reactions challenge the individual's ability to maintain a positive self-image in the middle years. However much the midlife woman feels the same person with the same needs and desires, she is faced with others' changed perceptions of her. She is judged by her age and is expected to conform to a social image of a woman of middle years.

> Feeling young, or rather refusing to resign myself to the scrap heap that society seems to want to put older women on, is not easy. There is no doubt about the effect the media has on us all, and for me, the challenges to this image I have of myself have come through my children. My 12-year-old daughter began menstruating and although we had talked about this, when she told me I stared at her as if seeing her as she was for the first time. I realized she was not my little girl any longer, but a young woman. And if she was now capable of having children what did that make me? Six months later, I was again bumped up the generational ladder when my 14-year-old son introduced me to his very attractive 15-year-old girlfriend. As they both looked at me, I wondered what they were seeing—an "old woman"? There was an unspoken expectation about who I was and how I should behave. I was quite unnerved by this experience.

The requirement that a midlife woman conform to a social stereotype applies to all aspects of her behavior, especially her sexual behavior and her clothing. Whereas men dress in essentially the same type of clothing from youth to old age, symbolizing the fact that they maintain their social status, women's clothing changes. The young woman is encouraged to display her sexual assets by wearing tight-fitting and revealing clothing. The woman in her middle years who continues to wear such clothing, however, becomes an object of ridicule rather than admiration. She must conceal rather than display, as if her body now becomes a source of personal shame. If she does not, she invokes a harsh judgment. In common language, she is expected to "act her age," and there is a whole repertoire of negative language that can be applied to the woman who does not. She is "over the hill," "no spring chicken," "past her prime," and "mutton dressed up as lamb."

I was looking for something to wear to an evening event. Everything was very short, tight and glitzy—in my youth it would have been called "tarty." I came across a wonderful fifties-style frock with a full circular skirt and strapless bodice. It was black velvet and I thought I looked great in it. When I asked the shop assistant how you would stop your breasts popping out the top, she said gently: "It really is a frock for a younger woman." I was totally deflated.

I'm torn between feeling comfortable with my weight and feeling cross with the stereotypes and wondering if I should take it off. I get annoyed with clothes—there is a gap for older women. I'm not ready for middle-aged frocks.

Sexual disqualification

Social proscriptions about personal style stem from a requirement that women submit to becoming sexually invisible. As Paula Weideger writes in her book *Female Cycles*, the woman at midlife is "forced to hide or disguise her sexuality. . . . Part of the menopausal disguise is the denial of sexuality."(3) This is consistent with the social determination that female worth is judged according to reproductive ability. When young women flaunt their sexual attributes, this is tolerated and even encouraged as appropriate mating behavior. In older women, where it has no reproductive function, it is viewed as disgracefully sexual, a desperate and inappropriate attempt to obtain sexual gratification. If older women seek sexual partners, they are required to be discreet about it and not resort to the methods employed when they were younger.

The fact that my sexual attractiveness has diminished is a terrible blow. I have noticed men's reactions and had to see myself as an aging woman. It was a blow to my self-esteem and took a lot of getting used to. I've had to accept that I can no longer have the presumption that there could be an attraction. In friendships with men there was always a sexual element, the possibility that you would be sexually attracted. That is no longer true and it is a loss. Youth and sexual attraction are strong bargaining points. They are assets which allow you to be more confident and articulate.

The caveat needs to be made that these restrictions apply primarily in the heterosexual community. There is far more freedom among lesbians in terms of allowable behavior. Nevertheless, midlife lesbians also encounter the same judgments about being older as do heterosexual women from society at large, and also have additional problems because of the social unacceptability of lesbianism.

> I feel great about getting older most of the time (I will be 60 this year); other times it seems a hoot that I will soon be that old because increasingly I feel younger in many ways, and healthier in nearly all ways, than I ever have. I am aware that one of the most unhealthy things in my life is that lesbians are invisible, so that if I make myself visible there is a lot of resistance, ridicule, whatever. One reason is that to many people with heterosexual privilege "lesbian" means "sexual," and an older womon [sic] who is sexual is a contradiction in terms for so many. That whole myth/mind-set is so abusive of lesbians, and of womyn. It is hard to be healthy if you are invisible at any age or gender.

Messages from the media

Many women mentioned the damaging effect of media stereotypes of midlife women. Women's magazines constantly exhort women to think about their appearance, to take off weight, and to admire glamorous media stars like Joan Collins and Jane Fonda. Their principal merit appears to lie in how "well preserved" they are, rather than in any actual accomplishments. It is their lack of wrinkles and the prolongation of their sexiness we are asked to admire.

Women's magazines consistently present demoralizing images of midlife women, dwelling on the awfulness of midlife weight gain and facial lines. "Elizabeth Taylor then and now—winners and losers in the battle with Father Time" was the cover caption on a *New Zealand Woman's Weekly* in 1990.(4) Inside, a major feature, written with particular savagery, examined the aging of "some of the silver screen's most spectacular beauties." Brigitte Bardot "still holds her head high despite the ravages of the Riviera's harsh sunshine . . . her face—always partly covered by dark glasses when she appears in public—is lined and the lips which once pouted provocatively from the big screen, have a sad downward curve." Ursula Andress "admits that she has too many wrinkles to play love scenes on the screen" and Liz

Taylor has the temerity to be marketing a perfume called Passion: "The name does not sit quite as happily with the 58-year-old grandmother who inspired it as it might have done a year or two back." Taylor's sin is not only to be middle-aged but also to be plump.

In articles such as this, aging is depicted as a battle in which women are compelled to engage, but from which it is only possible to emerge victorious at considerable cost. Angela Lansbury, we are told, has had four face-lifts. She says, "Cosmetic surgery is one of the most helpful things women can do to fight the process of age. Plastic surgery shouldn't be the secret of just actresses and socialites. Now it's available to anyone who can afford it." Phyllis Diller has had cosmetic surgery nine times in 14 years: "Some people call it vanity, but I call it pride. It has to do with how you feel about yourself— self-esteem. I never thought about plastic surgery until I saw myself on the tube one night, and thought, 'Oh, my God, look at that monster.' The very next day I called my doctor and told him I needed a face-lift."(5)

Submitting to surgery or extreme dieting, such as liquid diets, is seen as a normal pursuit of midlife women, rather than the midlife equivalent of the young woman's anorexia nervosa.(6) Both are potentially life-threatening reactions to rigid judgments about female worth. The anorexic tries to gain control in her life by starving her body into the "right" shape, the midlife woman seeks the same end by resorting to surgery.

Beyond the preoccupation with fighting normal aging, the media otherwise portrays midlife women as ruthless, even twisted shrews, or treats them as invisible.

> As I age I feel that society/the media is phasing me out. Those in their twenties are it. We at midlife have had kids, got separated, divorced, found lumps, had positive smears, got melanoma. Things (usually bad) happen to us. When does the media portray well the new things women do at midlife? Women don't even get well rewarded for the things they do do (for example, the farcical New Year honors list).

The lesbian woman quoted earlier also wrote about the portrayal of midlife women in the media:

> Messages from the media I could go on about for hours: I began

counting in the middle of last year about how mothers were being represented on television dramas (the "better quality" ones that is), and we had four episodes of a menopausal-aged womon as monster, plus a series of ditto-aged womon as Christian fanatic mother, plus various others. I became enraged at how older womyn are treated on television ads, the misogyny directed toward older womyn, once one focuses on it, is horrifying . . . . In newspapers we tend to be conspicuous by our absence, as a rule.

Keeping in one piece

The women I talked to were actually more concerned about incapacity of some sort than the effects of aging on appearance. They worried about losing physical abilities, such as hearing, eyesight, and mobility, and also about losing mental powers. Becoming dependent on other people was another source of concern.

> I realize my eyesight—so acute, so infallible—is changing and fading. I sometimes find that figures in the distance are a complete blur. If I'm like this now, what am I going to be like in twenty years' time?

> I'm not concerned to look older, but I definitely care about my ability to do everything as in the past, so, for the first time since my twenties, I'm taking up regular gentle exercise.

> Of course I hate getting older. I fear I might be a burden to people. I know my time is limited and I want to go out with my boots on. I dread getting crippled, or worse, becoming senile.

> I worry about my forgetfulness. I talk about my menopausal memory loss. On the other hand I think my brain is storing so much information it gets overloaded and discards the unessential stuff. I also wonder whether the antihypertensive drugs I take have something to do with it.

Running out of time

Some women felt panicky and negative because of a feeling that time was running out. Whereas in youth the future stretched ahead seeming to offer infinite time to explore new fields, set goals, or change career direction, women in midlife have a sense of diminishing opportunities. As well, they know that openings are limited by their age. Many midlife women have taken time out from the workforce to have children, and never quite regain their position.

> There are heaps of things I want to do, one being a new career, but it's going to be difficult with a child at primary school and no money for retraining. I had a child at a point in my life when I was changing from commerce to psychology. Part-time work is easy to find in the commerce field so eight years later I'm still here. My age is compacting and limiting my choices, yet I have another 18 years of work left, or more!

> At 46 you know if you haven't made it, your chances are pretty slim, so I've had to accept that I'm not going to have a successful career. That I dissipated my energy and was not focused enough to take my career seriously. I made bad decisions early on through lack of confidence. I'm underqualified for the kind of work I'd like to do and age is definitely a problem. There are too many young Ph.D.s competing.

This sense of having run out of time seemed to apply mainly to women who had children relatively late and took time out from the workforce to do so. It seems difficult to catch up. Women who broke their working life earlier and therefore reentered the workforce when still young do not seem to have suffered in the same way.

> Now that I've got a Ph.D.—having that piece of paper gives me a lift. I like my job and I recognize that my experience far exceeds that of people I'm boss to and even my controlling superior. That makes me more confident. I've organized my job so I'm not too stressed, so I feel I've got more control in my life.

Welcome to the "empty nest"

There has been a persistent idea that midlife women will regret the end of their fertility and their most intensive mothering years. This woman describes such feelings:

It took some time to adjust to the diminution of the household. I wasn't used to two people—it seemed thin and quiet. I missed that richer texture of life with kids coming and going. I didn't expect that. I regretted not having had more children.

Her reaction was intensified by the accidental death of one of her children soon after he left home. In general, it seems that most women do not regret the end of their reproductive lives. For many women their thirties was actually their most difficult decade and they are relieved not to have unremitting demands that come with being the mother of young children. They have put childbearing behind them and have increasingly fewer responsibilities toward children.

I loved my family, mourned my lost children for years, but am now feeling the advantages of not being responsible for them—even at present calling on them for support, though I don't intend to get too much into the habit of this. So I think for me increasing freedom is the keynote. I have more time now and do pay more attention to my needs—physical, emotional, and spiritual—which I gave very short shrift to in the past. I never had time either. I was always running.

Teenagers can be demanding and difficult, and many women looked forward to regaining their privacy and tranquility as children left home. This also allowed more space to enjoy things with husbands or partners, where in previous years family activities had taken precedence.

My husband and I constantly make plans for when our last child leaves home. We will move into a smaller house which will enable us to spend more time at our beach cottage, and we will be able to travel overseas, something which has been impossible while the children were still at school.

The pluses of midlife

From talking to women and from the views expressed in workshops I have taken, I have formed the view that most women feel positive about being at midlife. The anxieties and pressures they may experience are caused mainly by the society they live in. Negative attitudes toward menopause, sexist prejudices about aging in women, and inequities in employment and financial security are the main problems they face. Midlife women have to maintain their sense of well-being in spite of this.

There are many aspects of their lives that women in this age-group value. They have a history: achievements they have made, abilities they can be proud of.

Midlife women have gained a maturity, experience, and confidence which younger women often lack. They know what they are good at and know that they can cope with most things. Having attained some seniority in employment and having fewer responsibilities toward children means they are freer to concentrate on themselves, and decide what they want out of the next third of life.

Having recently reentered the paid workforce in my first full-time job after 17 years of child-rearing and working for a variety of community groups, I feel stronger, happier and more energetic than ever.

I am more confident and have fewer traumas than in my thirties. I'm not so restless. Life is more settled and the children are older, which is easier. I enjoy things like gardening, reading, and music. We've got more money and material things, and I'm not out in the sexual marketplace, which was hell.

They are more secure in their own opinions and beliefs, and are less afraid of expressing them. Even the invisibility of midlife women had its positive side as it allowed some space free of pressures to think about what they really wanted to be doing. As the woman quoted above said, "increasing freedom is the keynote."

I don't care what people think about me as much. When I was younger I needed approval and admiration but this was very controlling. I couldn't just be myself. I'm actually a fairly forceful person, but I had to keep toning myself down. It doesn't matter anymore—I have nothing to lose by suiting myself.

I am now in my forties and able to bring together my beliefs, my values, and my philosophy with who I am. I can actually act out who I am and that is very exciting. It's possible because of my

status in my career. I've redefined what my idea of success is—
success is what I do with what I believe. I'm going into my middle
age without a partner and it feels great.

In one workshop I took for midlife women, the participants
became very enthusiastic about the idea of "having some fun." I had
made a passing reference to this; it was seized upon by women in the
group who agreed that they wanted to enjoy life, to be a little self-
centered after years of putting others first. They wanted to kick up
their heels and to hell with what people thought. Knowing that there
are only so many years ahead can be liberating, inducing a sense of
"now or never" about ambitions that may have been put aside. This
may be something as major as a career change, but it could also be
something relatively small, like taking up a sport, climbing a moun-
tain, or going nightclubbing.

Perhaps the last word should go to an 83-year-old. "To make a
success of old age," she said, "start young."

Part Two

MENOPAUSE

Chapter 3

The Construction of
the "New" Menopause

In the course of researching for this book I realized that beyond saying simply that menopause is the end of menstruation, there is no empirical definition of menopause. How it is viewed will differ subtly from woman to woman, and will differ substantially from society to society. Cultures construct the meaning of menopause according to their own social values.

Whether menopause is seen as a negative, positive, or neutral event will depend on such factors as social attitudes toward older women and the status accorded women's reproductive role. In defining menopause for herself, the individual woman will draw on the current stereotype of menopause in her own culture.

The Discovery of a New Disease

In Western cultures, the lack of an objective description of menopause has left the way open for competing interests to contest what menopause means—the principal protagonists being the medical industry and the feminist movement.

Two stereotypes of menopause are currently promoted to the public. The medical one describes menopause as an endocrinopathy or disease of the hormonal system, a "deficiency syndrome" resulting from loss of estrogen. From this standpoint the menopausal woman is in a pathological or diseased state and should be medically treated. By this definition, the meaning of menopause is removed from the individual woman or the collective control of women to become properly a matter for doctors.

Menopause is transformed from "a stage in the normal processes of aging into a hazard to health."(1) As an Australian gynecologist succinctly put it, "The postmenopause should be regarded as a sex-linked endocrine deficiency disease which requires careful evaluation, management and follow-up."(2) Dr. Don Gambrell, Professor of Endocrinology and Obstetrics at the Medical College of Georgia, had a similar description. The menopause, he said, "is a hormonal deficiency state and, like all endocrinopathies, should be managed as vigorously as need be and without a necessary limitation of time."(3)

The medical model of menopause has infinitely expanded the period of menopause. As we are judged "estrogen deficient" until we die, menopause is no longer a matter of months or years, but a life sentence. It is a permanent condition to be permanently managed.(4) "I wish to impress on you that the menopause is not a short event in a woman's progression through life," says American endocrinologist Dr. Robert Greenblatt, "but a condition to be endured from the moment the ovaries begin to falter to the very last of life."(5)

Medicine argues that menopause under its control is more normal than an "untreated" one. Since women are "deficient," what they have lost must logically be "replaced." The word *replacement* in the term "hormone replacement therapy" implies that a normal condition is being regained by the drugs. As one doctor put it: "Hormone replacement therapy is a replacement—it's not a treatment. It's a replacement for the hormones you actually lose . . . it is a method of making the 20 years that occur after menopause more natural. That's what we doctors are aiming at. To make life more natural."(6)

In reality, the medicated menopause is a mutation and an artifice, remodeling the experience of menopause. The cessation of periods is no longer a marker of menopausal transition, for hormonal treatment prolongs menstruation indefinitely. Even loss of fertility is not a foregone conclusion, for postmenopausal women have even been induced to have pregnancies with the aid of hormones and donated ova.(7)

The definition of menopause as disease is a function of the ideological underpinnings of medicine. Medicine is oriented toward illness. Like the explorer seeking new continents or the hunter stalking game, the doctor tracks down disease. His mission is to diagnose and treat. The explorer names his new territory despite the fact that its inhabitants may already have a name for it. Doctors discover and name diseases regardless of the wishes of the people who are host to them.

The original people of the land and the carriers of the disease are colonized, and naming rights become the possession of the discoverers, to bestow as they think fit. In the medical literature, doctors frequently argue that it is the professional not the woman who must determine when she is menopausal. She cannot know since by virtue of being both "patient" and woman, she is simultaneously subjective and subordinate. The professional, on the other hand, believes he is able to specify her condition objectively according to scientific criteria. To facilitate this process, woman's belief in her own ability to define menopause must be undermined. Her experience and her reality must be taken from her.

In the case of menopause it is not just individuals who are singled out for the disease label, but all women of that age. Unless we die before menopause, none of us can escape it. We are all doomed to become estrogen deficient and therefore diseased. This medicalization of a woman's normal experience is not just confined to menopause. Reproduction and childbirth are other social aspects of our lives that are defined as medical events. Premenstrual tension is another disease label widely given to women. Medicine is inherently sexist. The male is the norm in medicine and woman the other. Virtually any experience or capacity that differentiates women from men has been deemed by medicine to be pathological. Aging in men is normal; menopause is not. Our biology renders us abnormal.

Biology as Destiny

Although medicine touts itself as rational and objective, it is in reality deeply influenced by the prevailing ideology and power structure of the society within which it operates. Whether it is to support the racist regime of apartheid South Africa or the antisemitism of Nazi Germany, medicine has always come to the aid of ruling elites by redefining powerless groups as biologically inferior, thereby justifying their subordinate position.

In the case of women, medicine has reinforced social beliefs that women's proper roles are as mothers and wives, and that women should be narcissistically obsessed with physical appearance. Women who are not—lesbians, career women, unmarried women—are labeled deviant, destined to become psychologically disturbed. When it comes to menopause, woman's distress can be explained by the diminution of all her "natural" roles.

Consequently, although medicine is claimed as a science, doctors have seen no contradiction or irony in venturing into all areas of women's lives, including sexuality, relationships, social roles, and appearance. In his book on menopause for physicians, for instance, Dr. Wulf Utian enjoins his colleagues to give advice on "total body care, including advice about oral and dental hygiene, cosmetics and care of skin and nails."(8)

Estrogen deficiency may have been defined in the laboratory by measuring the hormonal output of menopausal ovaries, but the medical stereotype of menopause owes everything to the wider social context in which it has been developed. Medicine merely supplied the scientific justification for the social stereotype. Integral to the medical model is the equating of women's biological role with the meaning of her existence. Through this perspective of biological determinism, woman is her hormones. Her life is defined by her fertility. Her most "normal" period and the apogee of her whole life is her fertile years, between puberty and menopause.

According to Dr. Robert Greenblatt, "Each woman passes through three epochs in her progression through life. The first, from birth to adolescence, is in preparation for the second, the years of fecundity. The third ends her potential for reproduction. Thus, she enters the menopause, the permanent cessation of menstruation. Now, in her advancing years, she is protected from the stresses and tribulations of childbearing, for which, unfortunately, she pays a price, the loss of estrogen production by the ovaries."(9) Thus, the purpose of female existence is defined as reproduction, with childhood a preparation for it, and old age a rest from it. By this definition, women have only a biological purpose in life and no social purpose at all. Their status is determined by the state of their ovaries. The contribution of women to the spheres of the arts, sport, work, and political and social endeavor are all utterly denied by this description.

Frances McCrea, an American sociologist, has identified four themes that underlie the medical definition of menopause. These are: "(1) women's potential and function are biologically destined; (2) women's worth is determined by fecundity and attractiveness; (3) rejection of the feminine role will bring physical and emotional havoc; (4) aging women are useless and repulsive."(10)

Every one of these themes involves a social judgment about the status and proper role of women. There is no area that demonstrates the entrenched sexism of medicine more sharply than that of menopause. The defining of a normal bodily state as diseased, the suggestion that women become worthless with the loss of childbearing capacity, the overlay of chauvinistic attitudes about the importance of sexual attractiveness—even the language of menopause—are inherently misogynous.

Diseases have other purposes besides identifying pathologies which need to be cured. They have commercial potential, and they can also be a form of social control. The act of labeling someone with a disease provides a tool for disempowering her or him. Whether a schizophrenic or an "estrogen-deficient woman," the person becomes the disease label. She or he is stripped of individual identity and self-determination. Salvation for the patient lies in dependency on the physician who bestowed the label. In the case of the woman with problems at menopause, the solution does not lie in the woman's own abilities, nor in social change to improve the conditions of her life, but in what the doctor has to offer. Only he can remove the stigmata that have been placed on her. He holds the cure to her disease.

The new view of menopause as disease is socially controlling in another way. The definition of the midlife woman as deficient strikes a blow at her sense of completeness as a woman. It exploits her fears about aging and is personally eroding. Medicine is meant to be neutral and detached, but in this case science reinforces negative social attitudes about the menopausal woman's waning value in the sexual marketplace. It legitimates the social prejudices by providing a "scientific" basis for them. In its worst excesses (and these will be illustrated later in this chapter) it is more akin to pornography or sexual terrorism than science. The current medical model of menopause is neither scientific nor neutral. It is ideological—a strategy for enforcing women's compliance to medical treatment and acceptance of their social role.

Hot Flashes or "Power Surges"— The Gospel According to Feminists

Feminists have fought against the redefinition of menopause as a disease. Frances McCrea explains that this and other similar struggles to preserve the right of groups to collective self-definition are "stigma contests" whereby subordinate groups reject their deviant label.(11) At stake are status and prestige. Stigmatized groups attempt to retrieve their "spoiled identity."

Against the negative medical stereotype, feminists have sought to rehabilitate menopause by insisting on its normalcy. Thus some feminist writers have claimed that menopause should be a period of renewal and spiritual awakening, a time to be more contemplative and self-centered. They have adopted the term "postmenopausal zest" to describe this stage in women's lives and assert the belief that having shucked off their maternal responsibilities midlife women now have the chance to branch out and achieve things they could not previously. At their most celebratory, feminists have attempted the redemptive feat of reclaiming words like "hag" and "crone"—words for which there is no real male equivalent and that symbolize the visceral revulsion toward aging women that exists in Western society.

These attempts by feminists to assert the naturalness and dignity of aging in women have been only partly successful. Medical orthodoxy is always difficult for laypeople to counter because they lack credibility. But to some extent feminists have been the instruments of their own failure. In seeking to reduce the stigma of menopause, some feminists have described menopause in a way rather removed from women's lives. They have created a kind of mythology: an idealized vision of a trouble-free, even joyous, transition from young to old which is actually unrecognizable to many women. Women live in the real world where for them aging is a relentless process of sexual disqualification and the deterioration of one of their assets—their physical beauty. While the feminist stereotype might be attractive, it is difficult to reconcile with the attitudes women encounter around them. As well as this, some women do encounter difficulties at the time of menopause, and there is no place for this in the feminist canon. Feminist ideology runs the risk of denying women's actual experience. The effect can be that women blame themselves for not coping better.

Modern women are left in some confusion about what to expect at menopause. The medical stereotype has been widely promoted through the mainstream media and is available not only to menopausal women but to those around them—husbands, family, friends, and coworkers. Will it be all doom and gloom, a period when one's feminine attributes inexorably wither away as the doctors say? Or will it be a time of celebration and rebirth, as delineated in the gospel according to feminists? At the very least, women are anxious about menopause, wondering whether they will be spared its worst depredations. This is particularly true of middle-class women who have been most exposed to these ideologies.

New Drugs Need New Diseases

Until the 1960s doctors were not much interested in menopause. It was simply something their female patients went through and if women came to them with complaints, they were likely to be told it was just to be put up with. Perhaps this lack of interest stemmed from the fact that there was nothing much doctors could offer: there were no operations, no complex tests, and no wonder drugs. Medicine exhorts doctors to act, to "do something." As long as menopause was a condition about which nothing much could be done, doctors ignored it.

Medicine can create diseases to provide a market for new products developed by the pharmaceutical industry. There are two alternate scenarios in the development of drugs: biomedical scientists can go looking for a cure for a known illness, such as cancer; and new compounds are sometimes synthesized in the laboratory without anyone being initially clear what purpose they can be put to. The end result is a drug in need of a disease. The more broadly the disease can then be defined, the greater the treatable population and the greater the potential sales. Well people and others experiencing social problems are obvious targets.

Menopause—All in the Mind?

Medical interest in menopause was initially stimulated by the advent of the psychotropic or mind-altering drugs—the tranquilizers and antidepressants. Medical journals in the 1960s are littered with advertisements for products like Valium, Librium, and amitriptyline, for whom the principal target was women. This was the period when myriad housewives suffered from what Betty Friedan dubbed "the problem that has no name."(12) The symptoms were lethargy, boredom, anxiety, crying spells, irritability, and insomnia—all classic hallmarks of reactive depression and anxiety psychoses.

It was not until the women's movement came along with its analysis of sex roles that the real causes of this widespread malaise were pinpointed. In the aftermath of an economic depression and a grueling world war, men and women had wanted a period of settled life, a haven from the vileness and inhumanity of the world, where children could be safely reared and the emotional needs that had been put aside for so long could be met. At the center of this dream of domestic peace was the woman—the housemother, busy in her apron, attending to her husband's and her children's needs. Their happiness was to be her fulfillment.

Women fell victim to propaganda, promulgated through women's magazines, that they should have no ambitions beyond their quarter acre—true feminine nirvana lay in the home. Women's dissatisfaction with this limiting role did not at first manifest itself as individual objection or collective rebellion, as it later would, but obliquely as mental and emotional symptoms reported to doctors. This is where the psychotropic drugs came in—"mother's little helper," in the immortal words of the Rolling Stones.

Psychotropic drugs were first used in mental hospitals in the 1950s, but there was a bigger market waiting to be tapped and the pharmaceutical companies were not slow to realize it. By the early 1960s psychotropics were widely promoted to doctors as being ideal for middle-aged women and able to "cure" the "symptoms of menopause." Advertising for these drugs developed a stereotype of the menopausal patient as beset with psychological devils, anxious about her femininity and her waning attractiveness, and grieving for the loss of her fecundity. There was even a psychiatric label to put on her—"involutional melancholia"—a major depression of midlife. This condition is now considered never to have existed, but in the postwar years it was a powerful tool for diagnosing the menopausal woman as ill and in need of treatment.(13) Drugs could help her to be serene in her role and no longer troublesome to her husband.

In developing this stereotype of menopause as a time of mental illness, medicine was able to draw on the work of psychoanalytical writers. Earlier in the century, Freud had viewed menopause as neurotic, and other psychoanalysts amplified the theme. By the 1940s menopause was described in their work as a negative crisis period for women during which they mourned the end of their feminine attractiveness and their childbearing capacity. The Freudian Helene Deutsch, whose book *The Psychology of Women* was very influential, defined menopause as obsolescence: woman had "reached her natural end—her partial death—as servant of the species." Menopause spelled the loss of the meaning of a woman's life. "The woman is mortified because she has to give up everything that she received in puberty."(14)

In the late 1940s Therese Benedek began to introduce the endocrine deficiency argument into the psychoanalytic equation. She argued that menopause was "a progressive psychological adaptation to a regressive biological process" at which women could succeed or fail according to their prior adjustment to the feminine role. Just as "masculine protest" could result in premenstrual tension during the reproductive years, the menopausal woman who failed to weather "the desexualization of the emotional needs" could become hostile and regressive, exhibiting behavior which seemed "a repetition of puberty."(15)

The psychoanalysts invented terms such as "midlife crisis" and "empty nest syndrome" to explain the emotional feelings women were supposed to suffer at this time. There is a complete acceptance in this literature, as there was in the medical world, that women's feelings of self-esteem were entirely bound up in the feminine role, so that any perceived diminution of it must create emotional trauma. Biology was destiny and woman's biological clock had run down.

Psychology provided the rationale; pharmacology provided the tools. With these twin weapons, medicine could go to work on menopause. New vistas of "treatable" populations opened up. It was possible to interpret virtually any emotional or physical complaint made by a midlife woman as stemming from the menopausal neurosis she was suffering.

In Britain, doctors began warning of "the relentless march of the psychotropic drug juggernaut."(16) Every study of psychoactive drug use conducted during this period in both America and Britain showed that women were far more likely than men to be using them.(17) In Britain, by 1972, 45 million prescriptions were being written out annually for psychoactive drugs at an annual cost of £24 million. These drugs were 17.7% of all drugs prescribed. Many were written out for vague complaints such as "neurosis," "depression," "to calm me down."

A major survey of general practitioners' prescribing of psychotropic drugs published in 1971 showed that the use of minor tranquilizers (Librium and Valium) had increased by 110% in a five-year period, and the use of tricyclic antidepressants (amitriptyline, imipramine—Tofranil) had increased by 320%. During the study period, 17% of all women (compared to 8% of men) had been prescribed psychotropic drugs; the median age for women using them was 44 years.(18)

The epidemic scale of prescribing psychotropic drugs to housewives eventually led to its discreditation, but not before the way had been prepared for acceptance of the next category of drugs that would "treat" menopause. The psychotropic drug era began the process of reorienting menopause from a normal biological event to that of a disease that could respond to medical treatment.

The Hugh Hefner of Menopause

This reorientation process was elaborated in the seminal work of Dr. Robert A. Wilson, who almost single-handedly cemented the idea of menopause as disease. Wilson was a prominent New York gynecologist who in the 1960s launched a crusade to rescue women from the "living decay" of menopause. The "tragedy of menopause," he claimed, "often destroys her character as well as her health." From this fate women could be saved by using estrogen from "puberty to grave."(19)

The discovery that prompted Wilson to undertake his mission was the development of a cheap estrogen preparation. According to Drs. Howard Judd and Wulf Utian, it was estrogen that changed the status of menopause from "a side issue of nuisance complaints to an issue central to the subject of aging in women."(20)

In the psychotropic drug era, medicine had regarded menopause as a disease of the mind; the new medical model deemed menopause to be a disease of the body. Robert Wilson incorporated the psychological explanation into his mythology of menopause, but he gave it a physical cause—a deficiency of estrogen. He argued that tranquilizers were unnecessary for the menopausal woman: all her complaints could be dealt with by simply abolishing menopause, making her "feminine forever," a feat he proposed could be accomplished with hormones.

Wilson was not just a doctor but also an evangelist and entrepreneur. In the book *Women and the Crisis in Sex Hormones,* Barbara and Gideon Seaman describe how Wilson founded a private trust, the Wilson Foundation, in 1963 for the purpose of promoting estrogens. Funding to the tune of $1.3 million came from the pharmaceutical industry. In one year (1964), Wilson received $17,000 from Searle, $8,700 from Ayerst Laboratories, and $5,600 from the Upjohn Company. All these companies made hormone products that Wilson claimed were effective in preventing or treating menopause.(21)

It is tempting to speculate as to why Wilson embarked on his crusade. Obviously he made money from drug companies and from the thousands of women who flocked to his practice (by 1966 he said he had treated 5,000 women with estrogen), but he also had a messianic vision of himself as something akin to a medical saint. He actually talks about himself as a martyr for science, describes scientific research as "a form of worship," and refers to his coworkers as "converts." But what also comes through in his writing is the egotistical desire of an aging and paternalistic man to "save" women from their fate. If Wilson had been a saint, he would undoubtedly have been Saint George, slaying the monster of physical decay to rescue the midlife damsel in distress. Wilson sought and acquired a good deal of public prominence; there would undoubtedly have been women who saw him as their savior. If female adulation appealed to Wilson, he would certainly have got it.

In *Feminine Forever*, published in 1966, Wilson promoted his ideas to women. The book sold 100,000 copies in the first seven months and was widely excerpted in such popular women's magazines as *Vogue*. Journalists picked up on the theme so that over the late 1960s and early 1970s more than 300 articles promoting estrogen appeared in women's magazines.

Even before he began promoting estrogen to women, Wilson had taken his message to the medical profession. In several articles in medical journals Wilson expounded his thesis that menopause was a disease. Although some of Wilson's peers dismissed him as a crank, other influential doctors supported his claims. The highly regarded Dr. Robert B. Greenblatt, now Emeritus Professor in the Department of Physiology and Endocrinology at the Medical College of Georgia, wrote a foreword to Wilson's *Feminine Forever* in such colorful language that it closely rivals Wilson's own florid prose.

For most women, Greenblatt wrote, "the effects of estrogen deprivation are physically and emotionally devastating; for a fortunate few the damage is minimal, the scars only slightly visible." Women regarded "the threat of declining femininity, of waning romance" with dread. Woman, he continued, "will be emancipated only when the shackles of hormonal deprivation are loosed." Enter Dr. Wilson, who "like a gallant knight has come to rescue his fair lady not at the time of her bloom and flowering but in her despairing years . . . . Dr. Wilson, with boldness and clarity of purpose, sounds the clarion call, awakening a slumbering profession to a woman's needs."

Dr. Wilson did indeed go about the task of converting his medical colleagues with considerable vigor. As medicine had kept women alive beyond the viability of their ovaries, he said, medicine had a duty to set things right by medicating women into the preferred hormonal state. Wilson expounded his views most fully in a paper written in conjunction with his wife, Thelma, a nurse. Entitled "The Fate of the Nontreated Menopausal Woman: A Plea for the Maintenance of Adequate Estrogen from Puberty to the Grave," it was published in 1963 in the *Journal of the American Geriatrics Society*.(22)

The picture of menopause that emerges from this paper and other writing by Wilson is worth looking at in some detail because Wilson's stereotype was eventually adopted almost in its entirety by the medical profession. It has survived essentially unmodified to the present day. This was underlined for me when I discovered a paper bearing a title remarkably similar to that of Dr. Wilson's but published a quarter of a century later. This time it was "The Fate of the Untreated Menopause," written by Dr. Wulf Utian and published in 1987.(23)

Although Dr. Wilson published his first treatise in a scientific publication, his language is far from objective. The first few sentences set the tone:

> The unpalatable truth must be faced that all postmenopausal women are castrates. There is a variation in degree but not in fact, men do not live as long as the so-called weaker sex. However, they age, if free from serious disease, in a proportional manner. The pituitary-adrenal axis and thyroid are relatively intact until very old age . . . From a practical point of view, a man remains a man until the very end. The situation with a woman is very different. Her ovaries become inadequate relatively early in life. She is the only mammal who cannot reproduce after middle age.

This last statement, which it is tempting to dismiss as ludicrous and irrelevant, is still regularly quoted by medical writers as evidence of women's obsolescence after menopause. Having lost her reproductive capacity, the woman is redundant. She has outlived her ovaries and therefore her biological usefulness. If she was truly adapted like a dog or cow, she would die with fully functioning ovaries.

It is a revealing viewpoint. First, it displays a willful ignorance of the difference between human development, where the child is dependent for years, and the animal state, where the offspring can rapidly fend for themselves. Women have a stage at the end of their lives where they cannot reproduce precisely so they can rear their children to maturity before they die. This cycle has evolved to protect the species.

But Wilson's view hints at what is a persistent theme in the medical literature on menopause. The woman's identity and status is completely determined by her biology. Her reproductive capacity defines her womanhood: having lost that, she is no longer female. She is a "neuter," a "eunuch," and a "castrate." All these words are used by Wilson.

Wilson developed a huge list of "serious consequences" of the decline in estrogen. Among the physical consequences he lists coronary attacks, strokes, heart disease, hypertension, osteoporosis, "tough, dry, scaly and inelastic" skin, flabby "atrophic" breasts, and shrinking labia. Among the "psychic manifestations" he includes depression, mood swings, a "vapid cow-like feeling called a 'negative state,'" irritability, frigidity, absentmindedness, and even suicide. To underline the extremity of the menopausal state he claimed that menopause was a "mutilation of the whole body," and that "no woman can be sure of escaping the horror of this living decay."

According to Wilson, these "desexed women" are everywhere once you notice them.

> Once the veil is lifted, it is remarkable how quickly the previously uninitiated can detect these unfortunate women—our streets abound with them—walking stiffly in twos and threes, seeing little and observing less. It is not unusual to see an erect man of 75 vigorously striding along the golf course, but never a woman of this age . . . . Before this moderately advanced age is reached, the more intelligent woman instinctively knows that her loss of physical attractiveness is entirely out of proportion. She sees the marked skin changes, the disfiguring fat deposits, the atrophy of her breasts and the beginning disappearance of her external

genitals. If married, an irritated or inadequate vagina may bring more unhappiness. All this has a profound effect upon her psyche.

The menopausal woman is not just a tragedy for her own sake but is dangerous to her family and indeed the whole of society. "There is ample evidence," says Wilson authoritatively, without giving any evidence at all, "that the course of history has been changed not only by the presence of estrogen, but by its absence. The untold misery of alcoholism, drug addiction, divorce and broken homes caused by these unstable, estrogen-starved women cannot be presented in statistical form."

"Menopause," concludes Wilson, "is borne bravely by women, but is really hardly endurable."

In *Feminine Forever,* Wilson is deeply muddled about his role as a physician. He doesn't just cross the boundary between objective scientist and member of the male sex, he leers across it. There is something unpleasantly voyeuristic about his desire to ensure that all women are walking around with plump juicy genitals. Wilson's views as a man determined his clinical judgment. He was the Hugh Hefner of menopause.

Wilson had strongly traditional views on such matters as women's role, their sexual behavior, even their appearance and dress, and he saw it as a part of physicians' business to address these matters. He even believed that career women would need stronger doses of estrogen, as if involvement in the male world of business would have depleted their hormones. His homilies to his female readers commonly spring from his own sexist fantasies and erotic objectification of women. "There is hardly anything lovelier to see or touch," he wrote, "than the skin of a young woman of about twenty—so smooth, pliant and delicate."

And there is his description in *Feminine Forever* of a typical man's behavior at a party, grazing among the female guests, part of Wilson's effort to explain that normal men do not see breasts as women's principal attraction.

Roving about at a party, a footloose male might scan his surroundings at floor level, searching for a pair of trim legs. A slow upward sweep of the eyes thereupon assesses the general posture of his object of interest. As a physician professionally trained in the art of observation, it has not escaped me that what turns male heads at a gathering is not a woman's face or even her figure. It is an erect, graceful, posture that invariably commands attention . . . .

Once his interest is aroused, a man usually takes a rather systematic inventory of a woman's appearance. He assesses her face, though beauty in a classical sense does not seem to rank high as a sexual attraction, then he examines the way she dresses, reacting strongly to the indefinable quality of chic, which, by the way, has little to do with being fashionable. There are women who look more chic in dungarees than others do in a Dior model gown. The critical survey then proceeds to her hands, teeth and throat. By that time the investigating male is doubtlessly edging closer in order to hear her voice. Eventually, his eyes limn the contour of her breasts. But this, in most social situations, has low priority. I wish more women would realize that.

Wilson's views on women's clothing provide revealing insights into his views on the proper relationship between husband and wife and the role of the doctor:

Perhaps a doctor should stick to prescribing medicine instead of prescribing fashion. Yet I cannot in good conscience ignore the matter of dress. Trivial as it may seem, it is part of the total aspect of sexuality and marital adjustment. In particular, the recent trend of stretch pants for casual wear seems, to me at least, diabolically designed to stamp out mature sex. If the average woman could contemplate the vista she presents from behind, she would no longer wonder at her husband's lack of ardor. Clothes are part of a woman's charm, and they should be chosen with precisely that in mind. Too many of today's fashions strike me as distinctly anti-sexual, because, by revealing, they destroy charm and the sense of mystery that stimulates men. If a woman lacks the sense or taste to dress attractively, I believe her husband should insist on a suitable style of dress for her. This may contribute considerably to marital harmony.

The Legacy of Dr. Wilson

It is tempting to dismiss Wilson as over the top, and some doctors did, except that he was enormously influential. Dr. P. A. van Keep of the International Menopause Society said in a paper published in 1990 that as far as he was concerned HRT began when he read the paper by Robert Wilson.(24) Neither was his influence confined to America.

A survey conducted in 1969 by the International Health Foundation looked at women's knowledge of the use of HRT for menopause in each of five European countries. The differences in knowledge were entirely explainable by the availability of Wilson's book and the extent of publicity surrounding it. In West Germany, for instance, the publicity around HRT was on a scale unmatched before or since for any other medical topic. Leading experts quickly endorsed Wilson's views so that the 1969 survey found that a huge 71% of West German women knew that hormone treatment was available for treatment of menopausal symptoms. Comparable figures were 47% in Italy, 36% in Great Britain, 54% in France, and 57% in Belgium.(25)

Dr. Wilson's influence can be seen in the way his definition of menopause has been accepted and repeated. Even Dr. Wilson's phrases seem to have gained the status of common currency. For instance, who has been reading whom here?

Dr. Wilson, 1963: "The nipples become flat and nonerectile."(26)

Dr. Utian, 1987: "The nipples become smaller and flatter and lose their erectile properties."(27)

Drs. Karen Brown and Charles Hammond, 1987: "The nipples become smaller and flatter; they lose their erectile properties."(28)

And from a self-help guide for women written by a woman gynecologist in 1987: "The nipples may become smaller and flatter and lose their erectile properties."(29)

(Note: there is no firm evidence that estrogen is responsible for breast changes as we age, nor that taking estrogen will make any difference to the breasts.)

Another example: in defining menopause as disease, Dr. Wilson compared it to diabetes. Diabetics lack insulin; the menopausal woman lacks estrogen. Both, he said, can be replaced.

This comparison has proved enduring. Writer after writer has compared menopause to diabetes. It is an attractive comparison to make with the lay public because it has a certain superficial logic. In a newspaper article in 1987, Professor Colin Mantell, head of the Department of Obstetrics and Gynecology at Auckland University

School of Medicine, used the diabetes analogy to argue for increased use of HRT. "If it is known that a person is insulin deficient," he said, "we prescribe insulin without hesitation. Similarly with thyroid deficiencies. Yet many doctors hesitate to prescribe hormone replacements in menopause, when the women are quite often suffering dreadful symptoms simply because of hormone deficiency."(30)

Wilson as the Marquis de Sade

Wilson's approach to menopause has been carried on by his disciples. He invented a language for menopause which many who have come after him have adopted. It is not a scientific language but an emotive one, full of derogatory attitudes toward women. I have already given some examples, but the following description of a woman's breasts after menopause displays most graphically the negative stereotype Dr. Wilson strained to convey in building his case for the awfulness of menopause.

> After menopause, when estrogen and progesterone sink to a low level, the breast begins to shrivel and sag. Once the supply of those two nourishing hormones is cut off, the breasts become pendulous, wrinkled and flabby. Often the skin of the breasts coarsens and is covered with scales. The breasts lose their erotic sensitivity and sometimes do not even respond to painful stimuli. Only estrogen replacement therapy can prevent this premature decline of a woman's symbol of femininity.

Dr. Wilson may at times have been the Hugh Hefner of menopause, but in this mode, he is the Marquis de Sade! No midlife woman can read this misogynous description without wincing, just as I'm sure a man would if a doctor attempted a similarly highly distorted description of balding heads or beer bellies.

This biased disabling language has continued as part and parcel of the discussion of menopause by doctors. It is commonplace in medical writing on menopause to read such words as "sexual decline," "fading sexual attractiveness," and "the aging ovary."(31) "Slowly the vulva shrivels, becoming a dry narrow slit in some old women," say Dr. Derek Llewellyn-Jones and Suzanne Abraham in their handbook for women.(32) In both the medical and lay literature, there is a constant use of words such as "shrink," "atrophy," "wrinkle," "sag," and "dry." The picture is one of inevitable shriveling up. It does make you wonder how the many plump, upright, full-bosomed, or just plain large older women you see in daily life managed to survive this process of desiccation.

The repeated use of the word "deficient" in discussion of menopause reinforces the picture of older women as lacking, inadequate, incomplete, and defective. The dictionary defines a "deficiency disease" as "any condition, such as pellagra, beriberi, or scurvy, produced by a lack of vitamins or other essential substances." The menopausal woman, then, is like the sufferer of scurvy or beriberi. The comparison with diabetes accords the menopausal woman the same health status as a diabetic, who must inject herself or himself with insulin or become dangerously ill. Estrogen has been defined by medicine as essential to a woman's good health and to her womanhood.

Modern doctors have also followed Dr. Wilson's lead in advocating that doctors should intervene in all aspects of their menopausal patients' lives. In a 1989 article in *Postgraduate Medicine,* Dr. Robert Wells, who runs a menopause center at Long Beach, California, took a leaf out of Dr. Wilson's book in offering some advice to physicians in handling their midlife patients. The woman who is "clinically menopausal," he said, "needs hope. She needs to know she is not alone. She needs to be reassured that her problem is physical, not psychological. She needs to know she is not going crazy or experiencing early Alzheimer's disease. She needs to be encouraged to stop clinging to the past and to accept new challenges, to set new goals, to get excited about the future. 'Upgrading'—a change of hairstyle or hair color, a new outfit—may add excitement and heighten self-esteem." Offer your midlife patient HRT, he advised physicians, and you "will likely win a lifelong friend and admirer."(33) Sound familiar?

All We Need Is . . . Hormones

The idea of menopause as a disease of estrogen deficiency that needs treatment is firmly in place. In 1990 the *New Zealand Doctor,* a glossy publication given free to general practitioners and widely read by them, included an eight-page pull-out supplement entitled "How to Treat Menopause," which espoused what is now the orthodox medical position on menopause. It began with the statement: "As the life

expectancy of women lengthens so do the years spent in the estrogen-deficient state of menopause. One-third of menopausal women
suffer from symptoms severe enough to seek help." This supplement
contained articles on "symptoms" and "the effects of estrogen deprivation," while two pages were devoted to osteoporosis and one to
HRT. There is only a passing reference to the fact that many of the
so-called "psychological aspects of menopause" might have very little
to do with endocrine changes in the body.(34)

In 1990 one New Zealand general practitioner described menopause in terms very reminiscent of Dr. Wilson's a quarter of a century
previously:

> For some reason all the glands in the body have adapted to the
> new life expectancy except for the female ovaries and these pack
> up completely at the age of 50 in everyone. There is no exception.
> I say 50, 51, 52—not much longer than that and the poor female
> sex is then left in effect castrated. The female hormones mean
> an awful lot to women and they are left on their own so they
> have to fend for themselves without these very very necessary
> hormones and we feel rather sorry for them.(35)

In 1987, as guest speaker at a major gynecology conference organized by the New Zealand Obstetrical and Gynecological Society,
the outspoken Dr. John Studd, consultant gynecologist at King's College Hospital, London, called menopause "a multisystem deficiency
disorder" which affects the skin, skeleton, pelvis, bladder, heart, and
brain. He called menopausal women "these wretched women" undergoing "general atrophy." When women going through menopause
had complained to him about thinning skin and hair, "I used to think
it was the self-indulgent manifestation of their own misery," he said,
"but it is true."

As we shall see in the chapter on hormone replacement therapy,
there is absolutely no proof that HRT can accomplish the miracles
claimed by Dr. Wilson. It is not an elixir of youth and has only been
proven effective for a limited number of conditions. Yet it has become
commonplace for doctors following in Wilson's footsteps to make
somewhat exaggerated claims for the properties of the drug.

In an unpublished paper on hormone replacement therapy, Dr.
Graeme Overton, an Auckland gynecologist who runs clinics for
menopausal women at National Women's Hospital and in private

practice, listed a huge array of symptoms of "estrogen deficiency," all of which he said could be "alleviated or improved" by treatment with hormones. No research references are provided to back his claims. He gives 12 physical symptoms, 10 psychological symptoms, as well as effects on sexuality—a menopausal menu virtually identical to that developed by Dr. Wilson. The skin of the menopausal woman, he writes, "becomes thinner and loses its elasticity and firmness. Hair may become thinner and breasts usually shrink and droop as tone decreases." Even this, he claimed, would respond to HRT.(36)

Dr. Neil McKenzie makes similar extravagant claims. He argued that women must be given the choice of using hormones. He described how people coming into his surgery said: "'I'm getting osteoporosis now. I'm getting sexual dysfunction. I'm having problems with my appearance. I can't be a model anymore.' . . . Women do take a pride in their appearance and in the way that they look, the way that they function. The very very essence of life. It's absolutely vital for them to be given a chance." Dr. McKenzie said that he took a photograph of each woman as she went on estrogen: "That's the only way we can really prove to them that they are going to feel and look better. I show this photo as the years go by and compare it with how they look."(37)

Dr. Wilson also left a legacy of advocacy for HRT with the mainstream media. Dr. McKenzie was interviewed at length on Radio New Zealand in 1990. Dr. Studd, whose visit to New Zealand was funded by a company that markets estrogen products, presented his views on the television news and in the daily newspapers. Dr. Overton was featured in a full-page article in the *New Zealand Herald* in 1987. A photograph showed him holding a packet of HRT, over the caption "Dr. Overton . . . nature can be unkind."(38) Despite the fact that the photograph showed his own thinning hair and wrinkles, in Dr. Overton's view nature's unkindness was toward women.

The new promoters of estrogen may not promise it will keep women "feminine forever," although in claiming hormones can do things for hair, skin, and breasts they come perilously close to doing so, but like runners in a relay race, they pursue the same line. The baton may have changed hands, but they are still heading in the same direction. Although initially some members of the medical profession regarded Dr. Robert Wilson as unacceptably entrepreneurial and extreme in his views, his ideas have now entered the mainstream of medicine. In the main medical reference works, menopause is now variously listed under "Ovarian Dysfunction," "Diseases of the Endocrine System," and "Endocrine Disorders."(39) Wilson's myth of the menopausal woman as diseased and in need of treatment is now firmly in place as the medical model of menopause.

Chapter 4

Will the Real Menopause Please Stand Up

So if menopause isn't a deficiency disease, what is it? That question is surprisingly difficult to answer. The medical journals are certainly not much help. They are so obsessed with the subject of estrogen that they have virtually abandoned any other aspect of research into menopause. Journals that are supposed to be about menopause are now devoted to studies of hormones. Of 227 papers published in *Maturitas: The International Journal for the Study of Climacteric* between 1978 and 1985, 96 were related directly to hormone therapy and only seven to nonhormonal medication.(1)

It is precisely because hormones are being promoted as a cure-all for the "symptoms of menopause" that we need to be exact about what the symptoms are. Taking hormones may seem very attractive if we believe they can eliminate a whole smorgasbord of problems, real or potential. If they can only deal with a limited range of estrogen-related symptoms, the wisdom of taking steroids for years may be thrown into doubt. To arrive at a balanced perspective we need to examine menopause in some detail, so we can see what is hormonal and what is not.

One of the problems bedeviling such a discussion is the necessity to distinguish menopause from aging. Being menopausal and being a midlife woman are not exactly the same thing. Menopause is an event of midlife, it is not synonymous with midlife.

Men age and go through midlife and experience the stresses and rewards that phase of life brings. Women do too, but for women there is a tendency to conflate the troublesome aspects of these processes with menopause. Menopause gets blamed for any difficult aspects of midlife. For women, menopause focuses attention rather unavoidably on the fact that they are getting older. One manual for women expressed this idea of menopause as a marker for old age rather brutally: "Women who would have boasted in their teens about the start of menstruation as a sign they were grown up dislike admitting they are menopausal. They fear it is official confirmation that they are old, ripe for a bus pass and a pension."(2)

If men are forgetful, and find themselves putting the milk into the cupboard rather than the fridge, they may laugh it off as old age or as too trivial to worry about. Women may blame it on menopause.

On top of this, there are added meanings to aging for women that don't exist in the same way for men. Menopause brings the end of reproductive capacities whereas many men could keep on reproducing indefinitely. This end of fertility will only have a negative meaning in a culture that equates fecundity with women's worth. As well, our culture makes a cult of youthful femininity, so that physical aging in women is linked to sexuality and self-esteem much more closely than aging is for men. To some extent, menopause is seen as a symbol of depreciating sexual worth.

Many of the current ideas about menopause are also completely out-of-date. Women's lives have changed so dramatically in the past 20 years that their experience of aging must have also. Home and family are no longer the sole or even principal sources of identity. Work and a career are important to women in the 1990s in a way that was not true of the midlife woman of previous years. Yet the current menopausal stereotypes are still based on these old ideas that husbands and children are the be-all and end-all of women's lives, whereas women have moved on and lead much fuller lives.

It is not inevitable that menopause means what it means in this culture now. As part of a process of understanding the content and boundaries of menopause, it is important to disentangle fact and social fiction, and especially to understand what can be put down to hormones, what is caused by being a woman in late-twentieth-century Western society, and what is simply part of aging. This is not an easy task, but is an essential one if we are to understand menopause.

One of the perils of undertaking such a reevaluation is the danger of undermining women who do have problems at midlife. There are women who do have a very difficult menopause—who truly do have "raging hormones"—and it is important not to deny that reality. Yet other women might prefer to blame their midlife complaints on menopause, whether they are menopausal or not. This takes the problems outside their control; they are caused by "the change" and are not the result of other things in their life that may be difficult to do anything about.

Despite this, not challenging current ideas about menopause leaves the medical model intact, with the potential to harm women. The idea of menopause as a deficiency disease or inevitable time of trial is, I believe, not good for women. It sets up a potential obstacle in our future, and a generally negative stereotype of older women. It also lays the ground for the "treatment" of menopause when in reality there may be few in need of treatment.

The Meaning of Words

There is even some confusion around the language used to talk about menopause. Strictly speaking, menopause is simply the last menstrual period, just as menarche means the very first menstrual period. *Meno* comes from the Greek word for month, and *pause* from the Greek word *pausis*—halt.

But the whole process a woman goes through—the slowing down and eventual cessation of estrogen production, the menstrual changes leading to the end of menses, and the vasomotor effects such as hot flashes—all of which can take as many as 15 to 20 years—is called the *perimenopause* or *climacteric*. The origin of climacteric is the Greek word *klimakter*, meaning the rung of a ladder. As a metaphor for this event in women's lives, it doesn't have a negative connotation. The idea of progressing upward and achieving something is an antidote to the negativity often surrounding menopause. *Premenopause* is the word given to the period before the midlife woman has any menstrual changes.

Neither the words climacteric nor perimenopause are in popular use. In both lay and medical usage, menopause is now used to cover the whole period, and this is the way I have used it in this book.

A woman becomes *postmenopausal* when the whole process is completed, not just when the last period occurs. Just as a woman can have menstrual changes for some years before menstruation finishes, other signs such as hot flashes can continue for months or even years after bleeding ends. At some point in this process, the woman's reproductive capacity will end. This does not necessarily coincide with the last period; it may precede or postdate it, which is why women are advised to continue contraception for a year after the last menstrual period.

It is usual in the writing about menopause to see a discussion of the so-called "symptoms" of menopause, a term which is not really accurate. It reflects the fact that medicine sees menopause as an illness, which is not the view taken in this book. Menopause is a normal life event just as menarche is. This is not to deny that some women find menopause difficult, just as some girls have problems with their periods, but the majority do not. Natural bodily processes and physiological changes such as menopause should be defined by what ordinarily happens, not by the experience which is different. A better word than symptom would be "signs" of menopause, meaning indicators or signals of a normal event.

Another term that is inaccurate is the popular expression "change of life." True, the menopausal woman's reproductive status does change from one in which she could have children to one in which she cannot, but realistically most women have completed their families some years before they become menopausal, so the social change predates the biological change by some years. Change of life is an expression born of an era when women's role in life and status in the community was defined by her reproductive capacity and role as a mother. This is far less true in the 1990s when women have other sources of identity, and society holds less rigid ideas of women's proper purpose in life.

Women's lives vary far more in the 1990s than those of their mothers. The old set pattern of work-marriage-motherhood-menopause is now completely out of date. Women are more likely to stay in the workforce, taking time off to give birth, but having far more continuous working lives. The age at which women have their first child is increasing, with a significant number of women delaying their first pregnancy into their thirties. "When I started to get hot flashes, I went looking for books on menopause. They were all talking about children leaving home and grandchildren. I have a four-year-old."

Women are quite likely to have more than one marriage, and to have children in more than one relationship. In the past, children often married from home, or left home to their own apartment and married from there. A current trend is for children to leave, then come back from time to time. Arrangements between parents and adult children are much more fluid.

The idea then that there is a definite end to the mothering role about the time of the biological event of menopause, leading to some kind of "change" is now irrelevant for most women. Menopause is an event in their lives, and their lives before and after are not significantly changed by it. They "go through" menopause, but this biological marker does not signify a change in status or an entry into a stage in their lives significantly different from the year before.

In many ways women's lives do not change at all. The idea of change implies a major shift in the meaning and experience of life. In fact, the most major change women cope with in their lives is becoming a mother for the first time. At this stage, women must adjust to a considerable loss of control over their lives. Maybe we should rename first-time motherhood as "the change"!

Problems with the Research

In 1973, when epidemiologists Sonja and John McKinlay reviewed all the available research on menopause, they concluded that there had actually been remarkably little and that most of the research that had been conducted by that date was seriously flawed. Doctors had defined the symptoms of menopause and developed ways of treating patients based on their own subjective experience, not empirical evidence. The bulk of the literature on menopause, they said, consisted of unsubstantiated opinions not backed by data.(3)

In the nearly 20 years since the McKinlays made their comments, the quality of research has improved, although there is still not a great deal of it. The McKinlays themselves are conducting a major project in Massachusetts, monitoring a large group of women and interviewing them at regular intervals. Some of this has been published. It is generally true that the most useful information is currently coming not from the work of gynecologists and endocrinologists but from that of sociologists, anthropologists, psychologists, and epidemiologists.

There are still question marks over almost every aspect of menopause. Wulf Utian called menopause "an enigma in the human female life cycle" and this is quite true.(4) There is no universal agreement on what menopause actually is. The number of symptoms given for menopause by various writers varies from 1 to more than 40. Some research shows that only the hot flash can be accurately called a menopausal symptom, while others give an enormous list, which includes not only physical symptoms but also a large number of mental conditions, such as depression, anxiety, forgetfulness, and difficulty in concentrating, as well as sexual problems such as loss of libido. Because of this lack of agreement on basic concepts, it is very hard to know how much weight to give to the findings of individual studies or how to compare them.

It is not even clear how many women find menopause difficult. Determining this is a particularly thorny problem because the answer you get will vary according to how you define menopause and what you call a problem. For instance, the statement is often made that a certain percentage of women—usually around 20%—have menopausal symptoms "severe enough" to seek medical help, but what does this really mean?

An article in *New Zealand Doctor* said that one third of menopausal women were in this category, but it then went on to list at length the "symptoms" these women had, not all of which are in fact proven to be caused by menopause. For instance, the article said 15% of women who went to a doctor had muscle and joint pain even though there is no evidence such problems are caused by menopause. It also claimed that another 20–45% of these women had emotional problems such as "depression, anxiety, insomnia, tiredness, loss of libido, loss of concentration and loss of self-esteem." The article noted that these may or may not be related to menopause, and I will discuss this later, but their inclusion is typical of a tendency to make menopause a kind of rag bag for any problem, physical or mental, being suffered by women in this age group.(5)

It reminds me that I have been twice to my general practitioner to discuss very heavy menstrual bleeding which developed in my early forties. From my reading about menopause, I had gotten the impression that women's periods became lighter as they got older, and as I knew heavy bleeding could be a symptom of various diseases, I thought I should have it checked. I was reassured by my doctor that heavy menstruation like mine is not uncommon for women as they get older—nothing needed to be done. The bleeding would inevitably stop at menopause—all I had to do is wait!

I wonder now, if my doctor was to be involved in research on menopause, whether I would be included in the statistics of women with symptoms "severe enough to seek medical help." I certainly wouldn't include myself in such a category. Raewyn Mackenzie, who ran menopause groups for the Family Planning Association, said that many women came to the groups looking for reassurance that what was happening to them was normal. They didn't need medical help, only information, as I did.

It also has to be borne in mind that the more menopause is defined as a medical problem and the more women accept this, the more they will seek medical help, believing that this is the appropriate place for them to go. Parallel to this, the more doctors are encouraged to see menopause as a disease and therefore part of their territory, the more proactive they will be in soliciting reports of problems from their patients.

Women are, in general, more likely than men to report emotional problems to their doctors, because it is more socially acceptable for women to admit to emotional distress. At the same time, several studies have shown that doctors have a tendency to label health problems as emotional in women, where the same problems would be regarded as physical in men. All these factors could influence the reported incidence of menopausal problems.

The study of menopausal women is also complicated by the existence of the stereotypes of menopause discussed in the previous chapter. If the researchers themselves hold such stereotypes, they will be biased. A sociologist who studied midlife women in Israel said that the three members of the research team—two men and one young woman—discovered that they had brought to their work a number of erroneous assumptions. When they discovered that the women they studied did not regret the loss of fertility, whether they were traditional Muslim Arab villagers or modern Central European immigrants, regardless of the women's childbearing history, they realized they had overvalued the importance of fertility and childbearing because of their experience in their own culture.(6)

Menopausal stereotypes can also affect the women who are the subjects of the research. As sociologist Pat Kaufert puts it: "In menopause research . . . the potential for bias is multiplied because most women have preexisting stereotypes of what they should expect to experience."(7) Kaufert gives the example of a study she carried out on Canadian women looking at attitudes toward menopause. Although depression and irritability are not established as symptoms of menopause, they are widely described as such in both medical and lay literature. Consequently in Kaufert's study, 82% of the women agreed with the statement "Women become depressed and irritable at menopause."

There are other reasons why the medical research that has been undertaken on such things as the incidence and range of women's complaints needs to be handled with caution. Much of the research does not discriminate between women who have had a surgical menopause because of the removal of the ovaries or a hysterectomy which can compromise the ovaries, and women who have had a natural menopause. Women who have an artificial menopause can often have more severe menopausal symptoms and more depression than women whose periods stop naturally; they are also more likely to go for medical help, so this can bias any results. Much of the research also muddles pre-, peri-, and postmenopausal women, whose experiences might in fact be rather different.(8)

Another difficulty is that the research has been largely carried out on women who are patients of gynecologists or psychiatrists or who have sought help at menopause clinics, so they are not typical of all women. They are not a "well woman" sample. Nevertheless, this "woman with problems" has provided the stereotype of the menopausal woman.

Sydney psychologist Susan Ballinger studied the difference between women who sought help from a menopause clinic at which she worked and menopausal women who were recruited at local shopping centers. She found that there was no difference between the groups in the incidence of the classic symptom of menopause— hot flashes—although the flashes tended to be more severe in the clinic patients. The big difference between the two groups was in depression and other psychological symptoms. The explanation Ballinger offered for this was that the clinic patients not only had significantly more stressful events in their lives—such as relationship breakdowns or the death of parents—but they also perceived the events as more distressing than the nonpatient women. They were also more likely to have been depressed before the menopause. Ballinger concluded that the clinic patients "did not *cope* as well with stressful life events." She wondered whether the definition of menopause as a disease offered these women a socially acceptable excuse for reporting symptoms that otherwise might be labeled as "neurotic."(9)

How "Sick" Is the Menopausal Woman?

If you believed everything you read about menopause in the lay press, you would form the impression that menopause is inevitably traumatic, a picture which is sometimes difficult to reconcile with what you know about your own friends and other women you meet.

"There is a popular belief," says Patricia Kaufert bluntly, "that perimenopausal women are neurotic and hypochondriac."(10) She calls this belief "free-floating," in other words, there is nothing concrete to back it up in the way of evidence.

For instance, an article in the Auckland Star began with the wildly exaggerated claim that "many New Zealand women spend a third of their lives coping with the somewhat debilitating symptoms which occur after menopause. Most women do not enter the post-menopausal period without some degree of discomfort, whether it is physical or emotional."(11)

In this same mode, British journalist Jill Tweedie gave a highly colored depiction of menopause in one of her columns: "My Great-Aunt Florrie always said it was hard being a woman: you were Unwell from the age of puberty and all the Unwellness came together at 50 to make one giant Unwellness. We sit there leaking estrogen like old car radiators leaking anti-freeze, we get a whole clutch of alien symptoms, our bones crack if a moth bustles past."(12)

The picture one gains from articles such as these is that menopausal women have more illness and visit the doctor more often. In the medical literature, the range of women who are said to seek medical help for menopause extends from 20% in a London study to around 44% in a study in Aberdeen, but these figures look far less alarming when they are put in the context of how often other people go to the doctor.(13)

In New Zealand, researchers at Auckland University School of Medicine surveyed 90% of Hamilton general practitioners over a 12-month period to see who went to the doctor for what.(14) They found that among midlife women (35–64 years), 8 visits per 100 women were made for menopausal symptoms. By contrast, among women 15–24 years, there were 19 visits per 100 women for menstrual problems, and among women 25–34 years, there were 16 visits per 100 women for menstrual problems. In other words, young women were twice as likely to go to the doctor about menstruation than midlife women were about menopause, but we don't define menstruation as a disease—yet!

Among the entire group of people 15–64 years, there were 26 visits per 100 women and 20 visits per 100 men for high blood pressure, and 11 visits per 100 women and 6 visits per 100 men for being overweight. There were actually more visits for both men and women for the common cold and more visits by women for candida than for menopause.

The Massachusetts Women's Health Study also completely contradicts the picture of the menopausal woman as in poor health and as a frequent user of health services. As mentioned, Sonja and John McKinlay are part of a group of epidemiologists who have been following 2,500 women enrolled in their study when aged between 45 and 55. These women were randomly selected from the general population so they provide a representative cross section of midlife women. The McKinlays looked at how the women perceived their own health, what physical and psychological symptoms the women reported, whether their health restricted their normal activity, and how much they used health services. The results showed that apart from women with surgical menopause and hysterectomies, menopause did not cause poorer health status, either physical or psychological, or more use of health services.(15)

In short, the menopausal woman is not as "sick" as we have been led to believe. Contrary to the stereotype, she is not normally a big user of health services. There is a subgroup of women of this age who *do* use health services more—women who have had their ovaries and/ or uterus removed. As some of this surgery was probably unnecessary in the first place, it seems that the picture of midlife women as "sicker" is partially iatrogenic, that is, caused by doctors themselves.

What Do Women Think of Menopause?

There is often an assumption in the medical literature that women themselves regard menopause as something to dread. In reality, there is a range of attitudes among women even in the same community, although overall it would be true to say that women are matter-of-fact about menopause.

In 1985 a group of people working on menopause—anthropologists, clinicians, epidemiologists, psychologists, biologists, and sociologists—met in Finland to discuss their research. At the workshop the issue of what women themselves thought about menopause was discussed and the following report was made:

> In a comparison of results between participants, all noted that while a few women did have problems, most dismissed menopause as a significant event. The consistency of this finding was remarkable, given the number of studies represented at the workshop, the number of countries in which they had been done and the differences in their methodologies. This particular comparison suggests that labeling menopause as a crisis in women's lives may be a medical phenomenon, following from the representation of menopause as a disease or deficiency condition. Concern was expressed over the accelerating medicalization of a process most women accept as normal.(16)

In the Massachusetts Women's Health Study, midlife women were asked about their attitudes toward menopause. Three quarters of the pre- and perimenopausal women said they would either feel relieved when they went through menopause or they had no particular feelings at all. Only 2.6% expressed regret at the prospect of menopause, while the remainder (23.4%) had mixed feelings. Women who had already gone through a natural menopause were also asked about their attitude toward this event in their lives. Eighty-one percent of the women were relieved at having gone through menopause or they had no feelings about it; only 1.6% were regretful and 17% had mixed feeling.(17)

In an earlier study by one of the same researchers, this time of women in London, it was discovered that the majority of midlife women regarded menopause as presenting no change, or they were relieved about it, even though some 18–30% anticipated or had had some difficulty with it.(18)

In New Zealand, the Society for Research on Women (SROW) had similarly positive results when it surveyed the lives of a group of midlife women in 1986. A total of 56% of the women had not given it much thought or expected no particular problems, 42% expected mild problems, and 3% expected severe problems.(19) The reason these results are not quite as positive as the Massachusetts findings is explained by the method of selection of the women. The Massachusetts women are a representative cross section of their community, whereas 40% of the women in the SROW study had attended a Family Planning Association clinic for menopausal symptoms. One would expect more negative attitudes from these women, which would affect the results. The SROW researchers note that 9 of the 13 women who expected severe problems came from the clinic group.

Another survey of women's attitudes was carried out in New Jersey by psychiatrist Sandra Leiblum and psychologist Leora Swartzman in the mid-1980s. This study was particularly aimed at seeing if education and employment status affected attitudes, and at how the "deficiency disease" model of menopause had affected women's views.(20)

The researchers found a great diversity of opinion among their research subjects. Over half the women agreed that menopausal difficulties were caused by hormones and that menopause should be viewed as a medical condition and treated as such. The non-college-educated women were much more likely to take this view. But despite this endorsement for the medical model of menopause, the women had very conflicting views about treatments. Their opinions were divided about HRT: well over 60% thought that "natural approaches" were preferable.

The women also revealed other interesting attitudes. The overwhelming majority thought that women felt just as womanly after menopause and only very small numbers thought that libido decreased or that men found older women less desirable.

So how do we explain these apparent contradictions? It seems that women are aware of the medical view of menopause, they may even accept it to some extent, but this has not altered their underlying view that menopause is a normal process which should if possible be handled without medical treatment. They don't think menopause is a big deal and they don't dread it.

In Manitoba, Pat Kaufert found that women had varying attitudes to involving their doctors in their menopause. Although most thought their doctor might be helpful, only a third had reported they were having hot flashes to their doctors and many had never even discussed menopause with the doctor. Kaufert explained these results by saying that this indicated that women were still exercising control over how they handled menopause. They were choosing whether to disclose their condition to their doctor and for what reason. "This may change," she said, "as the argument about the health care costs to society of not protecting women against osteoporosis becomes more strident, but at present women may still choose whether or not to treat their menopause as a medical event and whether or not to take estrogen."(21)

This is an astute remark, for in the five or more years since this research was conducted, the campaign to promote osteoporosis as a menopausal symptom has markedly intensified. It had hardly got underway in the mid-1980s. This reorientation of menopause to include a lifelong and potentially crippling bone disease—preventable of course by hormones—may swing the pendulum in favor of women accepting the medical model and the need for treatment.

What about Midlife Men?

Another way of looking at women's "problems" at menopause is to look at what is happening to men of the same age. Of course men aren't going to get hot flashes, but if men have some of the same mental problems that in women get blamed on menopause, it would cast some doubt on the proposition that hormones are to blame.

Although men in midlife are just as likely as women to have spreading waistlines, thinning hair, and wrinkles, you don't hear a lot about it. Magazines for men do not often give beauty tips or dieting programs, or bombard their readers with dire messages about all the catastrophic illnesses waiting to strike them down in their "prime." There are no medical journals devoted to aging in men, and midlife men's health problems, such as cardiovascular disease, do not get labeled as a "men's problem." In the United States over 20% of all midlife deaths are men who die of heart disease, compared to about 9% for women. This is potentially a much more preventable condition than many of the cancers that are the major cause of death for women this age. Lung cancer kills over twice as many midlife men as women. Approximately 132,000 men were diagnosed with prostate cancer in 1992, with a five-year relative survival rate of 77.6% for white men compared to the 79.3% rate for white women with breast cancer.

Despite this, compared to women, men are allowed to simply get on with their lives. This lack of attention to men makes it very difficult to compare them to women for health status. John McKinlay, principal researcher in an unusual research project—the Massachusetts Male Aging Study—says that the ratio of published medical studies of older women to older men is probably in the order of 100 to 1.(22)

McKinlay says that for a number of reasons, including "an aggressive medical-industrial complex," interest is now starting to be shown in older men and even in the idea of hormone treatment for men. There is talk of a "male menopause" or "andropause," as the Europeans call it. McKinlay's work does show that men's hormones change in midlife, though whether this is an increase in estrogens or a decrease in androgens is not certain. But McKinlay sounds a warning note about the possible consequences of this new research interest in men. "The medicalization of normally aging men," he says, "that is the treatment of a typical physiological process as pathological, with the consequent labeling and associated clinical management (treatment), present ethical and public health policy challenges."

Such a warning, though directly applicable to women, is rarely sounded about the female sex.

Researchers in Oxford conducted an interesting and rather rare study which compared midlife women and men.(23) The study aimed at ascertaining which of women's complaints really were symptoms of menopause by comparing them to a control group of men of the same age. People in the study were asked a lot of questions about their lives without knowing it was really a study of menopause.

Overall, the study confirmed the findings of other researchers that hot flashes and night sweats were closely associated with menopause, but these were the only symptoms to show a clear relationship to it.

Many of the mental and somatic (bodily) symptoms commonly ascribed to menopause did not differ greatly between men and women, or the peak of their occurrence in women preceded menopause, and were, said the researchers, the result of chronological age.

Both sexes reported similar rates of formication, or crawling sensations on the skin. They also had similar rates of headaches, dry skin and hair, panic feelings, depression, aching muscles and joints, and difficulty with intercourse.

Loss of interest in sex increased with age for men, but not for women, as did men's bladder problems, which by the mid-fifties surpassed women's.

Women reported more problems with anxiety, loss of confidence, forgetfulness, and concentration, but the peak of prevalence of these symptoms was before menopause, so they cannot be ascribed to loss of estrogen. The pattern suggested they were more related to premenstrual tension and that they diminished at menopause, the rates becoming more like those of men. Irritability also diminished at menopause for women while in men it remained constant, once again suggesting a relationship with premenstrual tension for women.

These findings show that it is not accurate to label everything that is happening to women in their middle years as caused by menopause. Some symptoms are clearly caused by getting older and are shared by men and women, while others are actually more common in men than women. Men don't talk about these things and they have no "men's" magazines telling them they have problems. As well, the medical profession and researchers are not much interested in subjects such as men's loss of confidence and irritability. The one-sided focus on women has allowed many complaints to be defined as menopausal when they are clearly not, but are simply part of being human, and growing older.

The Many Faces of Menopause

There are as many different menopauses as there are cultures. This is what anthropologists mean when they say that while menopause is a universal physiological event, it is at the same time a cultural act affected by people's beliefs, expectations, and customs. According to anthropologists, menopausal stereotypes will differ from society to society according to the social meaning of being a woman who is no longer fertile and no longer menstruating.[24] It seems that if a woman's status increases or remains the same after menopause, she will make the transition with not too much trouble, whereas if she loses status, menopause will be experienced as a negative life stage.

Although Western medicine identifies various symptoms of menopause, in other cultures they may not be recognized or named as menopausal. About the only universally recognized sign of menopause is the stopping of periods.

American anthropologist Marcha Flint argues that the relatively high incidence of menopausal symptoms experienced by women in Western society is a result of the negative status given to aging women in our societies. Menopause acts as a kind of symbolic marker for aging in women, so the negative aspects of getting older become associated with menopause.[25]

When Flint worked among women of the Rajput caste of North India, she found that the end of menstruation was more like a liberation. The Rajput woman could emerge from the *purdah* that had severely restricted her life and enter society. She was freer to visit other households, and within her own household could now talk, joke, and even drink with the men—activities that had formerly been forbidden to her. Flint found that Rajput women looked forward to menopause and had virtually no symptoms. In societies like this, where there have been considerable taboos around menstruation, the end of menstruation can have positive consequences and may be anticipated eagerly.

Even hot flashes are valued in some cultures. In some parts of Wales for instance, a hot flash is seen as a sign of good health.(26) This contrasts with the embarrassment that American and British women have reported in studies.

In some societies older women earn respect and are consulted about decisions that need to be made. Among Lugbara women in Uganda, for instance, a woman at menopause becomes a "Big Woman" and she is given considerable authority among her kin. In traditional Maori society, the older woman becomes a *kuia,* an object of veneration and respect. It is the kuia who has the status to perform various rituals on the *marae* that younger women cannot perform. It is tempting to speculate that within traditional Maori culture, women may have experienced getting older in a positive way as it led to them having more power.

A study of women in Japan provided fascinating insights into the way menopause may be viewed differently by women in different cultures.(27) The researchers surveyed over a thousand midlife Japanese women. Until the end of the last century, Japanese women had no word for menopause; the word now used in both the medical world and among women is *konenki,* a word adopted from the German word *klimakterum.*

The hot flash which most Western women have during menopause is far less frequently noted by Japanese women. Only about 10% of the women noted this, and even fewer—3%—had night sweats. The researchers commented that this should make us cautious about assuming that any aspect of menopause is universal at any level, even biologically.

In Japan women have other symptoms they identify as menopausal—especially headaches, shoulder stiffness, ringing in the ears, and aches in the joints. The most frequently reported symptom was stiff shoulder, given by 52% of women. There is no equivalent for this in the menopausal syndrome as described in Western societies.

When the women were asked whether they saw themselves as menopausal, the researchers were surprised to discover that the women's self-definition did not always coincide with her menstrual status. Some women who had not menstruated for over 12 months, still said they did not have any sign of the menopause. Konenki in Japan is more closely tied to aging than to hormones, even by physicians. Changes in eyesight and gray hair were more likely to be seen as indicators of konenki than changes in periods or the end of menstruation.

Dumping Everything on Menopause

The main problem in trying to describe menopause is that everything negative that might be happening to women around this time of their lives has been labeled menopausal. With men, the same feelings and experiences are seen as part of normal aging. For instance, we all may have less energy as we get older. There may be more things in our lives to worry about, to make us anxious and give us sleepless nights. The event of menopause gives women a focus and label for the loss of former capacities and for problems.

As long ago as 1951 an astute writer noted that the presence of menopause could blind a physician to the real problem a woman might be seeking help for.(28) There was a tendency always to view the woman through the lens of her menopause.

Dr. Wulf Utian had this to say about doctors' attitudes toward menopause:

> The term "menopause" has traditionally been applied in so nonprecise a fashion that so-called "menopausal symptoms" have included virtually any complaint a middle aged woman cared to take to her physician . . . clinicians tended to divide symptoms presented by perimenopausal women on an empirical basis into "autonomic" and "metabolic" or, even worse, to simply itemize them in grocery-list style without any attempt at explanation. Clinicians were thus truly in the dark as to causation of symptoms and were inevitably forced to treat "effect" on an empirical

basis rather than "cause" on a valid scientific basis . . . the majority of clinical features ascribed to this period in the human
life cycle were therefore mere assumptions and could have been
no more than coincidental features in a generally aging population.

This medical mind-set is still in place and can have unfortunate
consequences for women in their middle years, as this woman describes: "I am 48 and I have no signs of menopause. My periods have
not altered in the least. But for the last 10 years I've been complaining
to the doctor about exhaustion. I was asked how old I was, and then
I was told: 'Of course, it's your age. You're perimenopausal.' Now
they've discovered I'm actually anemic and I've improved vastly with
iron. But it probably cost me my marriage."

Dr. Jean Coope, a British general practitioner with a special interest in menopause, described how this propensity for dumping
everything on menopause also affects women themselves:

> All that presents at menopause is not caused *by* the menopause.
> A large proportion of women who attend my surgery complain-
> ing of The Menopause and requesting hormones are suffering
> from some other problem. The first patient who came during
> the active promotion of estrogen treatment in 1973, complain-
> ing of tiredness and asking for hormone replacement therapy,
> had a hemoglobin concentration of 5.8 g/dl and was suffering
> from fibroids and menorrhagia [heavy periods]. The second pa-
> tient, "tired and wanting hormones," was mildly jaundiced. Both
> these women would have been made more ill by hormone treat-
> ment.(29)

There are problems with labeling aspects of normal aging and
all midlife problems as menopausal. First, it encourages an unnecessarily pessimistic view of menopause that will have repercussions for
all women. A more benign view of menopause might make it seem
less of an obstacle in our lives and less of a threat.

Second, if menopausal women are stereotyped as neurotic, emotionally unstable, and not in complete control, they may be seen as
less able to take responsibility and make rational decisions. This can
be used against us to dismiss legitimate grievances ("She's going
through 'the change,' you know") or to discriminate against older
women in areas such as employment.

Finally, when women do need help, they may get the wrong kind of help. Dr. Coope gave examples of women who needed medical treatment for physical problems to whom another doctor might have given hormones. There is also still an enormous amount of inappropriate prescribing of psychotropic drugs to women during midlife. Dr. John Studd, who founded the first menopause clinic in the United Kingdom, claimed when visiting New Zealand that some 40% of menopausal women in the United Kingdom were on antidepressants or tranquilizers.(30)

There may be aspects of a midlife woman's life that do need sorting out, such as an unhappy relationship, an unsatisfactory job, or boredom with her sex life. If she is diverted into thinking her dissatisfaction is all caused by menopause, she may not take the right action.

There are reasons then for trying to unravel what is known about the symptoms of menopause and for trying to identify what is conclusively hormonal, what is not, and the areas where the answer is not clear.

Chapter 5

Hormones at Menopause: What Really Happens When the Ovaries Retire

Until recently doctors thought that menopause began when all the eggs in the ovaries were used up; however, recent work has shown that menopause is probably not triggered by the ovaries, but by the brain. It seems that both puberty and menopause are brain-driven events.

Menstruation depends on a complex network of hormonal communications between the ovary, the hypothalamus, and the pituitary gland in the brain. The hypothalamus secretes gonadotropin releasing hormone (GnRH), which triggers the production of follicle-stimulating hormone (FSH) by the pituitary gland. FSH then stimulates the growth of the egg follicles in the ovaries to trigger ovulation. As the egg follicle grows before an egg bursts from it, estrogen is manufactured and released into the blood.

This chain reaction is not just a one way process. One of the ovarian estrogens in the blood stream—estradiol—also acts back onto the hypothalamus, causing a change in GnRH. Next, this altered hormone stimulates the pituitary to produce luteinizing hormone, or LH. This LH causes the egg follicles to burst and the ovum to be released. After the egg is expelled, progesterone is also manufactured by the collapsed egg follicle, now called the corpus luteum.

Ovarian estrogen and progesterone stimulate the growth of the endometrium, or lining of the uterus. Progesterone also causes the lining of the uterus to be shed at the end of a menstrual cycle, causing menstruation.

From about the age of 40, the interaction between the hormones alters, eventually leading to menopause. It is still not clear how. Menopause may start with changes in the hypothalamus and pituitary gland rather than the ovary. Scientists have conducted experiments where young mice have their ovaries replaced with those from aged animals, no longer capable of reproducing. They can then mate and give birth to baby mice. This shows that an old ovary placed in a young environment is capable of responding. On the other hand, when young ovaries are put into old mice, they cannot reproduce.(1)

Whatever the mechanism triggering menopause, as fewer egg follicles are stimulated, the amount of estrogen and progesterone produced by the ovaries declines. With the reduction of these hormones, menstruation becomes scantier and erratic and eventually ends.

In response to the lessening activity in the ovaries, the pituitary increases the release of FSH and LH so that the levels of these hormones become higher. The two major hormonal changes at menopause are the reduction in estrogen and the increase in FSH and LH. The true symptoms of menopause are caused by these hormonal changes. This does not always happen continuously, but often in a stop/start fashion. This explains the variations in menstrual patterns in perimenopausal women.

Estrogen production does not entirely close down at menopause. Although the ovaries stop producing estrogen altogether or produce very little, they continue to produce androgen, which can be converted into a form of estrogen called estrone, and the adrenal gland also produces androgen. The conversion of androgen to estrone takes place in fat, primarily fat on a woman's breasts and stomach. The more fat a woman has, the more estrogen she will continue to produce after menopause. The increase in fat around the abdomen and hips which many women experience at midlife could well be nature's way of ensuring that women have sufficient estrogen in the postmenopausal years.

The ovaries and adrenal gland also produce the male hormone testosterone, and this can cause increased facial hair in some postmenopausal women.

The lowering in estrogen levels has an effect on body tissue that is receptive to estrogen. The lining of the uterus is the most obvious example, but the genitals and reproductive organs are also affected. The ovaries and uterus become very much smaller, while the labia can lose their fatty tissue and become smaller. The vaginal walls can become thinner and less elastic. The vagina may become shorter and narrower and lubricate less easily. Lessened lubrication can occur early in the postmenopausal period, but the vaginal and vulvar changes occur very much later. It is not usually until 5 to 15 years after menopause that these changes, if any, become apparent—and they are not inevitable.

The loss of vaginal tissue can make a woman more vulnerable to bladder problems and prolapse, where one of the pelvic organs (such as the bladder, bowel, or uterus) sags into the vagina. This usually only occurs in old age.

Reduced bone tissue is another possible effect of loss of estrogen. This will be discussed in more detail in following chapters.

The Signs and Symptoms of Menopause

Despite the claims of some doctors who produce a lengthy menu of menopausal symptoms, only three signs can be directly attributed to the physiological event of menopause:

- menstrual changes

- vasomotor effects: hot flashes and night sweats

- loss of moisture and elasticity in the vagina

It is important to emphasize that apart from menstruation stopping, there is nothing universal about menopause. Patterns will vary tremendously between individuals. Some women have no symptoms at all. A recent Swedish study found that 47% of perimenopausal women were not having symptoms, and 21% of postmenopausal women had never had any.(2) There is no accurate way of predicting whether an individual woman will or will not have symptoms, or how mild or severe they will be. Some women speculate that they might have a menopause similar to their mother's. There is no way of knowing if this is true as no research has been conducted on this relationship.

Much of the research on menopausal symptoms has proceeded from the assumption that certain complaints are menopausal, without any adequate proof. As we saw above, many of the symptoms commonly described as menopausal were actually experienced by women at other ages too, and also, in some cases, by men. In the mid-1960s Sonja McKinlay and Margot Jefferys did one of the first major surveys to try and work out exactly what was menopausal and what was not.(3) They discovered that hot flashes and night sweats reached a peak at menopause and were clearly associated with it, but that six other symptoms often attributed to menopause—headaches, dizzy spells, palpitations, sleeplessness, depression, and weight gain—showed no direct relationship to menopause. Approximately 30–50% of women did report these complaints, but they were reported equally by women who were premenopausal, perimenopausal, and postmenopausal. There was no peak in incidence at menopause. In other words, these were midlife complaints rather than menopausal symptoms. This survey did not ask about any issues related to sexuality.

Twenty years later, in 1986, a group of researchers from King's College Hospital in London showed similar results.(4) Some 850 well women aged 45–65 years took part in a survey that covered many issues related to general health as well as menopausal symptoms. The women did not know the survey was about menopause; unlike the earlier survey, this one did ask about sex. Once again, this study confirmed that vasomotor effects are clearly caused by menopause, but that psychological effects were found across all groups. In addition, they found that vaginal dryness was much more common in postmenopausal women.

Changes in menstruation

During menopause, as estrogen levels change menstrual patterns usually also change, although in about a third of women normal menstruation occurs right until the periods abruptly stop. For other women, the following or a combination of them can happen. The periods can

- gradually diminish, becoming lighter and/or lasting for fewer days

- become heavier and longer, with more clots

- be erratic, stopping and starting with differing amounts of time between them

- become further and further apart

In her book *Menopause: A Positive Approach,* Rosetta Reitz reproduces a chart showing how her menstrual pattern changed during menopause. Over three years, she had variations in the duration of her periods from one and a half days to four days, sometimes with days of staining following the bleed. The gap between her periods varied from 20 to 212 days, or seven months.(5)

This kind of pattern is normal, as is virtually any other variation on the theme.

> I didn't realize for about a year that menopause had started. My periods, which had been every three weeks, went out to 28 days, then to 38 days, then I had no period for a couple of months. By the time I was 44 I was having four two-day periods a year. I used to have what I called my quarterly reports. Then they stopped altogether. I actually miss having my periods. I used to gauge my general health from the quality and quantity of my periods. When I was run down I'd have a three-week cycle, so I'd add iron and vitamin B and vitamin C to my diet.

> I've gone back to having bad cramps as I did when my periods first started. It's pretty heavy the first day, then it trails off very quickly. It looks brown and not very nourishing.

> Months would go by when I didn't have a period and I would think, this is it. Then one would turn up out of the blue—they'd be three weeks apart and three months apart. There was no pattern at all.

> I bleed a lot more now than I did right through my twenties and thirties when I was on the Pill. Clots and pieces of tissue come out. Only pads will cope with the flow. I have about five days' heavy bleeding, then another five or more when it's light. Sometimes it stops, but will start up again, especially if I have sex. I'm looking forward to the day it's all over—I'll have less laundry and will save heaps in sanitary napkins.

Although very heavy bleeding can occur at menopause, it should always be discussed with a doctor as it can be symptom of disease.

The age at which a woman has her last period can vary from her late thirties to her late fifties, but the average age is usually 49–51.

Hot flashes

The exact mechanism causing a hot flash is not known. It is not just a case of lowered estrogen, as it has been noted that women with lifelong low estrogen levels do not have flashing. Experiments have also shown that it is not caused by the levels of LH released by the pituitary.(6) It seems that the hot flash may be triggered by the hypothalamus, the part of the brain which controls body temperature and also influences the pituitary hormones. The hot flash may be triggered by a sudden downward setting of the central hypothalamic thermostat. To adjust the core temperature of the body to this new setting, heat loss mechanisms such as vasodilation and sweating are activated. This explanation tallies with the known fact that during a hot flash a woman's central body temperature falls.

During a hot flash, blood floods into the tiny blood vessels under the skin, the pulse rate rises, and skin temperature goes up, although the blood pressure is unaffected. The flash is over in two or three minutes, although the increased skin temperature and sweating can persist for longer.

Hot flashes can be very occasional and mild, but in a minority of women they can be drenching, dripping sweats accompanied by an intense feeling of heat which can occur many times a day. The experience of the following women show extreme differences in the intensity of hot flashes. In 1983 playwright Renée wrote:

> Six years ago I started having severe hot sweats; I use this term because "flash" seems to me to be too pallid a word for the drenching, debilitating experience. Every 35 minutes I had a hot sweat. Nights became a true nightmare. Changing the sheets, changing my clothes made me so wide awake that there was little chance of getting back to a restful sleep. I had a demanding job teaching, and it didn't make it any easier when drops of water fell from my face to the desk in the middle of a lesson or when my glasses fogged up just as I was taking roll call.(7)

On the other hand, many other women hardly notice what is happening:

> I seem to have gone through menopause. It's nearly a year since I had my last period. I think I have the occasional hot flash—I suddenly get very warm.

I had a nonradical hysterectomy in my early forties and had no symptoms whatsoever of menopause, not a flash, nothing, neither at the time nor later when my ovaries went into retirement.

Some women report that the hot flashes can be triggered by something, such as eating a particular food or being in constricted places, such as cars and planes.

I would have a hot flash when I stepped into the elevator at work on arrival each morning. They left me feeling exhausted for the first few minutes of every day and hot and sticky, wondering if I smelled badly to others. I learned to take my coat off before stepping into the elevator, to ease the problem. I had noticed that the slightest change in my temperature, caused by my walking through a patch of sunlight or putting on a dress in a shop, caused the hot flashes.

Hot flashes can be visible in some women and appear as a blush or patchy redness on the face, neck, and breasts. Some women report accompanying palpitations, nausea, or headache. Hot flashes can be followed by a feeling of tiredness or chill.

The number of women reporting hot flashes is around 55% to 70% and a slightly lesser number have night sweats. Sonja McKinlay and Margot Jefferys suggest that as the same women usually report both these symptoms, night sweats are probably a nighttime manifestation of hot flashes.(8) These researchers found that for just under half the women who had hot flashes, they caused acute physical discomfort and sometimes embarrassment. Another 20% were embarrassed about them but didn't find them especially uncomfortable. Discomfort and embarrassment were the factors that caused women to seek help from a doctor.

Other researchers have come up with lower figures than these. The Swedish study showed that hot flashes were moderate or severe for only 19% of perimenopausal women and 28% of naturally postmenopausal women (see the graph on page 107).(9) Of these women, 32–39% described their flashes as slight, and 40–42% didn't have them at all. This means that 72–81% were not troubled by hot flashes. This study found that women who had postsurgical menopause (hysterectomy and/or oophorectomy) complained of more severe hot flashes, and other studies have also demonstrated this.

Percent Experiencing Hot Flashes by Menstrual Status

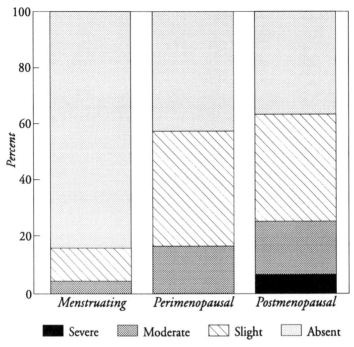

(Source: Adapted from Hagstad and Janson 1986)

Body size made no difference to the occurrence of hot flashes. Another study found that women who went through menopause at a young age were the most likely to have severe hot flashes and to be distressed by them.(10)

In some women hot flashes can go on for some years and can persist after menstruation stops. In the London study, 25% of women found that the hot flashes went on for five years after menstruation stopped.(11) Many women reported that they occurred daily, on the face and neck alone or on the whole body. Whole body flashes were more common in perimenopausal women; flashes on the face alone in postmenopausal women.

Although hot flashes are the main reason women seek medical help during menopause, the low rate at which women do so suggests that unless they are very severe, women are largely able to cope with them on their own. Pat Kaufert's study showed that most women saw hot flashes as normal and that having them didn't deter a woman from seeing her health as good or excellent.(12)

Some studies have suggested that stress can make vasomotor effects worse. Alternatively, it is suggested that hot flashes and night sweats could actually cause complaints about things such as sleeplessness, depression, lack of confidence, and irritability. After all, if you awaken during the night drenched in perspiration and even have to change your night attire and bedding as some women do, you are not going to get a restful sleep and this may make you tired the following day.(13)

One of the things women constantly say about hot flashes is that they find them embarrassing. If they happen in public, the woman tends to think everyone will notice even if they do not, and if they happen at an inopportune moment they can be unnerving, as these menopausal women explain.

> If I get a hot flash when I'm interviewing a client, I don't lose the interview, but I feel as if I almost will. In sensitive interviews, you can't write down what the person is saying without losing trust, so I have to concentrate hard.

> I've lost a bit of confidence driving. I'd be driving along in the car and this complete wash of hotness would come over me. I'd feel hot and bothered, then irritable and bad-tempered because it would make my blood pressure rise and this is a problem at the best of times. If I'm feeling nervous anyway, it will accentuate that. I remember one day when I had a hot flash when I was driving. I immediately slowed down to 25 miles an hour. I suddenly felt the car would tip or roll over if I went any harder. Gloria got irritated, I burst into tears. After that I got very nervy driving on the freeway.

Sex and Menopause

Writing on "Some Misconceptions Concerning the Menopause," Dr. David Youngs commented that there is a common misconception that "sexual interest and activity predictably decline" during menopause. Many doctors, he said, "work under the myth that as women become older, they become sexually abstinent."(14)

Youngs reviewed the gynecological and psychiatric literature and concluded that there was little support for this widely held belief. On the contrary, he said, the literature showed that sex "remains an important activity for large numbers of older women. There is also no clear evidence of a dramatic decline in desire or activity among this age group."

Where sexual activity of older women did decline it was the lack of an available partner rather than lack of interest. One study determined that when women discontinued sexual relationships, only 4% attributed this to their own lack of interest. Other researchers have shown that while most postmenopausal women are sexually active, those who were not were abstinent because they did not have a partner, or they or their partner had medical problems.

Another large cross-sectional study of women and men over 50, the largest since Kinsey's work in the 1930s, supports these findings. This study showed an overall decline in women's activity compared to men, but the decline was confined to women who lacked a partner. When married women were compared to married men, a small decline was seen between the fifties and seventies (from 95% to 81%), but the rate was the same in both sexes.(15)

The Oxford study, which compared men and women, found that a similar number of both sexes had difficulty with intercourse, although the numbers weren't high.(16) This suggests that sexual problems in midlife have more to do with aging than hormones. The same study also found that at 30 years of age more women than men were not interested in sex, and that although with women this increased only slightly with age, it more than doubled with men.

The Oxford study came to the unwarranted conclusion that the parallel between men's and women's difficulty with intercourse may indicate that when a woman had discomfort, this could cause it in the man, too. There is a persistent tendency in any discussion about sexuality and older women to assume that the men are able and eager lovers and that it is women who cause the problems. There is absolutely no evidence to back this up. Older men can have problems with arousal and erections, and they are not immune from sexual anxieties as they age. Jean Coope writes about the problem of the man "who has had a myocardial infarction or other major disease and is afraid to attempt intercourse for fear of a relapse."(17) She gives depression in both sexes and alcohol use with men as other causes of sexual problems.

Despite the lack of research evidence, however, midlife women encounter suggestions from their doctors and society in general that their libidos are inexorably on the wane. According to one theory, as a woman's self-esteem is dependent on her reproductive capacity, after menopause her sexual interest will dwindle. However, it is just as possible to argue that as menopause is actually a release from anxiety about accidental pregnancy, women will feel freer to enjoy sex without fear.

There is also a popular belief that a woman needs estrogen to be sexy, so that with less of it her libido will vanish. Women certainly need estrogen for vaginal lubrication, but there is no evidence that estrogen has any effect on feelings of arousal. If interest in sex or enjoyment declines around menopause, it is quite probably related to the social consequences of aging rather than hormones. If any hormones are implicated, it is more likely to be androgen than estrogen. This can especially be a problem for women who have had their ovaries removed.(18)

Before menopause, some women note that they are more sexually interested at certain times of the month. This varies with different women—for some it is midcycle, around ovulation; for others it is just before menstruation or at the end of it. These surges of interest are probably caused by changes in hormones during the cycle and may be lost at menopause, but there can be other compensations:

> I have no massive surge of desire in the middle of the month now, but I do find I'm more easily aroused right across the month. The old pattern was always difficult because most men don't feel madly interested three days at a time, so it's better to feel interested most of the time.

Vaginal discomfort

Of course, if a woman is having frequent night sweats or if sex is difficult because her vagina is dry, it will be hard to be interested and a few painful experiences may put the woman off sex. It can also affect sexual self-confidence.

> Lack of lubrication doesn't do anything for confidence at the beginning of a relationship. I've been questioned by lovers— Don't I turn you on? So they worry. If I'm in love with someone,

sex is on a different plane and I'm so emotional, it doesn't matter whether I'm lubricated or not. My clitoris is a better indication of whether I'm aroused or not. I always keep KY jelly in the car. If I think I may be going to have sex, I put some on beforehand. It takes me back to the old days of sticking in the diaphragm. It may be awkward the first few times, but after that it becomes part of lovemaking. It's cold, so that can be exciting and stimulating. At a certain point, my lover says, "Where's the jelly?" and that's exciting because of what's coming next.

Some women do have problems with vaginal dryness causing pain and discomfort but even so, the problem tends to be exaggerated. For instance, according to one recent publication: "You will almost certainly be forced to give up comfortable sexual intercourse 5, 10, or maybe 15 years after menopause because it will simply become too uncomfortable—or perhaps even impossible—if you don't replace your estrogen."(19)

On the contrary, in the SROW study, 70% of the whole sample had no or negligible trouble with vaginal dryness. Of the 55–60-year-olds, 37% had "quite a bit" or "a lot" of vaginal dryness.(20)

The Swedish researchers previously cited investigated the incidence of vaginal discomfort among the 1,750 women they surveyed (see the graph on page 112). A quarter of the perimenopausal women reported some vaginal discomfort, but it was mostly slight, while 39% of the naturally postmenopausal women reported some discomfort, 18% of which was moderate to severe.(21)

The King's College Hospital researchers came up with a similar result, but they also found that 84% of the women were satisfied with their sexual relationships and that this did not change with menopausal status.(22)

Sex, society, and the midlife woman

Some women *are* less interested in sex as they grow older, but this can have many causes. When we're constantly surrounded by messages that tell us that young is sexy, it needs an imaginative leap to believe that middle-aged or old is sexy too. The media constantly bombard us with images of young love and young sex, but how often do we see middle-aged lovers on the screen, especially naked or in bed? There is a gender bias built into this ageism. A Marlon Brando

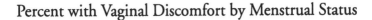

Percent with Vaginal Discomfort by Menstrual Status

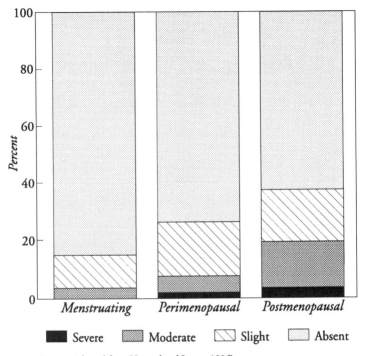

(Source: Adapted from Hagstad and Janson 1986)

with a Maria Schneider can be powerfully erotic but older actresses don't get cast as sex symbols. Brando's dynamism actually stemmed from his age in a way that a woman's never could. His age gave him power and sexual experience. The tension in *Last Tango in Paris* came from the juxtaposition of this with Schneider's youth and vulnerability. This film could never have worked if the genders had been switched.

Women notice such things. It takes a strong-minded woman not to internalize some of these messages. You have to feel attractive and desirable before you can behave as if you are. Fear of being judged unattractive can easily lead to lack of sexual confidence and unwillingness to take risks. Sex is exposing. To be satisfying, it requires emotional and physical intimacy; this is only possible if the woman feels safe. If she doesn't, she will naturally protect herself. One way she can do this is to avoid sex by losing interest in it.

Not all women have always found sex satisfying. There are differing levels of sexual interest, and not all men are wonderful lovers. In modern society, which pays much attention to sex, everyone is expected to want and enjoy sex. People are considered peculiar if they don't. This is a relatively recent development; previous generations did not expect everyone to have an intense sex life. Menopause can provide women who are less interested in sex with an excuse for retiring, thankfully. On the other hand, some studies have shown that women who enjoyed sex when they were young tend to also enjoy it as they get older.

The sexy older woman is regarded as a contradiction in terms. With the increase in divorce, some midlife women are likely to be single and in a bit of a quandary when it comes to meeting new men, while "spare" men in the same age group will be eagerly sought after by same-age and younger women. Other women find they are not prepared to put up with less-than-satisfactory men just to have sex. Women can decide to give up rather than risk "the meat market."

Sexual disqualification because of age is particularly a feature of heterosexuality and may not be such a problem among lesbians:

> Lesbian women tend to have a pattern. They either have women the same age right through life, or they are attracted to older women or, like me, younger women. I often find older women too conservative. I like going to nightclubs and dancing all night. I'm probably fitter than a lot of women my age. There is some ageism but far less than the heterosexual world. Some of us find older women very sexy—tough women are seen as sexy no matter what their age.

For those in long-term relationships there can be other difficulties. Domesticity can be a killer of passion. How do you transform the same bed with the same pajamas every night into an electric sexual encounter? Not easily. The midlife couple can become sexually bored even if they love one another. This is not fatal, but it does require some effort to deal with it.

> I read a book called *How to Make Love to the Same Person for the Rest of Your Life* and the author pointed out that when you were young you made appointments for sex. You've got to get away from the bedroom and nighttime. She said make dirty phone

calls to each other or go to hotels. It seems a bit silly at first but
it works. You've got to plan for sex. You have to treat each other
like lovers.(23)

Much of the medical writing about menopause ignores the issue
of the midlife woman's feelings for her partner. Sex is seen as an issue
of "libido" or "dysfunction"—a mechanistic approach that fails to
recognize that emotions have everything to do with sex. Some time
ago I worked with Dr. Rex Hunton who was at that time a psychiatrist with the Auckland Medical School's Department of Community
Health, but more importantly, interested in counseling for psychosexual problems. "The brain," he told me, "is the biggest sexual
organ." This comment struck me at the time; it seems very important
to acknowledge that what happens out of bed affects what happens
in bed. Medicine does not always recognize this. Because a woman
is in a long-term relationship with a man does not automatically
mean she loves him, or even likes him. Many midlife people can end
up stuck in a relationship which has survived because there were
children to bring up, but the spark has long gone. Sexual satisfaction
is unlikely in such a situation.

Depression and Other Mental Problems

There is a popular—and longstanding—misconception that depression is much more common at menopause. Despite numerous studies
that have demonstrated the opposite, the idea has been remarkably
persistent and shows little sign of going away. Depression and a range
of other mental problems are invariably listed among the symptoms of menopause. The stereotype of the menopausal woman is of
a woman who is depressed, anxious, and lacking in self-esteem.

There are currently two schools of thought on this association.
The estrogen-deficiency school argues that it's all diminishing hormones, while the social-circumstances school maintains that it's the
stressful things that are happening at this time of life: waning attractiveness, reproductive uselessness, children leaving home, disinterested spouse, divorce, and so on. "There is a tacit assumption in the
literature on menopause," says Patricia Kaufert caustically, "that a
woman loses her fertility, her children and her husband within the
same time span."(24)

There are also tacit assumptions that a woman minds not being able to conceive, mourns her children leaving home and that it is the husband who files for divorce. None of these is necessarily true! Midlife is certainly not all negative, as you could come to believe when you read the medical literature.

The McKinlays comment that while some commonly experienced life events such as illness, death of parents or spouse, divorce, unemployment, or caring for elderly relatives could be negative, others may not be.(25) Relief at losing the fear of conception, becoming a grandmother, newfound freedom when children leave home, a change in the quality of marriage, and realizing long-held aspirations could all be positive events. Whether the sum of these changes is negative or positive would be affected by socioeconomic status.

It seems that because depression is seen as a menopausal symptom, when a midlife woman gets depressed she and her physician are likely to assign its cause to menopause, even when the cause is something else. A good example of this scenario was given in a study of depression and mid-aged women by the McKinlays:

> Carol Harper is a single parent who works full-time to support herself and two adolescent daughters at home. She was hospitalized for a heart attack in the previous year and had her right kidney removed because of cancer. She wrote in her questionnaire that she "went to the doctor because of depression. Doctor said I was in the change. If I don't have a period by August 1984, I'll be through the change, and he prescribed valium."(26)

The reality is that people can get depressed, no matter what their age, sex, or menopausal status.

Depression and irritability are two symptoms which have high frequencies according to many surveys of community health. They are found in all age groups and among both men and women. It is to be expected that some women will be both depressed and peri- or postmenopausal at the same time. However, such a coincidence will add confirmation to the stereotype which describes these two as symptoms of the climacteric.(27)

The myth of the depressed menopausal woman

Recent research on this topic has shown that while depression can occur in midlife, it does not necessarily coincide with menopause. More than that, menopausal women have no more depression than anyone else. In fact, several studies have shown the highest rates of depression among women at around their mid-thirties.

A study of women in Glasgow by two psychologists found that life stresses caused the psychological (depression, anxiety, panic attacks) and "somatic" symptoms (physical symptoms such as aches and pains) usually attributed to menopause, and that the symptoms peaked before menopause rather than during it.(28) The life stresses were related to employment status, number of children under 15, and the quality of relationships with husbands, children, and other people.

While many of those who study the mental health of midlife women can end up putting forth a case for psychotherapy or drugs, one of the researchers in this study suggested that "macrosocial" solutions might be more appropriate than personal ones. By this he meant changes in society itself leading to the "emancipation" of women. He argued that equal education and employment, the availability of child care, and shared home-making responsibilities might lead to improved psychological health.(29)

The SROW New Zealand study showed no significant difference by age for a whole host of psychological symptoms commonly attributed to menopause, such as feeling tense, depression, not being able to make decisions, crying, worrying, panic attacks, or clumsiness. The age range studied was 35 to 60 years old.(30)

Depression is one of the subjects the McKinlays looked at in their large study of Massachusetts women. Unlike most other studies, which are cross-sectional—that is, they interview women at one point in time—this study is following 2,500 women prospectively, interviewing them at nine-month intervals over a period of years. This is generally considered to be a more reliable method of study, as it is less dependent on people's memories of events and feelings some time ago.

The McKinlays' study completely contradicts the view widely entertained in clinical circles that depression results from hormonal changes. They found that only women who were surgically menopausal had high depression rate scores, twice the rates of the other women. They concluded that "increased depression is not associated with the approach, or experience of, a natural menopause."(31)

Social causes of stress

The McKinlays found that social factors were far more important in explaining depression. Depressed women were more likely to be in poor general health. They also found that widowed, divorced, and separated women were the most likely to be depressed, single women the least, with married women intermediate. Having less than 12 years' education was strongly associated with depression. These women are more likely to be in dull, poorly paid jobs such as shop and clerical work, and to have lower socioeconomic status. Another predictive factor was someone causing worry, and that was most likely to be the husband and adolescent children.

On the other hand, they found "the small group of never married women are typically well educated and/or with stable career-oriented employment. They are also the least depressed." According to the stereotype, these single, childless women, who have never had a traditional home and family, should be worst off, not best! Although women who never have children may go through a process of reconciling themselves to this, the adjustment may happen before menopause:

> I had always wanted to have children but the right circumstances never seemed to be present. For years, when I was in my thirties, I used to worry that when menopause arrived I would feel very depressed because that would mark the end of the possibility of childbearing. But as my forties went by I noticed my desires for children gradually became less and less as I realized how little spare energy I had left to give them. Then I realized that I would not be depressed when I could no longer have them, although I used to joke I would have a child at 50!

In another paper the McKinlays looked more closely at stress caused by the multiple nurturing roles played by midlife women and came up with some interesting results. Contradicting the proponents of the "empty nest syndrome," far more stress was caused by adolescent children still at home (20%) or returning home after being away (24%), than children leaving. There was actually a reduction in stress among those where all the children had "flown the nest."(32)

I was anxious about being entirely on my own, but when my last child left home, I used to actually walk around the house wallowing in the quiet and the orderliness. After 30 years of childrearing I found the reality of being alone a real luxury. I didn't have to worry about keeping the fridge full of food, it didn't matter if I ate dinner at 10 at night, the amount of washing dwindled, there was less money stress—I could suit myself. On the other hand, the children all come and visit so I can still enjoy them but without having to work for them.

The same kind of finding was shown in the SROW study: "Not a single comment in the sections dealing with feelings about present life or present stresses mentioned dejection at children leaving home."(33)

In the Massachusetts study, one-quarter of the women were caring for an aged parent either in their own homes or in residential care. Half of these women found it stressful.(34)

Husbands were a major source of stress for 5% of women, whether the husband was living with them or was an ex-spouse. For women who were not in paid employment, those reporting ill health were most often those whose husbands caused stress. This was their most important finding, said the McKinlays, because

the literature is replete with reports of the positive effect of the presence of a wife on men's health. Almost no research has been reported on the impact of a husband on women's health. Separate analyses of the same data set indicate that approximately one-third of married women do not mention their husbands as members of their support network. It is a subset of these women who identify husbands as a source of stress.

Similarly, the SROW researchers were surprised to find that 10% of husbands caused a lot of stress, and that when it came to understanding and support for various symptoms, 20% of the women who replied said their husbands were not helpful, and another 24% said they were only a little helpful."(35)

In the McKinlays' study, a boss or coworker was never given as a source of stress, and other evidence indicated that work was not a major source of stress for the women. Continued employment, the McKinlays decided, had a beneficial effect unaffected by the transition through menopause. This may not just be a "healthy worker effect," they said, but work may have a beneficial effect in the face of the stresses from the nurturing roles.

Multiple nurturing roles did not stop these women from working, even when those roles were sources of stress. "Work," concluded the researchers, "with its clear expectations may provide a sense of satisfaction and self-worth not equaled by the familial nurturing roles, for which expectations are implicit and more ambiguous."

Another argument of the "menopausal depression" school is that women's self-esteem suffers such a blow at menopause that they get depressed. It is certainly true that for many women physical aging is hard to come to terms with, but this is not necessarily tied to menopause itself. The first wrinkles usually come earlier, and many women may have come to terms with this before their menopause. Or they may not have come to terms with this and menopause doesn't add to their despair. But other researchers have found that women who exhibit stress symptoms at menopause were women who have found life stressful in the past and who have often had a past history of emotional problems.(36)

Pat Kaufert looked at both psychological symptoms (depression, nervous tension, irritability, etc.) and self-esteem in groups of pre-, peri-, and advanced postmenopausal women. She found that while psychological symptoms and self-esteem were not related to menopausal status, they were related to each other. This meant that women did not lose self-esteem with menopause. Instead, there were women with low self-esteem in all three groups. But the women with low self-esteem were more likely to have psychological symptoms, whatever their menopausal status.(37)

A negative social image of menopause does pose a threat to women's sense of self-esteem. It seems probable that women with high self-esteem will be able to resist this, but that women with low self-esteem will experience menopause as an additional source of anxiety.

Another possible explanation

It would be a mistake to be too categorical about psychological symptoms at menopause and their causes. There have been many other examples of medical science catching up with women's experience after some time. Some normally stable and calm women are adamant that menopause caused uncharacteristic emotional upsets. They report mood swings, irritability, and panic feelings similar to those that women experience during premenstrual tension. Dr. John Studd poses the theory that similar feelings at menopause should be seen as part of a continuum—a continuation of premenstrual syndrome. This is hypothetical but worth thinking about. It is supported by researchers at Oxford who found an increase in PMS-like symptoms immediately before menopause.(38)

The causes of premenstrual syndrome are not clear. Dr. Studd puts forward four hormonal possibilities:

- estrogen excess

- progesterone deficiency

- estrogen/progesterone ratio

- falling estrogen/progesterone(39)

These factors could also apply at menopause. When talking about menopause there has been a tendency to point the finger at estrogen, when actually two hormones are involved.

Dr. Malcolm Whitehead thinks that women muddle PMS and menopause: "I think some patients get very wound up about their symptoms and they don't understand and often, increasingly in fact, women in their middle forties get very confused between menopausal symptoms and PMS."(40)

It is probable that the causes of the depression, irritability, and other mental symptoms some women report at this time of their lives differ from woman to woman. There could also be more than one. With the current information it is too simplistic only to blame menopausal loss of estrogen.

Fact, Fallacy, and Prejudice

Our journey through the menopause research shows that there is very little foundation for the stereotypes women encounter at menopause. The so-called menopausal syndrome is an unscientific mishmash of fact, fallacy, and prejudice. Menopause has become a catchall, a dump bin for everything that is happening to midlife women. The medical menopause is something of a con.

Despite the claims of the doctors who parade a long list of menopausal symptoms, the research shows that only three signs can confidently be attributed to the hormonal event of menopause:

- menstrual changes

- vasomotor effects: hot flashes and night sweats

- loss of moisture and elasticity in the vagina

The research also shows what most of us knew anyway: that women mostly cope with menopause in a low-key and commonsense way. They do not make a big deal of it. Neither do they regret it or regard is as a "life crisis," as is claimed in the medical literature. Most women are relieved to complete the passage to the other side, where they won't have periods anymore and they don't have to worry about pregnancy.

We have also seen that menopause is a many-faceted event, so although what I have said is true of most women, it is not true of all. A minority of women find menopause very difficult, either because they suffer from debilitating physical effects or because they feel psychologically not on an even keel. The evidence so far points to other causes for the psychological problems women have at menopause. The most plausible explanation is that these problems are coincidental to menopause, and are not caused simply by loss of estrogen.

In talking to midlife women while writing this book, I found that women's worries and anxieties were more about aging than about menopause. They were about having run out of time to do things they wanted to do, financial security, unsatisfactory relationships, and resentment at social attitudes toward older women. Researchers have also noted that aging is of greater concern to women than menopause itself.(41)

It is possible that as menopause is popularly viewed as an emotional crisis it allows some women to identify feelings of depression in themselves at this time; it gives them permission to do so, so to speak. Maybe the depressed feelings were already there and menopause provides a focus and a name to put to them.

There is also the so-called domino or cascade effect—that is, emotional symptoms that are a consequence of disabling physical symptoms. These will resolve once the physical symptoms are addressed in some way or will pass with the passage of time.

Even if it does emerge that hormones can cause psychological effects at menopause, women need to assert that this is normal and minimal in the vast majority of women, and is not a cause for treating all women as sick. The evidence supports the contention that most women can readily manage menopause by themselves.

Women need to reject the medical definition of menopause as a disease, for it is not only unsubstantiated and inaccurate but also damaging to our collective and individual psyches. Women should be able to make the passage through menopause like captains of their own ships, under their own control. For most women, this would mean simply incorporating menopause into their lives, rather than allowing it to define their identities or their experience of life.

On the other hand, some women may take the opportunity to undertake a major reassessment of their lives, their goals, and their futures. Menopause may be a "marker" of age, but a marker of a positive kind. It does remind us that we have lived nearly two-thirds of our lives, but that we have at least a third left. Time to take a few risks, to slow down, to speed up, to make our own decisions. Some could even take a lead from the woman in this poem by Fiona Kidman who has decided to "do it badly."

> i'm flashing
> myself, throwing
> up my skirts
> above my pants
> like an old whore
> on party night,
> showing blood
> to the moon;
> i am ready
> to let it leak
> down my legs
> plunge my fingers
> in this sticky
> coagulation
> touch it to my mouth
> and cover my face
> if necessary
>
> with scarlet juice

like dahlia stains.
look i've had all
these years of screaming and crying and hurting
and behaving badly
being inappropriate
and trying to hide the pain
and disguise the smell
i've had enough
of this bloody
thirty year flowering

before it's finished
can't i just show
you
my guts?

Part Three

OSTEOPOROSIS

Chapter 6

The Meaning and Marketing of Osteoporosis

Until recently most of us had never heard of osteoporosis, the condition where the bones in the skeleton progressively thin with age. In the past few years, however, the mass media, dancing to the tune of the advertising and pharmaceutical industries, have turned osteoporosis into a household word. Osteoporosis, said one doctor recently, is the latest "media disease."(1)

Making the public aware of health problems that have been overlooked is in general a good thing, especially because the health concerns of the group this condition primarily effects, the elderly, often get ignored. But in the case of osteoporosis, a little caution is called for. We need to understand the reasons for the media blitz.

Osteoporosis sells things. The dairy industry and the pharmaceutical companies that make calcium supplements and hormone replacements all vie to blow their trumpets on the osteoporosis bandwagon. When we read articles in the media about health topics, we tend to think that the originator of the article was the journalist or newspaper editor. What we don't realize is that commercial interests court the media and try to influence what is published. The public relations companies that promote particular products keep up a steady barrage of media releases and sometimes even bribes, such as paid advertising or glamorous media launches. Favorable information about products rolls off the faxes in newspaper offices. Pharmaceutical companies in particular depend on the mainstream media to get exposure for their products because they cannot advertise prescription drugs directly to the public, and an editorial article has the advantage of appearing objective. It has that "ring of confidence" that an advertisement can never attain.

For their part, journalists work under pressing deadlines. There isn't always time to do your homework. Public relations firms kindly provide the names of tame "experts" willing to testify to the wonders of the new product. Journalists are often grateful to have their work done for them and simply regurgitate the promotional line. The media proved itself only too willing to sell osteoporosis to the public. It made good copy, and women, in particular, were avid for information about this new disease they hadn't known they could get.

Osteoporosis suited a number of vested interests. It came to the rescue of the dairy industry at a time when sales were plummeting because of people's anxieties about eating saturated fats. Calcium was added to skim milk, thus transforming milk into a product that could be marketed as healthy—a preventative for osteoporosis.

In Britain, the initial targets for the new milk were mothers who wanted their children to have adequate calcium and women who were slimming. Next, older women were warned through women's magazines that their bones would become brittle if they didn't take extra calcium by way of the new calcium-fortified dairy products. In 1989 the dairy industry in Britain spent £10 million on a renewed promotional campaign. Targets this time were to be slimmers, pregnant and lactating women, and next "the gray consumer who can suffer from irreparable bone damage through lack of calcium."(2)

Makers of dairy products have not been the only industry working to raise the profile of osteoporosis in the public mind and to cash in on the widely publicized calcium/osteoporosis link. The makers of calcium supplements have also claimed their products will prevent osteoporosis and fracture, even though the benefits of this therapy are probably much more limited.

By 1986 Americans were spending $166 million annually on calcium supplements. Prior to the calcium craze and contributing to it, the National Institutes of Health (NIH) had recommended in 1985 that women should increase their daily calcium allowance, but by 1989 the NIH was warning that the promoters of calcium "promise more than calcium is going to deliver."(3)

Osteoporosis also came to the rescue of the makers of hormone replacement therapy. As we saw in a previous chapter, estrogen had originally been promoted in the 1960s and 1970s as a cure-all for the ills of menopause. It fell into disrepute in the mid-1970s after several reports published in medical journals established a link between the use of estrogen and endometrial cancer. But in 1980 the first of several studies on estrogen and osteoporosis provided a way out of the commercial doldrums for the makers of hormones. This research demonstrated that estrogen was effective in preventing menopausal bone loss, and the makers of estrogen were not slow in exploiting this new finding. As we shall see in Chapter 8, HRT was remarketed as a method of prevention for osteoporosis, but to be successful this strategy involved heightening public awareness about the condition. It was the estrogen industry that set the osteoporosis bandwagon in motion—the calcium crowd was then quick to hop on board.

The "Littler" Old Lady

The campaign to raise the public profile of osteoporosis has taught us to fear it. Terms such as "the silent epidemic" and "insidious," and the description of osteoporosis as "a silent thief" create anxiety that we personally might be marked for disablement without even knowing it.(4) The symbol for osteoporosis in this campaign has been the old woman with the dowager's hump. Distressingly bent over, she appears with monotonous regularity on book covers, in articles in the popular press, and in advertisements in medical journals—in fact, anything to do with osteoporosis. She is often shown as the final stage of a sequence of increasingly stooped daughter/mother/grandmother photographs implying that this is the eventual fate of normal middle-aged women. These images are often accompanied by alarming statistics, such as: "the crippling disease that strikes 25% of all women"; "leads to more deaths in older women than cancers of the cervix, ovaries and womb combined."(5)

These claims are suspect and need some explaining, but baldly stated and accompanied by the severely osteoporotic old woman, they imply that this is what will happen to those 25% of women destined to get osteoporosis—and we may be part of them.

In a culture where women are valued for their appearance, the image of the deformed old woman also touches on our worst fears about aging. The imagery is so powerful that we don't stop to think how often in real life we actually see a woman with a dowager's hump. Where are they all? Since one third of all women live into their eighties, and we are told that a quarter of all women will be struck by this "crippling disease," there should be thousands of women like this and we should see them every day. In fact, in our daily lives we only occasionally see a severely osteoporotic woman, and such deformities are relatively rare. But we don't always think this through; rather we are emotionally affected by the power of the imagery and the statistics.

Dr. Bruce Ettinger, Associate Clinical Professor of Medicine at the University of California and an endocrinologist at Kaiser Permanente Medical Center, addressed this question. "Women shouldn't worry about osteoporosis," he said. "The osteoporosis that causes pain and disability is a very rare disease. Only 5% to 7% of 70-year-olds will show vertebral collapse; only half of these will have two involved vertebrae; and perhaps one fifth or one sixth will have symptoms. I have a very big referral practice, and I have very few bent-over patients. There's been a tremendous hullabaloo lately, and there are a lot of worried women—and excessive testing and administration of medications."(6)

Fear and Pharmaceuticals

Of course, if we're anxious about a health risk, we'll be more inclined to do something about it. In the case of osteoporosis this means using products that we can either buy or obtain through visiting doctors. Pharmaceutical manufacturers, chemists, producers and retailers of dairy foods, the fitness industry, advertising agencies, the medical and mass media who run the ads, the companies that make the bone-measuring machines, the entrepreneurs who set up storefront bone-measuring clinics, and doctors all benefit from our anxiety about bones. There are many vested interests in the area of osteoporosis.

To target as wide an audience as possible, the publicity campaigns often distort the epidemiology of osteoporosis. Examining the examples given in the previous paragraph reveals that the full story is rather more complex. Twenty-five percent of women may develop osteoporosis, but, as Dr. Ettinger said, many will never know it. The disease will remain invisible and untroublesome for them. This statistic does not distinguish between those who have significant health problems because of osteoporosis and those who do not.

Turning to the second example, it is true that deaths occur in men and women who have hip fractures, but these people are usually very elderly and may not have had many years of life left anyway. This may sound callous, but it does help put the statistics into perspective. People who die from hip fracture are often very frail or ill from other causes and the existing quality of their lives may be poor. Doctors find it hard to quantify how much of the death was related to the fracture and how much to the other causes.

It is certainly arguable whether hip fractures lead to more deaths in older women than cancers of the reproductive tract. It all depends how you play with the figures! A different use of the mortality data might give the opposite impression. For instance, one might equally well make statements such as, "Heart disease kills nine times more older women than hip fractures" or "Hip fractures lead to only one-quarter of the deaths of older women caused by strokes." It is easy to take statistics out of context and use them for shock value.

If members of the public get assailed with suspect claims about osteoporosis, so does the medical profession. A recent advertisement in a medical magazine for one drug product shows a bent-up kiwi bird saying that this shows the "classic dowager's hump typical of an elderly woman suffering from osteoporosis."(7) The exaggeration is continued in the headline that states that "Every New Zealand woman can suffer from osteoporosis," which is as true or untrue as saying "Everyone can die of cancer" or "Everyone can be run over on the road."

Claims like these imply that it is the fate of all women to end up crippled by osteoporosis, and this is not so. Promises are also made about the products, which don't always stand up to close scrutiny, as we shall see, or the detrimental effects of using them are glossed over amid the extravagant claims. We should be suspicious about promotional campaigns that target one section of the population —women—when osteoporosis also affects men, although not as often.

Osteoporosis—Another Women's Disease

The osteoporosis campaign and the promotion of "cures" has been aimed almost entirely at women. Loss of estrogen at menopause has been highlighted as the major cause of osteoporosis for women and the condition has been defined as a woman's problem. In this campaign men have been invisible. This is a distortion. Men get osteoporosis too. When looking at hip fracture, which is the most serious fracture both in terms of effect on the individual and cost to the country, men have half as many hip fractures as women but are more likely to die as a result of them.

Yet we hear little about men and osteoporosis. The "male factor" in osteoporosis has been downplayed in the promotional campaigns because it doesn't fit with the redefinition of the condition as a woman's disease caused by loss of estrogen. This strategy was necessary to promote hormone replacement therapy. Just how this was achieved will be discussed in Chapter 8.

Typical of this approach is a lecture on osteoporosis prepared by the New Zealand Medical Association for use by general practitioners to the public. The lecture emphasizes osteoporosis as a woman's disease, saying women are "nine times more likely to develop it." This figure can only have emerged from some very creative manipulation of statistics, but it sounds impressive . . . and scary.

The lecture says that "estrogen deficiency is the most significant factor influencing the decline in bone mass"—a statement very much open to question but necessary to make if you are trying to build the case for hormone replacement therapy, as the lecture goes on to do.

Hormones and Hips

The inadequacy of the hormone "deficiency" explanation for osteoporosis can be seen by looking at hip fracture. Hip fracture is indeed a serious health problem. Many people are permanently disabled following a hip fracture and some people do die. These dire facts have been repeatedly used in writing about osteoporosis in both the lay and medical literature. Anyone reading these articles would have gained the impression that osteoporosis was the sole culprit when it came to hip fracture.

But the real story is much more complex than that. The bone loss that contributes to hip fractures in women is caused by old age as well as reduction in estrogen. Added to this, hip fractures are not just a matter of bone loss: there is not a dramatic difference between the bones of people who have hip fractures and those who don't. The key to understanding hip fracture is to recognize that people have to fall over to fracture, and fall badly. Unfortunately, there is not a lot of research on why some people who fall fracture when others do not.

Osteoporosis should more properly be seen as one risk factor among other risk factors for hip fracture, rather than the cause.(8) By seeing it that way, we would have to start thinking about how to prevent falls, for both sexes, rather than simply promote the idea of drugging the entire female population.

The first thing to be said before embarking on a discussion of osteoporosis and its prevention is that it is a highly complex area with contradictory research findings and a lot of unanswered questions. There are no simple answers. Literally thousands of medical research papers are published annually, and scientists themselves often differ significantly in what they believe. General practitioners, the first line in giving advice on health matters to consumers, are unlikely to have the time to keep up-to-date with this research. They are more likely to rely on other sources of information, such as nonresearch articles in medical magazines, presentations at medical seminars, and information from drug company representatives.

There are problems with those sources of information. The medical magazines, many of which are free giveaways, are highly dependent on drug company advertising to survive, and tend to steer away from outright criticism of particular pharmaceuticals. It is also not uncommon for the authors of such articles to have a relationship, even if indirect, with drug companies or to have a strong career investment in the subject. The articles themselves are often accompanied by advertisements for products that are supposed to treat the disease. Similarly, seminars sponsored or supported by drug companies are not always reliable sources of unbiased information. Scientists and doctors with views favorable to the company's products are more likely to be invited to speak than dissenters. The vested interest of drug reps is obvious.

General practitioners, then, are not always well placed to interpret and convey the highly complex and often contentious information about osteoporosis to their patients. This makes it especially difficult for laypeople to assess where the truth lies and what it means for them.

What Is Osteoporosis?

Osteoporosis means, literally, holes in the bones. Osteoporotic bones are thin, with decreased bone mass. Bone loss occurs normally in all people as they age, which is why there is argument about whether osteoporosis should be seen as just a part of aging, something that happens to everybody to some degree, or as a disease.

The strength of our bones as we get older is dependent on three major factors, which will combine differently in the individual:

- genetic inheritance, including race; this sets the possible size bones can reach, called peak bone mass

- environmental or lifestyle factors, such as inadequate diet, lack of exercise, and smoking, which compromise the strength of bones

- gender; the reduction of estrogen experienced by women at menopause accelerates loss of bone for a period of time

Osteoporosis does not necessarily cause problems. It is invisible and painless and, unless there are fractures, there are no symptoms. It is not the thin bones in themselves that cause problems, but the fact that thin bones can fracture more easily than dense, strong bones. The vertebral bones can fracture spontaneously or when the person is performing even such simple tasks as lifting a grandchild. Falls are an important factor in wrist and hip fractures. If a person with osteoporosis falls, she or he is more likely to break the wrist that is put out to break the fall, or break the hip bone that is hit with the fall.

Other factors can come in to play here as well. For instance, not everyone who falls fractures bones. Thin people with less padding around their hips are more likely to suffer fractures, and fractures are more frequent in elderly women who are taking sleeping tablets and psychotropic drugs. This is because they are less alert and less steady on their feet and therefore likely to fall badly. Fractures are not just a matter of thin bones. What all this adds up to is that osteoporosis is a complex condition with many factors contributing to how it will affect an individual.

Bone remodeling

Bones are not inert. They are living tissue made up of cells, the organic matrix, and minerals. Bones are constantly being broken down and reformed in a process called *bone remodeling.* It is estimated that adults have 10–30% of their bone replaced each year.

Bone tissue is made of tiny crystals of *calcium* and *phosphorus* embedded in a matrix or network of protein fibers, primarily *collagen,* a protein also found in skin and tendons. Calcium makes the bones hard and strong, and collagen fibers give bones their flexibility.

There are two basic types of bone tissue. The hard outer shell of bones is called *cortical bone;* the more porous, honeycomb-like inner bone is called *trabecular bone.* All bones are made up of these two types of tissue, but the relative proportions of each differ from one bone to another. The long bones of the arms and legs, for instance, are made up primarily of hard cortical bone with areas of trabecular bone at each end, while the vertebrae of the spine are mostly trabecular bone with a thin cortical shell.

In bone remodeling, new bone tissue is formed through a process called *bone mineralization,* while old bone is broken down or resorbed. Because of their greater surface area, bones with the most trabecular tissue are the most vulnerable to bone loss as we grow older.

Bone remodeling depends on the complementary actions of two types of cells. The *osteoclasts,* the bone-resorbing cells, dig microscopic pits along the surface of the bone. Next, the *osteoblasts,* the bone-forming cells, fill in the cavities and then produce the collagen framework or matrix of the bone. Finally, the mineral salts—calcium and phosphorus crystals—are deposited in this framework. This process is called bone mineralization.

The ingredients of strong bones

The *calcium* needed for bone formation is taken from the bloodstream. Adequate calcium is needed in the diet to provide supplies of calcium for building bone, but the process of calcium absorption and utilization is highly complex and not just a matter of sufficient dietary calcium.

Other substances in the body also play critical roles in keeping calcium levels in the bloodstream in the correct balance. The action of four hormones is necessary: parathyroid hormone or PTH, vitamin D, calcitonin, and estrogen. PTH, vitamin D, and calcitonin play such an important part in maintaining healthy bones that they are sometimes called "the bone hormones," while estrogen acts on bones in indirect ways through its relationship with PTH, calcitonin, and vitamin D.

Parathyroid hormone is produced by a tiny gland in the neck, which monitors the level of calcium in the bloodstream. If the level of calcium falls, PTH is released from the gland and acts to increase the supply of calcium in the blood. It does this in several ways, including signaling to the kidneys to stop excreting calcium in the urine; but another is to stimulate the breakdown of bone so that stored calcium is released into the bloodstream. This is clearly not good for the bones, but calcium is needed for other processes in the body, in the brain, in muscles, and for blood clotting, so the body sacrifices bone calcium to meet this need.

Another element needed for healthy bones is *vitamin D,* found in some foods but primarily derived from exposure to sunlight. Vitamin D is actually a type of hormone. It is present in an inactive form in the skin, is activated by sunlight, and then stored in a partially activated form in the liver. It is converted into its final activated form, called *calcitriol,* by the kidneys. Vitamin D helps increase the absorption of calcium from the small intestine, and it also increases resorption of calcium through the kidneys. Like PTH, vitamin D can also draw calcium from the bones if PTH levels are high in the body.

Calcitonin, the other "bone hormone," is secreted by the thyroid gland. It protects bones by inhibiting the action of the osteoclasts, the bone-resorbing cells.

The role of estrogen in maintaining healthy bones is not entirely clear. It has been suggested that estrogen blocks the bone-dissolving action of PTH so that after menopause, when estrogen levels fall, the bones are more vulnerable to PTH, which can then cause increased bone breakdown. More recently, estrogen receptors have been found on bone, suggesting that estrogen may act directly on bone in some way that is not yet understood.

Exercise is another critical factor in developing and maintaining strong bones throughout our lives. Exercise places physical stress on the bones and they respond by becoming bigger and stronger. This will be discussed in more detail in the following chapter.

Peak bone mass

During childhood, when our bones are growing, we produce more bone tissue than is lost through bone resorption. At adolescence, the increase in sex hormone production, specifically estrogens and progesterones in girls, leads to acceleration in the bone-building process. In young adults, new bone is formed at a rate that matches the loss of bone through bone resorption. The action of the osteoclasts and osteoblasts is precisely linked.

The size of bones varies considerably among individuals and is affected by many factors, principally heredity, race, and diet. Peak bone mass appears to be genetically set, in other words, we are probably born with a maximum size our bones can reach.(9) Environmental and lifestyle factors can then affect whether we attain the bone mass we are programmed to achieve. Exercise and a healthy diet enable us to achieve it. Reaching maximum bone mass potential in youth is important as then our bones will be heavier and stronger when bone mass begins to decline.

Bone loss

Peak bone mass is reached at somewhere around 30 to 35 years of age, possibly even earlier. After this age, the bone cells "uncouple" and osteoclasts begin to dominate. As a result, the rate of breakdown begins to exceed the rate of formation of new bone, and bone mass begins to decline. Until the age of about 50, this decline is only slight, the bone being mostly lost from the long bones of the arms and legs.

Gradual bone loss continues in men throughout their lifetimes, in women it is temporarily accelerated by the reduction in the amount of estrogen produced by the ovaries at menopause. This is why some researchers talk about a "biphasic pattern of bone loss," meaning there is a protracted slow loss of bone in both sexes, and an accelerated transient phase that occurs in women after menopause.(10)

Bone loss at menopause

The relative importance of aging and menopause to osteoporosis in women is not known.(11) It is wrong, then, to simply blame loss of estrogen for fractures experienced by postmenopausal women.

At menopause, the average loss is around 2% annually. The most rapid reduction occurs in the first five or six years following menopause. The amount of bone loss during this accelerated phase is the subject of debate. Dr. Lawrence Riggs of the Mayo Clinic suggests that 10–15% of cortical bone loss and 15–20% of trabecular bone loss can be attributed to menopause.(12)

Dr. Riggs also poses an interesting and so far unresolved question: if, by definition, all postmenopausal women are "estrogen deficient," why do only a few develop osteoporosis in the 15 to 20 years after menopause? He suggests that "additional factors must be present that interact with estrogen to determine individual susceptibility and select for the 5–10% of women destined for early vertebral fractures." He suggests two possibilities: first, that in some women the accelerated bone-loss phase lasts longer, and, second, that women with osteoporosis may have more increased bone resorption than other women.(13)

At around the age of 65, bone loss in women slows to the same rate as in men, around 0.2% per year.(14) While quite a lot of attention has been paid to menopausal bone loss, there are still many gaps in medical knowledge about the rate of bone loss in elderly women. Some studies suggest that bone loss ceases altogether at around age 70 in some individuals. One long study measured bone density in a group of women over 70 at two-month intervals for a period of years. It was found that bone density actually increased in 31% of these women, decreased in only 29%, and was unchanged in 40%.(15)

Fracture risk

Dense bones are strong bones. Loss of bone density makes the bones thinner and weaker, sometimes leading to fractures. The higher the peak bone mass attained, the less likelihood there is that fractures will occur in later life. People who only ever reach a low peak bone mass are at greater risk of fracture because the bone loss they suffer as they age can put them below what is called the "fracture threshold," an arbitrary level of bone density under which fractures are more likely to occur.(16) Bone density in women does not fall below the fracture threshold until about the age of 65.

Both men and women can develop fractures, but this is twice as likely to happen to women for two reasons: (1) the peak bone mass women attain is usually around 30% lower than men's, consequently when women lose bone they do so from a less favorable position; (2) the reduction in estrogen at menopause accelerates bone loss for a period of time.

It must be remembered that not all individuals are at the same risk. The factors that determine how strong bones will be are discussed in some detail in the following chapter, but individual differences in bone strength mean that the risk of fracture varies greatly. If bone measurements of the hip were taken of postmenopausal women, it would be discovered that 70% are at low risk, some 22% are at intermediate risk, and only 8% are at high risk.(17) The corresponding figures for the vertebrae are 72% at low risk, 21% at intermediate risk, and 7% at high risk. The risk of fracture in high-risk groups is obviously far greater than in the low and intermediate groups (see the table on page 139).

Types of Osteoporotic Fractures

Although osteoporotic fractures can occur in many bones in the body, including the ribs, ankle, and pelvis, there are three main types of fracture:

- wrist fractures, sometimes called Colles fractures

- vertebral fractures

- hip fractures, also called fractures of the proximal femur

These three types of fracture occur under different circumstances, at different ages, and in differing proportions between the sexes, so that research scientists argue that the causes may be subtly different. Different factors could affect bone at different sites in the skeleton.(18) While it is clear that loss of bone mass is the major factor in vertebral fractures, the relationship is not so clear with hip fracture and wrist fracture. Studies have shown that there is not a huge difference in the bone mass between people who have wrist fractures and those who don't or those who have hip fractures and those who don't. The tendency to fall and an inability to protect oneself from injury may be just as important in determining who will fracture wrist or hip.(19)

Distribution of Bone Mass by Site and Projected Lifetime Risk Among 50-year-old Women

	Hip %	No. of fractures	Vertebrae %	No.	Wrist %	No.
Low risk						
Proportion of women	70	3	72	10	79	20
Lifetime risk	4		14		25	
Intermediate risk						
Proportion of women	22	5	21	11	17	13
Lifetime risk	20		54		76	
High risk						
Proportion of women	8	4	7	6	4	4
Lifetime risk	42		90		90	

Adapted from NOF Scientific Advisory Board Report 1989

This table shows how the categories of high-, intermediate- and low-risk contribute to the total number of fractures in a hypothetical group of 100 women.

Because of the greater number of women deemed to be at low and intermediate risk for hip fracture, they would contribute eight of the total number of fractures, while the high-risk women–low in number–would only contribute four. The same pattern is seen with vertebral fractures, where 21 low- and intermediate-risk women would have such fractures, but only six would occur in the small group of women deemed to be at high risk.

Vertebral fractures are infinitely more common in women than in men, and of the osteoporotic fractures are most clearly linked to loss of estrogen. By contrast, hip fractures occur much later in life and are more closely linked to the loss of bone caused by the general aging process and to other factors relating to age, such as less physical stability.

These differences in the effect of menopausal loss of estrogen on bone density in different parts of the skeleton have led some researchers to postulate that vertebral osteoporosis is actually a different disease from osteoporosis in the hip.(20) The hypothesis is that wrist and vertebral fractures are related to menopausal loss of estrogen, while hip fractures are the result of an aging process that occurs in men and women. The fractures that occur earliest—wrist and vertebrae—are thought to occur because of a loss of trabecular bone. Trabecular bone is most vulnerable to bone loss as it has a greater surface area than cortical bone. Whereas the bones that fracture late in life—such as hip and pelvis—contain substantial amounts of both cortical and trabecular bone.(21)

Because of these differences in the various fractures, the question of whether a fracture at one site, such as wrist or vertebrae, will predispose that individual to later fractures in another part of the body is not easy to answer and is still being studied. In general, one type of fracture does usually indicate an increased susceptibility to other types, but it is not a strong relationship. A woman who has a wrist fracture, for instance, is only slightly more likely to have a later hip fracture. A man who has a wrist fracture, however, is six times more likely to have a hip fracture.(22)

Wrist fractures

Wrist fractures occur in the distal radius and begin to occur in women in their fifties. The incidence increases until the age of 65, then reaches a plateau. Studies have shown that women who have wrist fractures have not lost excessive amounts of bone density, although they do tend to be in the low normal range.(23)

Wrist fractures usually occur when the woman extends her arm to break a fall. In most cases they heal easily and do not lead to subsequent disability, but in a number of cases the fracture can result in a stiff or sore wrist.

Vertebral fractures

Fractures of the vertebrae typically occur in the first two decades after menopause when estrogen production drops. The bones of the spine—the vertebrae—are composed primarily of porous trabecular bone, making them particularly vulnerable to bone loss. The wrist and lower jaw also contain large amounts of trabecular bone, so that postmenopausal bone loss can affect them. Women at this age can have increased tooth loss because the jaw contains trabecular bone and the teeth can be loosened if this decreases.(24)

Vertebral fractures can occur spontaneously, as vertebrae simply collapse under the weight of the body, or because of everyday stresses such as coughing, lifting, making a bed, or sudden movements.

The vertebrae go through stages as they collapse. At first, the side of the vertebra toward the front of the body collapses, producing what doctors call a *wedge fracture*. Next, the side toward the back of the body can collapse as well, flattening the whole vertebra. This is called a *crush fracture* or a *compression fracture*.

Most women with vertebral fractures have only one or two, but a few women suffer more. If a number of vertebrae collapse, the spine compresses downward and shortens in length. This can cause a loss of height, each crush resulting in about a one-third inch reduction in height. A few women lose as much as eight-and-a-half inches, and this can cause transverse rolls in the skin of the abdomen, thickening in the waist, and a pot belly as the internal organs are pushed into a smaller space.

In the worst cases the whole spine curves over, causing the so-called dowager's hump. The rib cage is pushed down toward the hip bones, the lower spine curves inward, and the upper spine curves outward. The medical term for this is *kyphosis*.

Not all vertebral fractures cause problems to the women who experience them, and it is by no means inevitable that having had one vertebral fracture a woman will experience more. Women can be unaware they have had a fracture of the spine; it may be discovered only incidentally when the woman has a chest X-ray for some other reason.

There is sometimes a sharp pain at the site of the fracture when it occurs. Because the muscles around it may spasm, there can be pain for some weeks, but then the pain will go as the fracture heals. These fractures do not cause any more chronic back pain than that experienced by individuals without such fracture, except in severe cases.(25) It is only women with kyphosis who tend to suffer chronic pain from their condition. Their lives may be quite limited and their condition emotionally distressing. The alteration to their body shape and appearance can lead to a loss of confidence and self-esteem.

Hip fractures

Hip fractures are more accurately a fracture of the upper part of the thigh bone or femur. They are primarily a problem of people in their eighties and older. The femur contains a large amount of hard cortical bone and it is loss of this bone with aging that leads to the fracture. However, fragility of the bone is not the sole cause. Two other factors interact to cause hip fractures in the elderly:

- increased falls in the elderly

- environmental factors such as poorly designed living environments, wearing slippers when cold, and other factors related to being old such as medication use, lack of physical fitness, and impaired judgment

Old people fall quite often, and the older they get, the more they fall. Between the ages of 60–64, women fall at a rate of 19% per year; by 80–84 this has increased to 33%.(26) But just falling won't necessarily cause a fracture. Only 1–6% of falls in older people actually result in fractures and not a lot is known about the factors that protect those 94% of people who fall and do not fracture.(27)

It has been suggested that part of the increase in hip fractures as people age is explained by a change in the way people fall.(28) Old people may fall badly because their responses are poor, they are less likely to break the fall by putting out an arm, and they have less ability to absorb the impact. Factors which come into play here are weak muscles, disorientation, slow reaction time, and reduced fat and muscles around the bones of the hip.(29) On the other hand, active old people also fall. They are more likely to fall outside, where the hard ground increases the likelihood of their incurring a fracture.(30) Doctors and others working in this area argue that we could prevent some of these fractures by improving living environments and modifying other factors in the lives of elderly people.

Although both women and men can have hip fractures, women experience them at twice the rate of men. There are several reasons for this. Smaller bones are one reason, but medication rates tend to be higher in women, they may have less fat and muscle around the bone, and awkwardness in moving through lack of exercise could be another. A study of falls, which compared men and women, showed that women fell more often than men, and there were significant differences in the circumstances around the fall.(31) Men were more likely to fall outside, at greater levels of physical activity, while women had increased falls in winter and went outside less than daily. Women were also more likely to be using psychotropic drugs or hypnotics (sleeping tablets). Over 30% of the women in the study were using such drugs, mostly hypnotics.

Another study found that elderly women with the highest rate of hip fractures were more likely to have both low bone density and poor cognizance. In these women, whose mental ability and coordination were poor, the fracture rate during two years was 12.8%. On the other hand, women with the same low bone density but good cognizance did not fracture as often (3.4%), while in women with poor cognizance but good bone mass, the fracture rate was 6.2%. The researchers commented: "It probably takes a fall for an osteoporotic woman to fracture a hip, and with good cognizance a fall is less likely."(32)

The circumstances surrounding a fall event can affect the outcome. One medical journal gave this example:

> At one extreme, a resolute but imprudent elderly man ascends a shaky ladder, extends his head backwards, reaches an arm out to change a lightbulb; the ladder moves, and he falls to the ground. He may or may not suffer serious injury as a consequence, but he is essentially a fit person and his health is not likely to suffer seriously. At the other extreme, a weak, malnourished, ill old person walks slowly across the room; her legs give way and down she goes. Perhaps she sustains little injury, but may be so shocked and weakened by the experience that she is unable to rise, lies on the floor for hours until rescued, and becomes gravely ill.(33)

Hip fractures are the most serious of the osteoporotic fractures and can have devastating effects on the health of people who suffer them. They can take a long time to mend and operations for hip replacements are necessary for some. Permanent disablement can ensue, with many hip fracture victims never regaining their former level of mobility. A percentage of people even die. The deaths are not caused by the fracture per se, but by complications such as pneumonia or blood clots resulting from the prolonged bed rest often needed to recuperate from a hip fracture. People who do badly or die after hip fracture are likely to be very old, to be institutionalized, and to have preexisting illnesses or physical and mental disabilities. Hip fractures can also lead to a dangerous cycle of loss of confidence and reduced mobility, which can in itself lead to another fall.

An important factor in the outcome is "the long lie," as illustrated by the scenario above. People who are not found for some time after the fall do worse, and a delay in treatment can also worsen a person's outcome. In New Zealand (if not also in other countries), this is more likely to happen to women, as more than half of women over 75 years of age live at home alone. In the past, hip fracture victims were often seen as pretty hopeless cases when they were admitted to hospital. They went to the bottom of the waiting line, leading to delays in treatment, and were often given the cheapest possible operations.(34)

Medical management of hip fracture has improved dramatically in recent years. People are now mobilized as soon as possible after the fracture is fixed to try to avoid bed-rest complications. In some countries, multidisciplinary units specializing in the rehabilitation of elderly fracture patients are standard practice.

How Big a Problem Is Osteoporosis?

As noted above, osteoporosis has become a hot topic in the media in recent years. From pharmaceutical manufacturers to dairy farmers, many industries are "marketing" osteoporosis to consumers. The resulting advertising and public furor may be obscuring some of the truth surrounding the facts of osteoporosis.

Vertebral fractures

Vertebral fractures are most likely to occur between the ages of 50 and 70 with the average age about 65. One widely quoted study from Denmark showed that 4.5% of 70-year-old women had crush fractures and another 18% had wedge fractures, a total of 22.5%.(35) Dr. Bruce Ettinger studied crush fracture prevalence and concluded: "Our figure of 6.6% prevalence for women of a mean age of 68 years fits well with prevalence figures reported in studies done in other parts of the world, and controverts the popular opinion that vertebral crush fractures are a common clinical problem in elderly women. Multiple vertebral fracture prevalence is commonly found to be half that of single fractures."(36) The estimated lifetime risk for both kinds of vertebral fractures is 27%.(37)

These figures need to be treated with caution. The problem with statistics on vertebral fractures is that they fail to distinguish between fractures that give the woman little or no trouble, and those that are disabling and disfiguring. Many of the studies looking at the incidence of vertebral fractures have been done by looking at chest or spinal X-rays taken for reasons other than fracture problems. In other words, many of these women whose X-rays showed a vertebral fracture didn't even know they had one.

A Dutch group that conducted research on fractures commented: "The majority of women who had newly occurring vertebral fractures were asymptomatic; only three [of 37] of them were seeing their general practitioner for this reason."(38)

There are no figures that measure how serious a problem vertebral fractures are. We have no idea, for instance, what proportion of women develop kyphosis, although as Dr. Ettinger said, it is probably quite small. For an individual woman, being told you have a 22% chance or worse of a vertebral fracture by the age of 70 sounds rather grim. If we knew what proportion of these were actually troublesome, we might see it rather differently.

Hip fractures

There are approximately 250,000 hip fractures each year in people over 65 years old, due to osteoporosis. By world standards the United States has a high rate of such fractures; one study put American women first in a comparison of women from 12 countries.(39) A recent study in Western Australia showed that for every five-year increase in age the incidence rate of hip fractures doubles, with the really steep rises in incidence being for those over 75 years old.(40) These researchers found that at the exact age of 55, a woman has a 17% chance of sustaining a hip fracture before death, and a male a 6% chance. Because the chance of a hip fracture before age 55 was negligible, the researchers said these rates could be taken as an approximation of the lifetime risk. In most Western countries, the average age for hip fracture is 83.(41) Only 16% of men and 33% of women survive to the age of 85 years, although the number of women who live to over 85 is increasing, making hip fractures an increasing public health problem.

There is controversy about whether the incidence of hip fractures is actually increasing. It does seem to be in some countries. If there is an increase, some have speculated that this may be in women in particular cohorts—that is, women born in a particular era. Women who are now in the age group for fractures—the 60- to 80-year-olds—may have suffered deficiencies in their diets from having lived through an economic depression and rationing during the war. If this theory is true, women born since the 1950s should do better, except that these younger women may have restricted their diets for other reasons. The vogue for thinness that has exerted a powerful effect on women since Twiggy popularized the anorexic silhouette in the 1960s may have had an effect on the health of bones. Younger women are also more likely to be smokers. Sedentary lifestyles, a result of urbanization and affluence, may also have a negative effect on bone strength.

In terms of outcome, hip fractures are among the most serious: about one quarter of hip fracture victims die of complications within six months, and of those living independently prior to suffering hip fracture, 15–25% are still in long-term care institutions a year after the injury.

Individuals who have hip fractures have their survival reduced by about 12% compared to other individuals of the same age, and women who have a hip fracture are four times more likely to have another hip fracture than are other women.(42) In men, the risk of a second fracture is eight times that of men who have not had one at all.(43) In one study it was found that men had around double the fatality rate of women after hip fracture and that people, especially men, living in nursing homes did less well.(44) On average, people stay in hospital two to four weeks after a hip fracture. Up to two thirds will never regain their former mobility, and some will need permanent nursing care.(45) This is especially true of people who were ill or disabled prior to the fracture. However, figures from one multidisciplinary unit showed that three quarters of their hip fracture patients admitted to hospital from their homes did return home.(46)

Conclusion

Osteoporosis is a serious health problem for women who suffer fractures; however, there has been a tendency for the extent of the problem among women to be exaggerated. Caution is called for when looking at the figures for the incidence of vertebral fractures. Although a significant minority of women will suffer one or more vertebral fractures, many will not know this has happened to them. Despite the commercial interests' use of images of women showing extreme forms of osteoporotic deformity, it is difficult to know how many women actually suffer such disability. The indications are that it is not at all common.

For women who suffer hip fractures, the outcome can be devastating, with a considerable loss of mobility and independence. People who fracture their hips and then recover incompletely tend to be very elderly and in poor health. The blame for hip fractures, however, cannot be put solely on loss of bone density. An increased propensity to fall with old age and environmental factors, such as drug use, interact to place women at risk of hip fractures. Attention to such factors as medication and safer living environments could well reduce the incidence of fracture among the elderly.

Chapter 7

Preventing Bone Loss and Fractures

A person knows he or she has osteoporosis only if a fracture occurs. Unfortunately, by this time a good deal of bone has already been lost, and there are no known methods of treating a person so that lost bone can be regained. This lack of effective treatment methods has led doctors to look for ways of preventing fractures from ever occurring. Work in this area has primarily focused on ways of preventing bone loss in the hope that this will prevent fractures. Little attention has been paid to changing lifestyle and environmental factors to prevent falls and thus stop fractures occurring.

Predicting Risks

Much of the emphasis in the prevention of bone loss has been on "risk factors." Books and articles for women about osteoporosis tend to make predictions about particular factors that are said to place a person at greater risk of developing osteoporosis. Medical journals do the same, and doctors repeat these to their midlife female patients. These risk factors have been arrived at through studies of large populations and are really averages of factors that contribute to the risk of osteoporosis. The difficulty comes in translating these averages into useful predictions for individual women.

For a start, no consistent set of risk factors has emerged from all studies. Researchers have found that the presence of risk factors only goes a little way toward explaining variations in bone density or fracture risk.(1) Risk factors account for only about one-third of the variability in people's bones.(2) Added to this, as we have seen, low bone density is only one factor in hip fracture.

In practice, it is difficult to predict accurately from examining someone or taking her or his medical history who will or will not have a fracture later on. The so-called risk factors are rather imprecise: having none is not a guarantee a fracture won't occur, while having one or more risk factors does not mean you will inevitably break a bone. Risk factors are only part of the osteoporosis story, so applying them to ourselves as individuals can only give us a rough guide as to what to expect in the future.

Measuring bone density

The most accurate way of predicting fracture risk is by actually measuring bone density, although there are limitations to this as we shall see. While moderate or high bone density does not give complete protection against fractures, numerous studies have shown that low bone density does increase the risk of fracture.(3) This is especially true for vertebral fractures where there is the clearest relationship between decreased bone density and fracture.

One study of 1,237 women aged between 43 and 80 produced interesting results. It divided the whole group of women into quartiles, or fourths, according to their bone density found by measuring their bones. The women were then followed to see if they had fractures. It was found that women in the lowest quartile for spinal bone mass (that is, they had the lowest bone mass) were at three times greater risk of any fracture than women in the highest quartile. For vertebral fractures, women in the lowest quartile had an almost 14 times greater risk.(4)

Over recent years various ways of measuring bone density have been developed. The earlier methods measured bone density at only one site in the body, usually the forearm. Recent work has shown that bone measurement at one site in the body can reasonably accurately predict the likelihood of fractures of other bones in the skeleton.(5) Research is being undertaken on a form of ultrasound which measures bone density in the heel. If this technology is effective, it could make bone measurement more accessible, as the equipment is cheap and portable.

The newest technology and the most effective is *dual energy X-ray absorptiometry,* or DEXA. This is a noninvasive technique which measures the density of cortical or trabecular bone at any site in the body with great precision. The x-ray reading is translated into a computerized picture. An examination using this technology takes only two minutes and exposes the patient to a very low level of radiation— 1 mRem. Another technique is computed tomography (CT) scanning. It uses X-rays to measure bone density. Researchers are now adapting this technique to CT equipment already available in many hospitals.

While no blood or urine tests specifically diagnose osteoporosis, these tests may eliminate secondary causes of bone loss such as corticosteroids, heparin (an anticoagulant), and certain other medications; hyperthyroidism and hyperparathyroidism; kidney disease; and certain forms of cancer (lymphoma, leukemia, and multiple myeloma); or excessive excretion of calcium in the urine (idiopathic hypercalciuria).

Screening for osteoporosis

In countries with national health services, preventative screening is being discussed. Because of the very high cost of treating hip fracture patients, preventive strategies for osteoporosis have turned to the possibility of screening women in the first five years after menopause to check their bone density. But there are serious questions being asked about this approach. These are:

- Which group of women should be offered screening (especially when there are only a few machines)?

- What treatment can be offered to those shown to have low bone density?

- Will screening prevent sufficient serious fractures to justify the expense?

One suggested approach would be to offer screening to "high-risk" women only, "high risk" having been determined by general practitioners making a clinical assessment of women for risk factors. But as we have seen, it is very difficult to accurately predict by risk factors who those high-risk women are, so this would be an ineffective way of carrying out screening. Many of the women sent for bone measurement would turn out to have normal bones, while some of the women who didn't get sent would actually have bones within the high-risk range.

In some medical circles there has been debate about the idea of screening all women soon after menopause for loss of bone density, and there has been some promotion of this idea to general practitioners and to women.(6) But there are many problems with this proposal. For instance, doctors cannot agree on what constitutes abnormal bone loss and at what level of bone density treatment might be offered. There is no sharp dividing line for bone density between people who are at high risk for fracture and people who are not.(7)

As we have seen, the relation between bone mass and fracture differs for the three most frequent fracture sites. This means that while there is a strong correlation between low bone density and fractures of the vertebrae, low bone density is only one factor for fractures of the wrist and hip. Steven Cummings of the University of California notes that "patients with hip fractures do not appear distinctly more osteoporotic than persons of similar age . . . thus measurements of bone mass might not be a reliable way to identify those at greatest risk of hip fracture."(8)

Cummings also raises another critical and as yet unanswered question.(9) He asks whether a bone measurement at menopause can accurately predict what will happen to a woman 30 years later, which is when most hip fractures occur. So far the research has been of a much shorter interval; at the most, people have been followed for less than seven years. More research is needed before questions like this can be resolved.

Taking bone measurements will only give us part of the picture of an individual's risk of these fractures. This means that screening could only be partially effective in preventing fractures and would only be able to save part of the money spent on treating hip fractures, by far the most costly fracture in terms of expenditure of public money. This limited saving has to be weighed against the very considerable cost of buying more technology and undertaking screening.

In fact, no country in the world has yet tried such a mass program, and there have been no research trials of the effectiveness of this approach. Several recent major reviews of the question of screening for osteoporosis have concluded that mass screening cannot be recommended until a protocol for such a program is formulated and its effectiveness justified.(10) In New Zealand, a working party set up to advise the Department of Health on strategies for preventing osteoporosis agreed that there was insufficient evidence to support the institution of a mass screening program.(11) An American review also made the point that the strategies suggested so far "ignore men . . . who experience a significant number of age-related fractures even though their risk is lower."(12)

Screening all postmenopausal women also raises the question of what you would do for women whose bone density was shown to be low. There is really no point in measuring for bone loss unless you can do something about it. Hormone replacement therapy is being promoted as a way of preventing further bone loss, and women who already show significant bone loss could be offered HRT. But such an approach would result in large numbers of women taking a drug that is still the subject of considerable controversy regarding long-term safety, and we do not know how acceptable the long-term therapy needed would be to women. Even if a woman used HRT, this would not give her a guarantee that she would not have a fracture, as HRT can only reduce her risk, not eliminate it.

From a public health point of view, this approach would not significantly reduce the considerable burden to the health system of the cost of osteoporotic fractures. It would not prevent fractures in men at all, and it could only reduce the number of fractures in women if every single woman used HRT and used it for the optimal period of time, 10 to 15 years. Any less than that and the gain in preventing fractures would be far less. The National Osteoporosis Foundation in America recently carried out a detailed review of the feasibility of screening for osteoporosis. It determined that if all 50-year-old women had their bones measured and women with low bone density were put on HRT, the lifetime risk of a hip fracture for all women would decrease from 10% to 8% and for the spine from 25% to 22%, not a very large gain in public health terms.(13)

The review also shows how women with low bone density are actually a minority of the postmenopausal female population. The majority of women have intermediate or high bone density, and they can still have fractures, even if less frequently. Because there are far more actual numbers of women in these groups, they account for a far greater proportion of the total number of fractures each year than do women in the small high-risk group. One study showed that the

20% of women who were deemed to be high risk contributed 40% of all the fractures noted, while the 80% of women not judged to be at high risk contributed 60% of the fractures.(14)

To make a real dent in the cost of osteoporosis to the country, most postmenopausal women would need to be on HRT. A few doctors agree with this approach even though no one knows what the ultimate effect of that would be in terms of either public health costs or repercussions for individual women. Many women are not at all keen on the idea of long-term medication, as for most women it means a continuation of menstruation into old age. For this reason, some doctors argue that HRT will never be an effective preventive strategy for any but highly motivated women who are at clear risk.

Another suggested screening regimen is to provide bone measurements for women thinking of going on HRT; however, this is a very individualistic and inequitable approach. It means some women, probably middle-class women, would be provided with a service because they knew enough to ask or their doctors suggested it, while others did not. It would also be a highly inefficient use of scarce resources, because this approach would not necessarily reach the women most at risk.

At the moment, most countries have adopted the practice of offering bone measurement to men and women suspected of being at high risk because they have recognized major risk factors. This includes people with the following indications:

- vertebral abnormalities, where bone measurement is used to diagnose whether the abnormalities are being caused by osteoporosis or some other condition

- long-term glucocorticoid therapy

- amenorrhea in young women

- hyperparathyroidism

Risk Factors

As we have seen, there is no simple answer to the question of how to prevent osteoporotic fractures, either for individual women or for people designing health services. This takes us back to the subject of risk factors. Professor Bruce Riggs of the Mayo Clinic makes the point that although it is difficult to rank risk factors according to relative importance, the more that are present in an individual person, the greater the likelihood that bone density will be low.(15)

For individual women, eliminating or modifying risk factors in our lives is a sensible approach. While a few of the risk factors, such as race and sex, are outside our control, we can do something about many of the others. For most well women the three major modifiable risk factors are lack of exercise, insufficient calcium in the diet, and smoking. Improving diet and physical fitness and giving up smoking will provide significant protection against osteoporosis and will have many other health benefits.

Risk factors for osteoporosis can be divided into several categories (note: the question marks indicate that these risk factors are not yet proven).

Genetic and biological factors

- female sex

- family history of osteoporosis

- European or Asian ancestry

- light build and shortness

- fairness

- early natural menopause (?)

- childlessness (?)

Medical factors

- surgical menopause

- hysterectomy (?)

- glucocorticoid therapy for asthma and other diseases

- gastrointestinal disease

- hyperthyroidism

- hyperparathyroidism

- renal (kidney) failure

- rheumatoid arthritis
- extended bed rest/immobilization
- Depo Provera use (?)

Lifestyle and environmental factors

- lack of exercise
- extreme overexercising
- smoking
- vitamin D deficiency
- inadequate fluoride in the water supply (?)

Dietary factors

- low calcium intake
- anorexia nervosa
- chronic dieting (?)
- high alcohol consumption
- excessive coffee
- excessive salt (?)
- excessive protein (?)
- phosphorus (?)

By grouping risk factors in this way, it is possible to see that the genetic and medical factors are largely although not entirely outside our control, while the lifestyle and dietary factors are more within our control; in these areas we can have some impact on our future risk. If you have some of the unmodifiable risks, this makes attention to the risks you can do something about, such as diet and exercise, all the more important.

Most of these risk factors have their opposites—that is, conditions and factors that have a protective effect. For instance, lack of exercise is a risk factor, but regular weight-bearing exercises are protective. Some important protective factors worth emphasizing are

- fatness or obesity

- Polynesian or African ancestry

Genetic and Biological Factors

Sex and race

Being female is a strong but not absolute determinant of being at greater risk of fracture. While it is true that in most countries studied, women have higher fracture rates than men, this is not a universal phenomenon. In Hong Kong the incidence rate is very similar between men and women. Amongst the South African Bantu, men have a slightly higher rate; in Singapore, men have nearly double the rate of women.(16) These deviations from the usual trends, the reasons for which are largely unknown, highlight how incomplete scientific knowledge about osteoporosis is. They suggest that environmental factors may be important in determining who develops osteoporosis, and they also illustrate the narrowness of describing osteoporosis as a woman's problem caused by being female and losing estrogen at menopause. Perhaps if we knew more about why the rate of osteoporosis is so low in Singapore (in women it is around 15% of the U.S. rate), and why Singaporean men are at greater risk than the women, we might learn something useful for men and women in all countries.

Race and skin color are strong determinants of susceptibility to osteoporosis. The fact that bone density remains similar in people of the same race even when they have migrated from their country of origin argues for the importance of genetics in determining bone strength.(17) Women whose ancestors came from Northern Europe, China, or Japan are at higher risk than women whose ancestors came from Africa or the Pacific.

Like black women of African descent, Maori and Pacific Island women have bone density that is 20% greater than European women.(18) The reason for this is not entirely clear. A study comparing Maori and non-Maori people suggested that Maori women might be more likely to be engaged in hard physical work.(19) Other reasons suggested by researchers are that black people have bigger bones and bigger muscles. It is possible also that black women lose bone with aging at a slower rate than white women, perhaps because of hormonal differences between the races, and black women may have higher levels of calcitonin, the bone-protecting hormone.

Being nonwhite does not give absolute protection against osteoporosis. Some black women do have hip fractures, although usually at an older age than white women, and black women who have a surgical menopause or other major risk factors can have fractures. Heavy smoking, which is prevalent among Maori women, might also negate some of the genetic benefit.

Family inheritance

Our genes also set our peak bone mass and have a major effect on body size. It is the slight, birdlike, dainty women who have the highest rates of osteoporosis. Tall women are less at risk, and fat and obese women are also protected. This is thought to happen for several reasons.

Greater body weight results in added stress being put on the skeleton which will in turn encourage the development of stronger bones. Overweight people have more chance of reaching their peak bone mass in early adulthood and stronger bones have been found in the spine and hip in overweight postmenopausal women.(20) Fat may also increase the resistance of bone to PTH; also, the male sex hormone androgen can be converted to estrogen in fat.(21) As discussed earlier, at menopause, although estrogen production from the ovaries slows down, both the ovaries and adrenal glands continue to produce androgen. This means that overweight women produce more estrogen after menopause than do thin women. Then again, the bones of overweight people are more protected when they fall so they are less likely to fracture.

This is not an argument for being overweight since there are other health hazards in being overweight, but it is refreshing to discover something positive about fatness as fat people normally get so many negative health messages. It is also possible for very obese people to have thin bones if they have gotten to the point of being immobilized by their bulk.

At Auckland Medical School, Dr. Ian Reid studied 140 normal postmenopausal women aged between 47 and 71 to see which of the recognized risk factors correlated with bone density.(22) He looked at a whole host of factors, such as age at menopause, age at menarche, number of children, breastfeeding history, smoking, energy expenditure, dietary energy, height, muscle mass, and fat mass. His startling finding was that total body fat was the strongest predictor of how strong a woman's bones were. The fatter a woman, the stronger her bones. Being thin, he concluded, was dangerous when it came to osteoporosis. He raised the possibility that, in addition to the effects of fat on bones (as discussed above), fat cells may in some way act directly on bones. There is also the genetic argument that people inherit both their fat and their bone density from their parents.

The idea that osteoporosis in the family could be an indication that an individual may be at risk is commonly repeated, but there has actually been little research on this relationship.(23) If your mother or grandmother has severe vertebral osteoporosis, such as kyphosis, this may slightly increase your risk of developing osteoporosis, but it is by no means certain. A recent study compared bone density in the premenopausal daughters of postmenopausal women with vertebral crush fractures with normal controls. It found that the daughters did have lower bone density compared to normal women by 7% in the spine and by 5% in the hip.(24) They concluded that this was probably due to heredity—the daughters having a lower peak bone mass than the other women—rather than any excessive rate of bone loss with aging. Lifestyle, such as shared diet, could also contribute to the difference.

Age at menopause is also determined by family inheritance, and early menopause is thought to place a woman at greater risk of fractures because this means more years with low estrogen levels. Early menopause is usually deemed to be menopause before the age of 45; however, this relationship is still not proven. One recent study showed a low fracture risk among women who had a natural menopause before 45 years of age.(25)

In general, the more years you have estrogen circulating in your body, the better protected you are, although age when menstruation starts does not appear to affect osteoporosis risk.(26)

Reproductive history

Two or more pregnancies may give added protection, possibly because at this time there is increased calcium absorption in preparation for breastfeeding. Conversely, not having had children may put women at some added risk. Unfortunately, there has not been a lot of research about reproductive factors so there is no clear answer to the question of whether early pregnancy affects risk. Another unresolved question is whether the use of oral contraceptives may give protection, as has been shown by some studies.(27)

Medical Factors

Certain diseases, medications, and surgical procedures are important risk factors for osteoporosis. One study found that such factors were present in about 20% of women and 40% of men with vertebral and hip fractures.(28)

Surgical menopause

When a woman's ovaries are removed because of some disease such as endometriosis, she undergoes what is called a surgical menopause. The operation for removal of the ovaries is called oophorectomy. A chemical menopause can also happen when young women undergo chemotherapy or radiation therapy for cancer, such as breast cancer, although it is not inevitable.

Surgical menopause at a young age is a clear indicator for bone loss. When the ovaries are removed, estrogen production is virtually eliminated. In normal menopause, estrogen production dramatically slows down but is not entirely eliminated; the ovaries still contribute to the production of some estrogen even into the seventies. This fact is an argument for retaining healthy ovaries at all costs, even in postmenopausal women.

When women at midlife and older undergo a hysterectomy, often they have routinely had their ovaries removed on the argument that ovarian cancer becomes a risk as we get older. The unofficial guidelines doctors follow put the age for this at 40, 45, or 50. However, there is no strong case for removing healthy ovaries and some doctors question this practice. Dr. Wulf Utian describes the effect on the woman who has her ovaries prematurely removed as "an abrupt crash" rather than the "soft landing" where menopause occurs naturally.(29) He points out that statistics show ovarian cancer occurs only in 1 in 500 to 1 in 5,000 women, so it is not a common disease. Women facing hysterectomy would be well advised to check out what their doctor intends to do and to think carefully before agreeing to the removal of healthy ovaries.

Young women who have a surgical menopause are often advised to take hormone replacement therapy to prevent osteoporosis. Most studies of users of HRT show that women with a surgical menopause are more likely than other women to use HRT because they tend to have more problems with menopause. However, this may not be possible for all women who have had a surgical menopause—for instance, women who had estrogen-related diseases such as endometriosis, ovarian cancer, or breast cancer.

Hysterectomy

It is not at all clear whether hysterectomy by itself might add to the risk of osteoporosis for some women, especially women who are young when the hysterectomy is performed.(30) After a hysterectomy, the ovaries sometimes stop working efficiently, either temporarily or permanently.(31) This seems to occur relatively frequently, in about one-quarter to one-third of premenopausal women undergoing hysterectomy, and explains why some quite young women report hot flashes and other menopausal symptoms after a hysterectomy. Many studies have shown that women who have had hysterectomies are more likely to attend menopause clinics because of troublesome hot flashes, sweating, and vaginal dryness, suggesting that they have suffered a disruption in their normal estrogen supply.

Diseases and medications

Certain diseases increase the risk of osteoporosis. Women with rheumatoid arthritis have an increased risk of hip fracture.(32) People who have had part of their stomach or intestine removed because of disease may be at greater risk, probably because they absorb less calcium from their food. The same can happen to people with chronic diarrhea caused by ulcerative colitis, or Crohn's disease, and kidney and liver disease. Hyperthyroidism, where the thyroid is excessively overactive, and hyperparathyroidism, where the parathyroid gland is abnormally active, can cause osteoporosis, but these diseases are rare.

Chronic use of various medications may speed bone loss and therefore predispose sufferers to osteoporosis. Long-term corticoid therapy (for example, prednisone) can lead to rapid bone loss and fractures. This therapy is used by people suffering from chronic asthma, active hepatitis, inflammatory bowel disease, rheumatoid arthritis, and chronic obstructive pulmonary disease.

Asthma is a very common disease and is actually getting more common. In 1990 there were over 10 million reported cases of asthma. Since asthma deaths have also risen, most asthma sufferers are using steroid therapies, so it can be seen that this could be a significant risk factor for osteoporosis. Not all steroids users experience bone loss; when it does occur, it is often in the spine and ribs.

Depo Provera

A recent study showed that women who used the progestogen contraceptive injection Depo Provera suffered a loss of bone density which could put them at greater risk of fracture.(33) After measuring the bones of young women who had been using Depo Provera for over five years, it was found that they had 7.5% less bone in the spine and 6.5% less in the hip than women who had never used the drug. These rates of bone loss were half again or more than those of normal postmenopausal women. The researchers estimated that this would increase the lifetime risk of fracture in Depo Provera users by 50%, although the risk would differ for each individual according to other risk factors.

The loss appeared to take place relatively early in Depo Provera use, although just how early is not known yet. It did not seem to get worse with prolonged use. When the same researchers followed a small group of long-term users of Depo Provera who then stopped using it, they found that the women regained bone over a two-year period, but regained less bone in the hip than the spine.

It is not known whether the bone loss is more serious for very young users of Depo Provera, who have yet to reach peak bone mass, or for women who use Depo Provera immediately after a birth, when bone density levels are already lowered. Women who use Depo Provera up to menopause and who would have no chance to regain lost bone before estrogen production began to decline represent another group to monitor for worrisome effects.

It seems that the bone loss in Depo Provera users is caused by the drug's action in blocking the production of estrogen and causing amenorrhea. It could be similar to the effect on women of overexercising.

Upjohn, the maker of Depo Provera, was only permitted to start marketing in the United States in January of 1993, so there are not many American Depo Provera users at this time. Given the popularity of this drug in other countries, however, if the findings of the study discussed above are confirmed, it could soon have serious implications for the fracture risk of American women.

Lifestyle and Environmental Factors

Exercise

It can't be emphasized too much how important exercise is to bone health. Exercise and calcium are the twin strategies for maintaining bone strength into old age. The evidence that exercise builds strong bones and lack of it leads to weak bones has been gathered from a number of observations and studies. For instance, the bones of limbs immobilized in plaster lose bone density. Patients confined to bed or wheelchairs as well as astronauts under weightless conditions are known to lose bone fast, especially trabecular bone. In 1970, after 18 days in space, Soviet astronauts were unable to walk for nearly three weeks after landing. Now, Soviet astronauts are put on special exercise programs which have been shown to dramatically reduce the loss of bone.(34)

Studies of people playing various kinds of sports have shown that the limbs they use most have the strongest bones; for example, the bone in the racket-holding arm of tennis players is denser and stronger than that in the other arm. The difference in bone mass from one arm to the other can be as high as 35%. The amount of bone density in athletes is related to the level of stress exerted, so that weight lifters have the most dense bones, and swimmers the least.(35) Most of these studies have been carried out on highly trained young athletes. The increase in bone density of recreational athletes through exercise is less.

Further evidence for the importance of exercise comes from studies that have taken groups of sedentary postmenopausal women and introduced them to exercise programs. The best conducted of these studies have control groups of people carefully matched for age and health status who are not put on an exercise program. The difference in the two groups can then be measured.

Although there have been some conflicting results from such studies, a pattern does emerge. The groups that exercise lose bone more slowly than the controls, and in many studies have actually gained bone density. One recent study placed women in a wide range of ages into 45-minute exercise classes three times a week for four years.(36) At first, they did dancing, jogging, and brisk walking; in later years, work with light weights attached to the wrists and ankles was added. Over the study period, the control group put on weight, decreased in fitness, and lost bone mineral content from the ulna and radius of the forearm and in the upper arm. In contrast, the women in the exercise group either lost significantly less bone or actually gained bone at all sites. This applied to both premenopausal and postmenopausal women.

In another study, women aged 50–73 who had already had a wrist fracture were allocated to either an exercise or control group.(37) The exercise program was carried out for one hour twice weekly over eight months and included exercises in various positions as well as ball games. At the end of the time there was a marked difference in bone mineral content in the spine between the two groups.

It is not entirely clear how exercise encourages bone density but certain aspects are clear:

- Exercise builds muscles, and muscles put stress on the bones to which they are attached.

- Gravity and movement exert force on the skeleton; the upright position appears important in maintaining bone strength, as does mechanical load.

The type, amount, and consistency of exercise appear important, although much more research needs to be done to establish precise guidelines. Among older people, the most impressive results have come from carefully designed programs with specific strengthening exercises. It is also important that programs for older people are designed so that participants do not injure themselves in other ways! There is little point in exercising to strengthen bones only to end up off your feet with a torn leg muscle.

In general, weight-bearing exercise—brisk walking, running, stair climbing, cycling—that places stress on the long bones of the body is the most effective. The recommended amount is one hour, three to four times weekly.(38) Because it is not weight bearing, swimming has been seen as less beneficial in discouraging bone loss.

More recently, however, swimming has had a reprieve, with new research showing that it builds muscles.(39) Initial research also indicates that regular swimming does have a beneficial effect on bones, especially the bones of the spine and arms, at least in men. More research is needed.(40)

Other research has found that there is a correlation between the strength of the back muscles and bone mineral density in the vertebrae of healthy postmenopausal women.(41) More than that, the researchers at the Mayo Clinic who studied these women said that bone density and the strength of the back muscles were correlated to the amount of exercise the women were getting.(42) Women who exercised the most had the strongest backs and the healthiest spines.

A Canadian study investigated whether fitter women had less kyphosis (curvature) of the spine than unfit women.(43) All the study subjects were healthy white women between 50 and 60 years of age. The study found that fit women who had been involved in weight-bearing exercise (such as tennis, dancing, walking) about three times a week for five years did have a straighter spine than less fit women.

The researchers also noted that posture had a lot to do with straightness of the spine. Women with the most curvature had had poor posture since childhood: years of slumping forward had exaggerated the kyphosis.

To gain the most benefit from exercise, it has to be maintained over a lifetime. When we are young, exercise helps us reach peak bone density. In our thirties and forties, exercise will help us maintain peak bone density. After menopause, exercise helps us slow bone loss; in old age, exercise will preserve bones and help prevent falls. Unfortunately, the benefit to bones from exercise seems to be lost if the person stops exercising.

Because a lifelong commitment to exercising is needed, it is important to find a form of exercise we can enjoy, so that keeping to a program is not boring or a chore. Establishing a regular routine helps in sticking to an exercise program. Earmarking specific time minimizes the likelihood that other demands in our lives will take precedence over our need to exercise. Exercising with other people can make it more enjoyable. If it is a team effort, we are less likely to chicken out. Joining a club, such as a tennis club or a walking group, provides a regularity and structure that can make it easier to keep to an exercise program.

It is important not to set impossible goals for exercise. Most women are busy and find it difficult to set aside a large amount of time. Walking up stairs instead of taking an elevator, walking instead of driving to the shops, taking the dog for a walk, mowing lawns, and just generally keeping active will all help keep us healthy. If we cannot reach the targets for the optimal levels of exercise to help bone strength, we should not feel so discouraged that we don't exercise at all. Any exercise is better than no exercise, and exercise is beneficial in other ways besides building and maintaining bones.

Cardiovascular fitness can result from the same kind of exercise that is good for bones. Exercise gives confidence and makes us feel healthier and more alive. The endorphins released during exercise are an antidote to depression and induce a positive mental state. Exercise will develop muscles, which is also important in preventing fractures, for muscles support and protect bones against fractures. Fit, flexible people who maintain mobility and balance are less likely to fall or to fall badly when they do. A study of men and women over 50 in Britain showed that inactivity and muscle weakness were associated with higher rates of hip fracture, while increased daily activity, including standing, walking, climbing stairs, carrying, housework, and gardening protected against hip fracture.(44)

A New Zealand study that compared hip fracture patients with healthy age-matched people concluded that muscle strength and mobility were even more important than bone density for predicting hip fractures.(45)

Overexercising

While exercise is generally beneficial to the skeleton, there is no point in exercising too much; indeed, overexercising can be positively harmful. Too much exercise can cause bone fatigue and microscopic fractures and cannot increase peak bone mass much beyond the genetic limit.(46) For women, too much exercise can shut off the ovaries, stopping estrogen production and periods. In very young girls, it can stop the periods from even beginning. This is called athletic amenorrhea.

Bone mineral tests taken of women with athletic amenorrhea show that they have poor bone mineral content, especially in the trabecular bones of the spine. There have also been reports of thinning of cortical bone.(47) One study of a group of amenorrheic athletes showed they had bone density equivalent to that of a 52-year-old woman. So far no spinal fractures have been observed in these young women, but they do have other fractures such as stress fractures of the long bones. Although menstruation may return when these young women stop exercising to excess, the bone loss they have suffered may be partially irreversible. They may reach adulthood with very low peak bone mass and be at particular risk of osteoporosis in later life. Hormone treatment appears to be of only partial benefit and the possible benefit may decrease the longer the amenorrhea goes on.(48)

Young women most at risk are endurance runners, such as triathletes, and marathon runners, ballerinas, and gymnasts. Often they not only exercise to excess but also do not eat enough of the right foods containing calories and calcium to make up for the energy they are expending. Many actively work to stay thin. One study showed that 55% of young ballet dancers ate less than the Recommended Daily Allowance (RDA) for calcium. It was initially argued that leanness and lack of body fat were important factors in athletic amenorrhea, but this has not been borne out by research. Current thinking is that it is the strenuous exercise itself that induces the loss of periods. In experiments with female athletes, it has even been possible to induce amenorrhea through intensive athletic training.(49)

There are many similarities between anorexia nervosa and athletic amenorrhea, and researchers argue whether these young athletes are actually anorexic. The answer to that question is not clear, although a 1988 survey in *Runners World* showed that an alarmingly high percentage of the young female athletes who replied were dieting even when at peak training, were "terrified" of being overweight, and were preoccupied with being thin; 26% said they purged themselves using laxatives or diuretics.

Parents of young female athletes should make sure that they do not exercise so much that menstruation stops, and that calcium content in the diet is high—1,500 mg daily.

Although it is important to be alert to the dangers of overathleticism, it should not get in the way of encouraging young girls and adolescents to take up exercise, be it volleyball or pumping iron at the gym. Attaining peak bone mass is one of the keys to bone health in later life, and exercise encourages physical confidence and habits that will stand them in good stead for a lifetime. Tennis and other racket sports, hiking, walking, swimming, golf, running, dancing, and some martial arts, such as tai chi, are all forms of activity we can maintain into old age, even if we get slower at them.

Smoking

Several studies have shown that women who smoke have a greater risk of lower bone mass and higher rates of all three osteoporotic fractures than women who do not. Studies in Sweden have shown that at age 70, the skeleton of a woman who smokes is equivalent to that of an 80-year-old nonsmoker.(50) Smokers were also very much more likely to have suffered vertebral fractures, and even ex-smokers showed a greater risk than women who had never smoked (see the table below).

It seems likely that smoking in some way acts directly on the body, possibly affecting estrogen levels, to speed bone loss. Women who smoke tend to go through menopause earlier and have lower

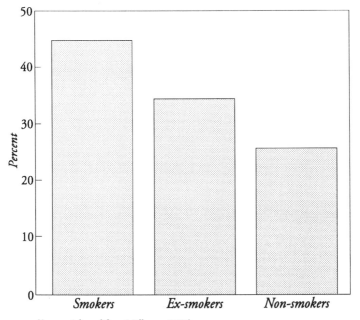

Vertebral Fractures (X-ray Proven) by Smoking Status (70–75 Years)

(Source: Adapted from Mellstrom 1989)

estrogen levels than women who do not. It is also possible that smokers have lower bone mass because of other factors common to them, such as being thinner.

Among women who take estrogen replacement therapy, those who smoke have lower concentrations of estrogen than nonsmoking women. In other words, the bad effect of smoking to some extent counteracts the good effect of estrogen on bones.(51) It may also be unwise for smokers to use hormone replacement therapy because no one is entirely sure what the combined effect of added hormones and smoking would be on the risk of stroke and cardiovascular disease.

With the dramatic increase in smoking among young women and the likelihood that at least some of these women will smoke for long periods of time, we may well see a marked increase in osteoporosis as these women grow older.

Vitamin D

Vitamin D is obtained from some foods, such as eggs from free-range hens, milk, butter, and some fish. People who reduce these foods in their diet to avoid saturated fats also reduce the amount of vitamin D they are obtaining from these sources. But vitamin D comes primarily from exposure to sunlight. In America adolescents and adults normally receive ample amounts of this vitamin from exposure to sunlight during their daily lives. Vitamin D deficiency can occur in people with liver or kidney disease or who use certain medications, but it is primarily a problem of elderly people who do not get outside much, particularly old people who live in rest homes or other aged-care institutions.

Studies have shown that up to half of elderly people in institutions have undetectable levels of vitamin D.(52) This is thought to be due to a number of factors: less of the right food, a decrease in the body's capacity to produce vitamin D, and not enough exposure to sunlight.

Supplementary vitamin D preparations are not necessary for normal adults. Calcitriol, or activated vitamin D, has been used to try to prevent further bone loss in postmenopausal women with osteoporosis, but the results have been conflicting.(53) Some studies of Calcitriol have actually shown an increased vertebral fracture rate; others have shown an increase in trabecular bone in the spine but also the worrisome possibility that the therapy might be having a deleterious effect on the hipbone.(54) Vitamin D preparations should always be used under medical supervision as too much vitamin D can cause severe side effects, including kidney stones.

Fluoride

More fractures seem to occur in areas where the water supply is nonfluorinated than where water is fluorinated to a relatively high level; but this is still being researched. As fluoride is known to stimulate the activity of the bone-building osteoblasts and increase the density of trabecular bone, experimental attempts have been made to use fluoride preparations to improve bone density in individuals with established osteoporosis. It is not suggested as a preventive for asymptomatic people. The various experiments carried out so far on people with osteoporosis have shown conflicting results. A recent French study showed a reduction in vertebral crush fractures in women who were given fluoride, but a Mayo Clinic study where women were given higher doses showed none. This might mean that fluoride is only effective in preventing fractures in people with established osteoporosis at a very specific dose. More study is taking place to determine if this is so.

Despite the lack of effect of fluoride on fracture rate in the Mayo Clinic study, bone density did increase in the spine in these women, adding to the suspicion that the quality of the trabecular bone stimulated by using fluoride could be poor. The Mayo study also showed an increase in other kinds of fractures. Fluoride is known to cause a decrease in cortical bone, so it could have a detrimental effect on the hip. Fluoride administered this way also causes a high level of side effects, and people in these studies frequently report stomach upsets and inflamed joints.(55)

Dietary Factors

Calcium

As we have seen, calcium is vital to bone health and adequate calcium throughout our lives appears necessary to enable us to reach peak bone mass and maintain the health of bones. Nevertheless, it is certainly far from clear how effective dietary calcium can be at preventing or slowing postmenopausal bone loss. Adequate calcium in young life may be the most important factor in ensuring healthy bones at midlife and in old age.

Total body calcium in women increases from about 25 gm at birth to roughly 1,000 gm at age 30. All this comes from what we eat. Calcium is excreted from the body through sweat, feces, and urine at the rate of about 150–250 mg daily. If insufficient calcium is absorbed from the diet to offset these losses, calcium will be withdrawn from the bones, which contain about 99% of the body's calcium stores.

The body cannot absorb all the calcium contained in the food we eat. Normally it absorbs only about 10–30% of the calcium in food. Therefore, the food we eat must contain sufficient calcium to meet the body's requirements.

Dieticians argue endlessly about what these levels are, which explains the considerable variations in ideal levels for calcium in the diets set by different countries. For example, the RDA in New Zealand is low compared to that in the United States and Australia.

Different levels of calcium are set for different ages. Adolescents and women who are pregnant or breastfeeding are usually considered to need more calcium than adults. As people age, they tend to excrete more calcium and are less able to absorb it, especially if their vitamin D levels are low, so that in some countries higher levels are also recommended for postmenopausal women. Research in many countries has shown that postmenopausal women frequently consume significantly less than the recommended daily amount. (See the table on page 171 for good dietary sources of calcium.)

Studies show that the usual intake of calcium for adult women (ages 25 to 74) in the United States is 450–550 mg per day. This is well below the current RDA of 800 mg per day for women and men who over 18 years old. Studies cited by the 1984 National Institutes of Health's Consensus Development Conference on Osteoporosis led the conference panel to offer the opinion that the RDA for calcium is too low, especially for postmenopausal women, and may well be too low for elderly men.

The panel recommended that premenopausal and older women receiving estrogen need about 1,000 mg of calcium per day for calcium balance, that is, to keep the amount of calcium in the bones constant. Postmenopausal women (all women past the age of meno-

Recommended Dietary Calcium for Girls and Women

	mg daily
Girls 12–15 years	1000
Women 16–53 years	1200
Postmenopausal women (54 and over)	800
During pregnancy	1300
During lactation	1400

Good sources of dietary calcium

Food	*Serving size*	*Measurement*	*Calcium (milligrams)*
Whole milk	1 glass	200 ml	240
Skim milk	1 glass	200 ml	320
Buttermilk	1 glass	200 ml	320
Soy milk	1 glass	200 ml	232
Hard cheese	3 cubes	40 g	320
Parmesan cheese	1 tablespoon		68
Cottage cheese	½ cup	130 g	80
Yogurt	1 container	150 g	180
Sardines	½ tin	50 g	230
Tofu		100 g	170
Canned salmon	½ small tin	50 g	50
Broccoli/silverbeet	½ cup cooked	80 g	70
Peanuts	1 handful	30 g	50
Fresh orange juice	1 glass	200 ml	120
Blackstrap molasses	1 tablespoon		137
Kelp		14 g	150

(Source: Adapted from information from the Arthritis Foundation of New Zealand)

pause) who are not on estrogen need about 1,500 mg of calcium per day. In addition, men who increase their calcium intake may prevent age-related bone loss as well.

For women who are pregnant or nursing and are 19 years of age or older, the panel recommends 400 mg above the normal requirement, or a total of 1,400 mg per day. For women who are pregnant or nursing and are 19 years of age or younger, the panel recommends 800 mg above the normal requirement, or a total of 2,000 mg per day.(56)

If the average American woman consumes an estimated 500 mg of calcium per day based on her current eating habits, then an additional 500 to 1,000 mg are needed; that is roughly the amount of calcium in two to four servings of other calcium-rich foods.

A word of caution about these recommended levels of dietary calcium: the reason for the differing levels set by various countries is that no one really knows how much calcium people need, especially after peak bone mass has been obtained, or what the minimum level is below which a person's bones might be compromised. So current recommendations for daily intake err on the side of generosity and should be met if possible.

There is a real danger in setting what appear to be rigid criteria for ideal dietary intake or exercise levels that then intimidate people. People should not be so daunted by the prospect of meeting the RDA that they simply give up. One mother of a teenaged daughter said she couldn't imagine how her daughter could meet the RDA for her age; it amounted, she said, to enormous amounts of milk.

The RDA is more approachable if we realize that we can meet it just by eating a varied diet. For instance, the teenaged daughter of my friend could meet the New Zealand RDA of 1,000 mg if each day she had a milkshake (480 mg), cheese in her lunchtime sandwich or salad (320 mg), a glass of orange juice (120 mg), toast for breakfast and bread for lunch (35 mg), and a leafy green vegetable for dinner (70 mg).

Dairy foods, especially milk, are by far the major source of calcium in most people's diets. Some other foods are rich in calcium, but huge amounts of many of them need to be eaten to match the amount in milk. Writing in the *Scottish Medical Journal*, one doctor noted: "A quarter pound of cheddar cheese contains about 750 mg of calcium, but the amount of other foodstuffs containing calcium equivalent to a pint of milk range through an entire 28 oz loaf to a can and a half of sardines to 4 lb of peanuts or four 8 oz cans of beans."(57)

People who cannot eat milk products must find their calcium in other food sources. Asian people, who do not use dairy products a great deal, get adequate supplies of calcium from soy milk products, including tofu.

Fat-containing foods have been on the firing line in a number of diet scares that have had widespread publicity in the popular media. The media is rather obsessed with the idea that something people are eating or using in ordinary life could be harmful, and any research suggesting such a link frequently attracts disproportionate media coverage. The problem comes when people make significant changes in their diet on the basis of such reports, oblivious to the fact that later research often contradicts or modifies the original research findings. This is not nearly so newsworthy and is less likely to attract headlines. If the substance or product in question is a cosmetic or something not necessary to our well-being, such changes in habits are harmless, but if the scare involves a crucial dietary item, the implications can be much more serious.

For instance, when people substantially cut back on fat-containing foods because of fears of cholesterol—fears exaggerated in the media—they may also be restricting their calcium intake (and, as we have seen, vitamin D). Perhaps they will avoid a heart attack, but they could get osteoporosis instead! Low-fat cheese and milk avoid a lot of cholesterol while ensuring adequate supplies of calcium.

The media have also highlighted a possible but unproven link between fat-containing foods and breast cancer in the context of a fear-inducing discussion of "epidemics" of breast cancer.(58) Some women may respond to this by restricting their fat intake, only to put themselves at added risk of osteoporosis. One hypothetical scenario emerging from this is that women then may be advised to take HRT for low bone density, thereby possibly increasing their risk of developing breast cancer as HRT itself has not been cleared of adding to that risk.

The sum of these scares over fat-containing foods is that people tend to avoid them. When it comes to excessive consumption of fatty meats, such as beef, or globs of butter and sour cream, this is probably a good thing, but unfortunately the baby has been thrown out with the bath water. The image of milk has been tarnished as part of the antifat campaign, despite counter-campaigns by the American Dairy Association ("Milk. It does a body good." "Got milk?") Still, there are reports that as part of their own wariness about fat-containing foods, some parents are not encouraging their children to drink milk.

The fetish for thinness also results in some adolescent women severely restricting their intake of dairy foods, thus seriously risking calcium deficiency and compromising their ability to reach peak bone mass. They could pay the price for this later in life with the increased risk of all the late-life fractures. Young women need to be made aware of the damage they are doing to their skeletons and encouraged to change their eating habits. Low-fat milk, cottage cheese, and tofu are low in calories and also good for bones.

Although not a lot is known about older women's attitudes toward milk, it seems that fear of fat may be turning midlife women off milk, too. When a group of British GPs set up a clinic for the prevention of osteoporosis, they found that many women were disinclined to increase their intake of dairy products because of a fear of gaining weight.(59)

Many factors affect how well we take calcium from the food we eat. Lactose helps calcium utilization, so foods that contain both, such as milk and to a lesser extent cheese and yogurt, are excellent sources of calcium. Oxalic acid and phytic acid inhibit calcium absorption from the intestine. Oxalic acid is found in some green vegetables, such as asparagus and spinach, and in rhubarb. This is a pity because both spinach and rhubarb are in themselves good sources of calcium. Phytic acid is found in the husks of grains especially oatmeal and bran and the seed coats of beans, making these something that vegetarians in particular need to watch out for.

Fiber, while good for most other health needs, can prevent calcium from being absorbed by speeding food through the intestine. It is primarily cereal fiber that has this effect rather than fiber-containing fruits and vegetables.

Excessive salt in the diet may increase calcium excretion.(60) In general Americans eat too much salt and it is recommended that the daily intake of salt not exceed one teaspoon. Vitamin D is also needed to efficiently absorb calcium.

The advice usually given by dieticians is to eat a balanced diet with sufficient calcium content to meet the recommended daily averages. It is important to eat a variety of foods and to eat fresh rather than packaged, processed, and takeout foods, which may contain substances that can be harmful in large quantities.

Calcium supplements

Because calcium is critical to bone health it has not surprisingly led to arguments that calcium supplementation might prevent bone loss in women—and men—as they grow older. Unfortunately, this has turned out to be difficult to prove, partly because of gaps in our knowledge of the role calcium plays at different ages. For instance, while calcium might be critical for adolescents, it may be less important for older people. It has been estimated that only about 20% of the variability in people's bones can be put down to calcium intake.

For many years there has been argument about the benefit of adults taking calcium supplements. A review of 43 studies relating calcium intake to bone mass, bone loss, and bone fragility showed an association in 26 studies, but none in the other 16, suggesting there was not a strong relationship. Most of the other studies that did not show a benefit were of women immediately after menopause; those showing a benefit tended to be of older women.

Recently several randomized, controlled trials have provided good evidence that calcium supplements can reduce the loss of bone everywhere in the body in postmenopausal women. Overall, the loss of bone was halved.

In one of these trials, 122 normal women at least three years beyond menopause (but on average 10 years after menopause) were given 1 gram of calcium each day for two years, while another group of matched women was not. The mean intake of calcium from their diets for the women in both groups was quite high—around 750 mg a day. (Many women have a daily calcium intake much lower than this.) When their bones were measured it was found that the loss of bone mineral density was reduced by 43% in the women taking calcium.(61)

Although this sounds impressive, the difference in bone density between the group that took supplements and the group that did not was quite small; although it might widen if there were more years of follow-up. The decrease in bone loss among the women using supplements was not as great as would be seen in women using HRT.

Other studies have shown a benefit to elderly women from calcium and vitamin D supplementation, while still others have shown that high fiber diets reduce the absorption of calcium taken as supplements.

What all the studies seem to indicate is that calcium supplements can do little if anything in the years immediately after menopause, when loss of estrogen is the major cause of bone loss, but added calcium can modify the age-related bone loss that occurs after menopause. And although these studies show a reduction in bone loss, there have been no prospective studies looking at the place of calcium supplements in preventing fractures in the spine or hip.

So is it worthwhile to take calcium supplements after menopause? That question is still hard to answer, but it seems clear that
the supplements cannot provide the sure-fire results often promised
by the manufacturers. Calcium supplements taken in midlife are not
going to do any harm, but they are not cheap either. A year's supply
at 500 mg daily (the recommended supplemental dose) would cost
around $125 annually. They certainly should not be relied upon to
prevent osteoporosis or fractures. The authors of the British study of
postmenopausal women mentioned above commented: "The calcium intake necessary for postmenopausal women may have been
overestimated, and prophylaxis with calcium supplements alone
seems to create a false sense of security. These supplements seem to
be of commercial rather than clinical benefit."(62)

Calcium supplements come in different compounds: calcium
carbonate, calcium lactate, or calcium gluconate. Supplements made
from these three ingredients vary widely in calcium content. Calcium
carbonate tablets are 40% calcium, the highest concentration available, and these are the most used form of calcium. Calcium lactate
contains 13% calcium, calcium gluconate only 9% calcium. To work
out how much calcium you are actually getting from taking supplements, you need to do some math. For instance, a 500 mg tablet
of calcium carbonate actually contains 40% of 500, or 200 mg of
elemental calcium. Some packaging will tell you the amount of elemental calcium contained in the product.

The body apparently absorbs calcium best when it is taken in
chewable or dissolved form rather than swallowed in a tablet. "Che-
lated" calcium has been touted as being more absorbable, but it seems
unlikely that it is any better than other forms, only more expensive.
Too much calcium is not a good idea, as it can cause kidney stones.
Calcium is best taken at night, when the body has no dietary source
of calcium and begins to use up its stores. Calcium absorption can
also be enhanced by taking it with milk, yogurt, or a meal.

Caffeine and phosphorus

Even moderate caffeine intake appears to increase the risk of hip
fracture.(63) Researchers in the Framingham study examined this
association and found that although there was no increased risk for
one or two cups of coffee or four cups of tea, there was for two-and-
a-half cups of coffee or the equivalent amount of tea. This association

has not been the subject of very much research, so this finding needs to be confirmed by further study. The researchers were not clear whether it was the coffee itself or something associated with coffee drinking that increased the risk. Some researchers have suggested that smokers are great coffee drinkers and it is the smoking not the coffee drinking that causes the damage.(64)

It is frequently claimed that soft drinks containing phosphorus accelerate bone resorption by increasing PTH levels, but there is as yet no clear proof of this.

Body size

Many women struggle to stay thin, or would like to be that way, but as far as bones are concerned there is no value in being slim. Of course obesity is unhealthy, but being rounded, plump, or simply large will not do you any harm. A study in Auckland, New Zealand, looked at a host of factors that might explain the strength of midlife women's bones and found that the single biggest predictor of bone strength was body mass or fat. In other words, women who were carrying a bit of weight had stronger bones than thin women.(65)

Anorexia nervosa

Anorexia nervosa in young women is a definite risk factor for osteoporosis, and bone measurements have shown that bone density can be very low in young women with this eating disorder. There have been many reports of multiple crush fractures in the vertebrae of anorexic women in their twenties, whereas these would not usually appear in normal women until they are in their sixties. Anorectics can also lose cortical bone. Lack of activity is another factor, as physically active anorectics have been shown to have greater bone mass than inactive anorectics.(66)

There appear to be multiple causes of decreased bone mass in anorexic women. Inadequate dietary calcium, as low as 400 mg per day, is quite usual in these women, while many have premature estrogen deficiency. It is quite common for anorectics to stop menstruating because the ovaries have stopped producing estrogen, and they are unlikely to reach peak bone mass. It is not clear whether these young women can regain the bone they have lost if they begin eating normally and menstruation starts again.

Chronic dieting

Various studies have been made of women's dieting habits, revealing that a large number of women are intermittently or permanently dieting for much of their lives. A 1990 Gallup Organization survey indicates that some 52% of Americans consider themselves over-weight, compared to only 31% in 1951. Among women, 62% are concerned about their weight, while among men, only 42% believe they need to lose weight. Interestingly, the U.S. National Center for Health statistics shows that actually only 27.5% of all Americans are 20% or more above their desirable weight, with 29.6% of all men overweight, but only 25.6% of all women.(67)

Not a lot is known about the effect of chronic dieting on bones. First in the firing line when we diet are often the very foods that help bones, especially milk. In any event, it is very difficult to consume sufficient calcium on diets of 1200 calories a day.(68)

Alcohol

Although it is not yet certain, excessive alcohol consumption may cause bone loss. Heavy drinkers certainly have more hip fractures. It is suspected that alcohol directly damages bone cells, but alcohol could also lead to fractures in other ways. Alcohol can damage the liver, which could impair its ability to metabolize vitamin D, and people who drink a lot are more likely to eat badly, smoke, exercise less, and generally have poorer health. Drinkers are also more in-clined to fall and this puts them at risk of fracturing a bone.(69)

Protein

A high protein intake increases the amount of calcium excreted in the urine, but the role of protein in contributing to bone loss is thought to be a small one.(70) Although dairy products are high in protein, they are also high in calcium and phosphorus, which more than offsets the effect of the protein.(71)

New Research into Osteoporosis Prevention

Researchers of osteoporosis are continually looking for new ways of preventing osteoporosis, and a number of drugs are being tried ex-perimentally. The use of Calcitriol and fluoride as preventive meas-ures against further bone loss in established osteoporosis have already been outlined. Hormone replacement therapy is discussed in a following chapter.

Calcitonin

We saw earlier that the bone hormone calcitonin protects bones from the dissolving actions of parathyroid hormone and activated vitamin D. It is thought to act directly on the osteoblasts, the cells that break down bone.

Calcitonin extracted from salmon and then synthesized has been successfully used to increase bone mass in people with established osteoporosis, although its effect on fracture rates is not known. Unfortunately, it is extremely expensive, and it has another disadvantage in that it cannot be taken orally. In the earliest studies, people had to be injected daily or every other day. More recently, experiments have been carried out using nasal sprays. Calcitonin administered in this way has also been shown to be effective in counteracting trabecular bone loss during early menopause. Its effect on cortical bone is not yet known.(72)

Calcitonin may turn out to be a useful preventive treatment, but its prohibitive cost will preclude widespread use until an alternative source can be found.

Thiazides

Thiazide diuretics used for the treatment of high blood pressure are known to slow the rate of bone loss in normal postmenopausal women. Women on long-term thiazide have fewer hip fractures. They are inexpensive and relatively free of side effects.

Bisphosphonates

Bisphosphonates are phosphate salts that work by binding to the surface of bone, strengthening it, and preventing reabsorption of bone and loss of bone density. These salts may be available for use by 1996. Studies have shown that bone loss and the incidence of vertebral deformity can be reduced in women with established postmenopausal osteoporosis by treating them with bisphosphonates such as etidronate. One trial showed that women who had already had one fracture gained bone density using bisphosphonates.

Conclusion

It is very difficult to predict fracture risk in individuals by applying risk factor criteria. Bone density measurements can predict vertebral fracture risk reasonably accurately but are less useful for predicting fractures of the hip because additional factors contribute to hip fracture risk. For this reason, this technology is not sufficiently effective as a tool for screening people at a population level to justify its widespread availability.

The woman "at risk" for osteoporosis appears to be small, inactive, thin, and European. Young women who have premature loss of estrogen because of oophorectomy, anorexia, or overexercising are at special risk, as are women using particular medications.

For women of Polynesian heritage, osteoporosis is not a significant health problem. For midlife European women, carrying some weight and keeping fit are probably the two most useful strategies they can adopt to prevent fractures. The benefits of exercise are multiple. Not only does exercise slow bone loss, it also strengthens the back, improves posture, maintains physical competence, and enhances self-confidence. Moderate midlife weight gain not only benefits bone structure but also may protect the person who falls.

It is not yet firmly proven that increases in dietary calcium beyond normal levels can bring similar clear benefits to the skeleton. The most important period for ensuring adequate calcium in the diet may be at a younger age, when peak bone mass is being attained. Young women, in particular, should be encouraged to keep their calcium intake at the recommended levels. Postmenopausal women should also maintain adequate dietary calcium, but, unless the diet is deficient, there is not a strong case for calcium supplementation.

Part Four

Hormone Replacement Therapy

Chapter 8

All Roads Lead to Hormones

One of the things that strikes a person researching the history of estrogen is that doctors fell in love with it. One writer accurately dubbed the relationship as "medicine's love affair."(1) Like lovers in the first flush of romance, doctors were blind to the possibility that estrogen might have faults.

When Dr. Robert Wilson pitched his bid for "estrogens forever," virtually nothing was known of its dangers. Even the claims made for its efficacy were based almost entirely on clinicians' casual observations in their own practices. The few clinical trials involved tiny study populations and were poorly designed, while some seemed to show that estrogen was no more effective than placebos at relieving menopausal symptoms.(2)

Whether estrogen worked was the burning question, not whether it was safe. Having decided that it did work, even on inadequate data, the question of safety was abandoned to the future. It was simply put to one side. After all, if hormones were "natural," how could they do any harm? Pharmacology was simply remedying nature's mistake. Civilization had succeeded in keeping women alive beyond their reproductive life spans, so civilization must deal with the consequences. It was all entirely logical once you had suspended disbelief.

Doctors threw caution to the wind and devoted themselves to saving middle-aged women from the depredations caused by estrogen deficiency. Those who favored estrogen, and it must be said that not all did, entered what one doctor in the 1970s called "this glorious new phase of medical practice."(3)

It would take a psychologist to interpret this unbridled medical passion for estrogen. Remember that the women being prescribed this potent steroidal drug were rarely "sick." Their lives may have been uncomfortable, but they were not in mortal danger and the "illness," if there was one, was self-limiting. No woman stays menopausal for ever.

Initially estrogen was only recommended for women with evident menopausal symptoms, and for a short time span. But time made doctors a little blasé and they were under pressure from the drug companies to extend both the indications for using estrogen and the time frame. So the asymptomatic woman also became a target for estrogen. For wasn't she "diseased" by virtue of being menopausal even if she was not complaining? Estrogen could "cure" her. By the same argument, why take women off the hormone when it was doing so much good?

The Genesis of a Technocracy

The enthusiasm seems to be partially related to changes in the historic role of medicine. In the postwar period, medicine had entered what seemed a Golden Age of technological transformation. Before the Second World War, medicine had been a relatively unsophisticated pursuit. Not long out of the era of leeches and bleeding, medicine in the twenties and thirties was more like a cottage industry. At its center was the family doctor, practicing an essentially hands-on art. Disorders were likely to be solved by a sympathetic talk and home nursing, while the pills and potions at the doctor's disposal were often made to his own recipe. Prewar drug companies were small-time concerns, making patent medicines that people could buy over the counter in pharmacies.

The pharmaceutical revolution changed all this. Immediately before the Second World War, sulfanilamide was discovered as an antibacterial agent; within five years, 1,000 sulfa drugs were synthesized. Next, the large-scale production of penicillin became possible, and in 1944 streptomycin was discovered. These breakthroughs led to an explosion of new antibiotic products, and the pharmaceutical industry expanded exponentially.

The development of hormone replacement therapy parallels the growth of the drug companies. The estrogen story goes back to the 1920s when Edgar Allen and Edward Doisey isolated and crystallized a form of estrogen from the urine of pregnant women. Allen and

Doisey named it *theelin,* later called estrone. This was given to meno-pausal women but had only restricted use because of the difficulty of obtaining supplies. But despite these limits, the Allen-Doisey dis-covery provoked a race between scientists in America and in Europe to discover an alternative, cheap source of estrone.

In America, a synthetic form of estrogen was developed called diethylstilbestrol (DES), which was widely used on women, espe-cially during pregnancy. But the final step in the estrogen saga did not occur until 1943 when an estrogen product was developed from the urine of pregnant mares. Called conjugated equine estrogen, it was manufactured by Ayerst Laboratories under the brand name Pre-marin (derived from PREgnant MAResʼ urINe). It was cheap and simple to administer and had fewer unpleasant side effects than the previous estrogens.

Across the Atlantic, the German pharmaceutical company Scher-ing had also been in search of a cheap estrogen. Scheringʼs first es-trogen product was an injectable form of estrogen called Progynon, introduced in 1928 and developed from human placentas. Later Schering collaborated with German university biochemists to search for a commercially viable source of estrone, although it was the Americans who were to make that breakthrough. But Schering suc-ceeded in synthesizing other forms of estrogen: the potent estradiol in 1933 (marketed as Progynova), and in 1938 the synthetic oral estrogen ethinylestradiol, mainly used in oral contraceptives.

In the postwar years, America, Germany, and Switzerland emerged as the giants of the drug world. As part of the rebuilding of West Germanyʼs economy, the pharmaceutical industry capitalized on its existing chemical, pharmacological, and technical knowledge base. By 1965 there were more than 2,000 manufacturers of phar-maceutical products in West Germany with over 60,000 registered drug products, while by the early 1970s there were only 800 compa-nies in America.(4) The growth of the Upjohn Corporation was typi-cal of the American boom. Begun by a physician to manufacture concoctions for his own patients, Upjohn expanded from a small company with 12 scientists in 1938 to a team of 400 scientists in 1970.

The major modern drug companies did not all emerge from a pharmaceutical background. They had varied and sometimes curious backgrounds; drug discoveries could sometimes result from other work. For instance, Merck, CIBA-Geigy, and Pfizer are the outgrowths of chemical firms that had been making dyestuffs, fertilizers, explosives, and similar products.(5) Merck's synthesis of cortisone was part of a wartime program sponsored by the U.S. Office of Scientific Research and Development.(6)

Whatever their origins, modern pharmaceutical companies have been spectacularly successful. One of the leaders, Hoffmann-La Roche, had sales of $1.2 billion in 1970. A major portion of its profit came from sales of Librium and Valium. Roche's cash position was so lush, banks and other industries came to borrow from it. Worldwide sales of the American drug industry leapt from $1,430 million in 1950 to $8,070 million in 1972; annual profits from $129 million to $734 million in the same period.(7)

The drug boom opened new doors for doctors. They now had oral contraceptives and intrauterine devices to offer their patients instead of primitive rubber condoms and diaphragms; there were mind-altering drugs and hypnotics to prescribe to depressed and insomniac patients instead of the traditional brandy in milk at bedtime. In the postwar years, "science" was accorded special status. The laboratory was the powerhouse driving society into a new age of rational progress. All the problems of society were explicable by the scientific method and could be solved by the timely application of science's brainchild—technology.

By harnessing the power and prestige of science, medicine moved into a new "modern" era, rendering the "healing hands" approach obsolete. Medicine could develop as a technocracy in which the experts were armed with chemistry and machinery. The new paradigm of medical excellence was the hospital doctor, guarding godlike his battery of equipment or engaging in arcane practices in the hospital laboratory. More than one writer has described modern medicine as taking over the customary function of the church, with the hospital, aseptic and glistening with stainless steel, as "the modern cathedral," the symbol of the new religion.(8) The general practitioner had insufficient status to aspire to be a priest at medicine's altar, but as an acolyte he did have access to drugs—the communion wafers and holy water of the new religion—to offer as salvation to his suppliant parishioners.

The modernization of medicine was mediated by the pharmaceutical companies; they provided the tools that made this transformation possible. "The phenomenal success of modern medical treatment seems to have depended almost wholly on non-clinical, often non-medical scientists, frequently working in, or in close collaboration with, the pharmaceutical industry," said Lord Platt in 1967.(9) Medicine was grateful.

The two industries—pharmaceutical and medical—forged a symbiotic relationship that has remained unchallenged by any of the pharmaceutical disasters that have followed. When babies were deformed by thalidomide, when teenaged girls developed cancer because their pregnant mothers had been given DES, when young women on oral contraceptives died from strokes, or thousands of menopausal women developed endometrial cancer from estrogen, medicine did not blame the drug companies or themselves. These were simply points on the learning curve, steps by which science could progress to a new, more refined level. Women sterilized by IUDs could leave a legacy of a different kind to society; their experience led to the development of second-and third-generation models of IUD, ones that were "anatomically engineered."(10) Medicine could even congratulate itself for being clever enough to spot the mistake and mature enough to take heed of it. Never mind feeling guilty about the people on whose bodies the mistake had eventually been discovered. Lucky folk, they had provided the "clinical experience" that enabled medicine to move on.(11)

Hormone Hype

In this mood, doctors were ripe for Dr. Robert Wilson's menopausal miracle and the promise that they could transform a sow's ear into a silk purse. In the 1940s and 1950s many doctors had been cautious about estrogen, as there had been reports of the hormone causing cancer in laboratory animals since the 1930s. But Wilson boasted of the thousands he had safely treated and his message was endorsed by highly respected doctors like Robert Greenblatt. More than that, women who had been primed by Wilson's book and the glowing reports in women's magazines came asking for it.

The women were oblivious to the fact that the articles they were reading were often planted by the makers of hormones and that they were being manipulated—exactly how we shall see later. But these campaigns were successful in generating consumer pressure. The result was that in the 10-year period between 1963 (the year Wilson published his first major medical paper on estrogen) and 1973, dollar sales of estrogen quadrupled in America. By 1975, with prescriptions at an all-time high of 26.7 million, estrogen was one of the top five prescription drugs in the United States, with an annual market value of $70 million.(12) By this date, six million American women were regularly using estrogen.(13) Similar trends in sales figures, though not as dramatic, were noted in other countries. In Sweden, for example, sales of estrogen rose from 3.65 defined daily doses per 1,000 women in 1973 to a figure three times greater in 1977.(14)

In the United States there was negligible government control of the marketing of these products. The drug companies had grown in the short space of a decade from small-time manufacturers of cough syrups into burgeoning multinational corporations. It took the federal authorities some time to catch up. Drug control legislation had been passed in 1938 after the deaths of 93 people who had used sulfanilamide prepared with a toxic solvent. The new act specified that drug manufacturers had to provide evidence of safety (though not of effectiveness) to the Food and Drug Administration (FDA), but in reality only minimal standards were applied.

Numerous new drug products were introduced into the market with inadequate testing. In 1960 the first oral contraceptive, Enovid, was allowed into the U.S. market on the basis of clinical studies involving a mere 132 Puerto Rican women who had taken it continuously for a year or longer.(15) Three young women who had died while the study was in progress had not been autopsied to establish why they died. Despite the lack of evidence for safety, within a short time "the greatest mass pill experiment in history" was underway.(16) DES was also introduced during this period and so widely used from the 1940s to the early 1960s that it has been estimated three million children were exposed in utero.(17)

It was the thalidomide tragedy that forced the passage of legislation to tighten FDA drug controls, despite the determined opposition of the drug companies.(18) The cautiousness of a single vigilant FDA official had prevented thalidomide from being approved for use in America. While evidence was being sought for the drug's safety, reports about thalidomide's neurological and teratogenic effects began to filter through from Europe. Thalidomide was never approved by the FDA, but the narrowly averted disaster prompted the U.S. Senate to finally approve significantly strengthened drug legislation. The new act, signed by President Kennedy in October 1962, required evidence of safety, and all new drugs had to be tested on animals before they were used on humans. Henceforth drug advertisements had to display information about contraindications, effectiveness, and side effects.

But estrogen had slipped through the net before these more stringent requirements were put in place. By the 1940s estrogen was being regularly advertised in medical journals with no restrictions on the claims made for it.

Ayerst, Squibb, Abbott Laboratories, Schering, Upjohn, Roche, and Lederle were just some of the drug companies who marketed estrogens for menopause. Early on, Ayerst's Premarin was established as a market leader; in America and many other countries it has remained the most used estrogen. This represented big money for Ayerst's parent company, American Home Products. In the mid-1970s it was estimated that Premarin had 75–80% of estrogen sales in the United States. Premarin was cheap to produce and the profit margin was 80% before tax.(19) In 1972 American Home Products' total sales were $1,587 million; it was estimated that Premarin accounted for about 10% of this.(20)

Premarin was also available in various mixtures with other drugs, such as male hormones (testosterone), vitamins, and tranquilizers. Ayerst's Mediatric comprised a formidable cocktail. In liquid form, it contained not only estrogen but also testosterone, a variety of vitamins, methamphetamine hydrochloride (otherwise known as speed), and 15% alcohol!(21)

Menopause according to Ayerst

The advertisements for these products, carried in abundance in medical publications, mirrored the stereotype of the menopausal woman developed by Robert Wilson. Wilson's work is even quoted as a source in some of Ayerst's advertisements. The major themes in these advertisements were women's anxieties about aging and the emotional instability of the menopausal woman. The physical symptoms of menopause, such as hot flashes, were not highlighted; indeed, some advertisements stated that they were not as important as women's inability to cope with life. As the same medical journals were punctuated with advertisements for psychotropic drugs for menopausal women carrying the same images, there was an overwhelming message that at this time of life women were dangerously on the edge, in imminent danger of losing emotional self-control. Menopause was depicted as a crisis of self-esteem, at which time women feared the redundancy of their reproductive and sexual selves.

One advertisement for Menrium, an estrogen/Librium mix ("because menopause is a state of mind too"), claimed that menopause "arouses anxieties about getting old, unattractive . . . being useless and unwanted."(22) Another Menrium advertisement repeated this theme that the menopausal woman "suddenly sees the specter of old age."(23) A Premarin advertisement from 1976 borrowed its image of the menopausal woman from that described by Freudian Therese Benedek a quarter of a century earlier. The advertisement carried the banner "Adolescence . . . all over again" above the photograph of a typically anxious woman: "Emotional displays, anxiety, tears, depression, sexual problems, instability and loss of concentration: at the menopause, many women find these long forgotten echoes of their adolescent selves. At both times, these problems are created by the dramatic change in estrogen production. Yet unlike the adolescent who anticipates a rewarding womanhood, the menopausal woman sees only the inevitability of old age waiting her."(24)

The idea is conveyed that the menopausal woman is a burden to other family members. One advertisement showed a drab woman beside her long-suffering husband under the slogan "for the menopausal symptoms that bother *him* most." Abbott Laboratories' advertisement for Ogen depicted a woman dressed for travel clutching her airline ticket but unable to get up from her chair. Her impatient husband is looking at his watch. "Bon voyage?" read the copy. "Suddenly she'd rather not go! She's waited thirty years for this trip. Now she just doesn't have the 'bounce.' She has headaches, hot flashes, and she feels tired and nervous all the time. And for no reason at all she cries."(25)

According to one doctor, "the lush advertisements for estrogens convey the message that estrogens are a cure-all for the anxious, wrinkled, sexually frustrated older woman who has to compete in this era of cocktail parties, sexual freedom and errant husbands."(26)

The readiness with which doctors absorbed these messages and translated them into prescriptions was shown by a study in Seattle in 1974.(27) In this study, 51% of women over 50 had used estrogen for over three months' duration, with the median use being 10 years. The researchers found that estrogen users were more educated and affluent than nonusers. This class difference in the use of HRT has been a persistent theme in the history of this hormone. Middle-class women were and are the prime targets for estrogen use, presumably because they can afford the constant visits to the doctor required of hormone users. As well, middle-class women may be more inclined to regard physical attractiveness as a marketable asset and may be more anxious to attempt to preserve it.

The researchers in the Seattle study found that estrogen users were only slightly more likely to have had troublesome hot flashes than nonusers. They commented that the level of usage was way above the known frequency of severe menopausal symptoms, suggesting that both prescribers and women users had succumbed to other promises being made for estrogen. In this study, the most used product was Premarin, used by one in three women, while another one in five were taking a Premarin combination product.

The scramble for hormones

It is worth speculating about how such astonishing levels of drug use were achieved so swiftly in well women who, on the face of it, appear to have been almost reckless about the possible risks to their health. The first thing to be said in explanation is that the propaganda went all one way. Although a dwindling number of doctors refused to prescribe hormones, their doubts were only privately expressed to individual patients. At a public level, doctors' criticisms were confined to the pages of medical journals. This created a public information vacuum into which the pro-hormone faction happily stepped. Bluntly stated, estrogen was sold to women.

Sometimes the pharmaceutical companies had a direct hand in the propaganda. Dr. Wilson was not the only person whose efforts were supported by them. In 1973 Sondra Gorney and Claire Cox published *After Forty*, another book extolling the virtues of estrogen. On the dust cover of the book, Gorney was identified as the Executive Director of the Information Center on the Mature Woman in New York. The book did not reveal, however, that the center was a "service for media" provided by Ayerst Laboratories, manufacturers of Premarin. Ayerst hired Sondra Gorney to provide free filler items praising HRT to magazines, newspapers, and other mass media. These were widely used, usually without any indication that the supplier of the material was Ayerst.(28)

As we have seen in a previous chapter, Dr. Wilson's *Feminine Forever* was widely read by women, and he and his family courted the mainstream media. His message traveled fast. He was written up in *Time* magazine as "the youth doctor," and his book was translated into foreign languages. Even in faraway New Zealand, *Feminine Forever* was speedily marketed, the book was soon available in public libraries, and its title soon became a generic term for the promise of estrogen.

Wilson was seen by many of the medical fraternity as unacceptably entrepreneurial, especially in promoting drugs directly to women, something pharmaceutical companies are forbidden to do by health authorities in most countries. Wilson's behavior cut across the traditional relationships between drug companies and doctors, and doctors and patients. He behaved like a salesman or middleman for hormones, pitching his message at other doctors' patients.

Wilson has not been alone in this. One of the astonishing aspects of the hormone story has been the willingness of serious research scientists to behave like missionaries for estrogen, making what are often extravagant claims in the lay media. Almost every book for women about HRT is endorsed or cowritten by an eminent medical person, regardless of the extravagance of the language used in the writing.

Dr. Lila E. Nachtigall, Associate Professor of Obstetrics and Gynecology at New York University Medical Center ("one of the most prestigious and respected medical centers in the world," says Dr. Nachtigall) and a published researcher on osteoporosis, joined forces with health writer Joan Heilman to write the extravagantly entitled *Estrogen: The Facts Can Change Your Life (The latest word on what the new safe estrogen replacement therapy can do for great sex, strong bones, good looks, longer life, preventing hot flashes)*.(29)

Coauthors of one of the most evangelistic of the HRT manuals, *The Amarant Book of Hormone Replacement Therapy (HRT is the greatest treasure of a middle-aged woman's life. I've reached fifty but feel twenty . . .*), are British MP Teresa Gorman and Dr. Malcolm Whitehead, Senior Lecturer in Obstetrics and Gynecology at King's College School of Medicine and an internationally recognized researcher in the menopause area.(30) The Amarant Trust was named after the amarant, a mythical never-fading flower, "a symbol of immortality and enduring beauty." "There is a distinctly different quality about someone who has received this therapy and someone who has grown old naturally," the book enthuses. It is hard to imagine how Dr. Whitehead could have put his name to some of the extreme statements in this book, especially when they contradict what he has said in the academic literature. For instance, the Amarant book maintains that the endometrial cancers caused by estrogen are "less invasive, and therefore are less dangerous, than those which develop naturally . . . ," a proposition often repeated in defense of estrogen. However, in *A Modern Approach to the Perimenopausal Years,*(21) Dr. Whitehead says claims like this result from a misinterpretation of the relationship of estrogen to cancer.(31) Because HRT users go to doctors more often, their cancers were more likely to be picked up early. When the grade of cancer was taken into account, there was no difference in the prognosis for users or nonusers.

In Britain, Wendy Cooper's book on HRT, *No Change: A Biological Revolution for Women,* published in 1975, carried a foreword by Sir John Peel, KCVO, FRCP, FRCS, and the Queen's former gynecologist.(32) In introducing her contribution to the campaign, Cooper paid homage to Robert Wilson, whom she had visited in person. She went on to acknowledge her debt to the advocates of estrogen who had gone before her in terms that vividly illustrate the zeal of the hormone lobby: "The words of great men carry great weight and are powerful weapons in war. This book will be quoting from many such authorities. But in the battle of Biological Lib, women themselves also have a part to play."

The history of estrogen is distinguished by such proselytizing of women on behalf of estrogen. If women doubted the messages from their doctors, they also had to withstand the pro-hormone messages of women journalists and other female public figures, which were often all the more powerful because these women gave personal testimony about how HRT had changed their lives.

In Britain the upsurge in use of HRT is largely attributed to the efforts of Wendy Cooper. Estrogen was slower to take off in Britain, but Cooper is credited with creating an upsurge of interest among women. Some 500,000 prescriptions were written in 1972; by 1976 this had more than doubled, to a peak of nearly 1,300,000 annually.(33)

In *No Change,* Cooper describes how the campaign got under way:

Just once or twice in the life of a working journalist, there comes a story so exciting, important and demanding that it refuses to be written out or written off. You may present it in a dozen different ways for a dozen different papers and magazines. In the process *you* may become exhausted, but the subject does not. Instead of public interest and response declining, they increase. The law of diminishing returns fails to operate. In the end you have to recognize that instead of *you* running the story, the story is running you.

It has been that way with me with the story of Hormone Replacement Therapy (HRT) to eliminate menopause . . . in 1971 I began intensive research both here and in America. I published the first of a series of articles entitled "A Change for the Better" in April 1973 in the *London Evening News*. Since then there has been continuous demand for major features on the same subject, for radio and television programs and for talks; not just to women either, but sometimes, and surprisingly, to doctors.

By the time she wrote her book in 1975, Cooper reported she had received letters from 5,000 women about menopause and HRT. She herself went on HRT not because of menopausal symptoms— she had gone through menopause—but "as an insurance against future trouble." She had, she wrote "thrived on the treatment personally," although she isn't at all explicit about how. Cooper's work was enormously influential. In 1988 a study of over 3,000 British women using HRT showed that a quarter of the women had read *No Change*.(34) Further evidence on the impact of the mass media was shown by the fact that 48% of HRT users, especially in the higher socioeconomic groups, identified the media, family, or friends as their first source of information about HRT. Researcher Kate Hunt said that women's expectations and perceptions of HRT were colored by the information they received through the mass media. Added to that, the study showed "evidence of considerable patient demand": 21% of the women had initiated the prescription of HRT from their doctor.

The appeal through the media worked on women's fears about aging. Women were promised the preservation of their youthful appearance, a powerful inducement in a culture that worships feminine sexual attractiveness. The critique of the postmenopausal woman offered by these doctors and repeated in the media—the anxious, wrinkled, depressive—hit a nerve in women's psyches. For many women, their "looks" were their greatest asset. Although it is not possible from Hunt's study to know exactly why all the women began using HRT, only 18% gave vasomotor symptoms as their first reason for starting on hormones, and 3.7% gave sexual or vaginal problems.

The other reason for women's wholesale willingness to try estrogen was that they were oblivious to possible dangers. The concept of informed consent was not well developed at that time. Many may not even have been clear about what they were taking. In the Seattle study, a quarter of women who at first said they had not used HRT were found subsequently to have actually done so. This was established from interviews with the women's doctors and by showing the women actual pill packets.

Women were unlikely to be told of the absence of adequate trials or of any controversy about using the drugs. They had been delivered a sales pitch and like any sales pitch the product was depicted in an entirely favorable light. In *No Change* Wendy Cooper calls HRT "beautifully and ingeniously simple." Her book contains testimony from 37 doctors, only 2 of whom mention any possibility of cancer.(35) In the first edition of the book, Cooper is at pains to reassure readers about the improbability of any cancer risk. By this time it was known that the estrogen DES had caused vaginal cancers in the daughters of users. Cooper was anxious that "the sinister shadow hanging over stilbestrol" not be projected "onto other innocent estrogens."

Embarrassingly for Cooper, within months of the publication of her book came reports that menopausal estrogen was not so innocent; studies had shown that users of estrogen had high rates of endometrial cancer. In the second edition of *No Change,* a discussion of this development is relegated to an appendix at the back of the book, and Cooper criticizes the study design. Besides, she says, only 5% of the women who developed cancer had "serious" cancer.

The Hormone Bubble Bursts

Warnings about the dangers of estrogen had been made sporadically for nearly 30 years. In particular, it was known that estrone, the form of estrogen in Premarin, could be associated with the development of endometrial cancer. As early as 1947 Dr. Saul Gusberg, a young cancer researcher at Columbia University, reported that at the hospital where he worked there was a steady stream of estrogen users requiring diagnostic curettage for abnormal uterine bleeding. The pathology reports from those curettes showed overstimulation of the endometrium. Gusberg had collected 29 cases of endometrial hyperplasia (overgrowth) and 9 of cancer itself. He called the ready use of estrogen "promiscuous" and warned that what was going on was a human experiment.(36)

Gusberg's warning caused some slowing down of postmenopausal estrogen use, until interest was restimulated by Robert Wilson. But even Wilson recommended the use of progestogen with estrogen therapy to induce a menstrual bleed and prevent the development of endometrial hyperplasia. In England, a combined estrogen/progestogen regime was the most favored therapy from the beginning, saving many British women from the disastrous consequences of the American experience.

But for every doctor who counseled caution in the use of unopposed hormones, there had been others ready to explain any dangers away. One American doctor said in 1974:

> The concept that endometrial cancer may be caused by unremitting stimulation of the endometrium by estrogen is certainly not new. At one time this supposition was so strong that some gynecologists advised women who were continuing to menstruate after age 50 to either undergo a hysterectomy or permit induction of menopause by radiation. Today, women over 50 who are menstruating are congratulated for still being young. When we consider that most women are under the influence of their own estrogens for about 40 years, it seems illogical to suppose that a few more years of ovarian function would be harmful or, for that matter, that a few years of estrogen therapy could be harmful.(37)

The two papers that shattered the hormone dreamworld were published in the 4 December 1975 issue of the *New England Journal of Medicine.* Harry Ziel and William Finkle had compared endometrial cancer cases with controls to measure differences in the prior use of estrogen. They had been prompted to do so by an increase in endometrial cancers registered in a health insurance scheme at the Kaiser Permanente Medical Center in California. They found that 57% of the women with cancer had used estrogens, whereas only 15% of the controls had done so. The risk of endometrial cancer, they concluded, was increased 7.6 times in women using estrogen.(38)

The study also showed that long-term users were at greater risk. While in the early days of estrogen use, doctors had tended to prescribe it for short periods only, eventually they had succumbed to slogans encouraging indefinite use, such as Ayerst's "Keep her on Premarin." "'Estrogens forever,'" said one doctor a year before the crash, "enjoys the status of a cult."(39)

Ziel and Finkle's study showed that worshippers at the altar of eternal youth had paid a heavy price. They found that women who had used conjugated estrogens for seven years or longer were 14 times more likely than nonusers to develop endometrial cancer. The researchers observed cuttingly: "The endocrinologist who gives estrogen as treatment for the menopause is hoping to prevent senescence. His patient is readily deluded by her wish to preserve her figure and by her physician's implication that estrogen promises eternal youth. In a rational approach to therapy, risk is weighed against benefit."(40) Rationality had long since fled the hormone scene.

The second study, by researchers at the University of Washington, similarly matched endometrial cancer patients with controls, this time other cancer patients, and came up with similar results.(41) They found that the risk in estrogen users was 4.5 times that of controls. Commenting on these research findings, the *British Medical Journal* pointed out that this kind of increase would result in between 4 and 8 women per 1,000 postmenopausal women with a uterus developing endometrial cancer against the normal incidence of 1 in every 1,000.(42)

The *New England Journal of Medicine* research findings were given further confirmation in the same month when figures released from the California Cancer Registry showed that among white women over 50 living in California, there had been more than an 80% increase in endometrial cancer between 1969 and 1974.(43)

There were doctors and others who tried to explain away this unpleasant news. Some maintained, as Wendy Cooper had, that as the cancers were picked up at an early stage when there was a good prognosis, it was not as serious as it appeared on the surface. This argument glossed over the effects on the women concerned of major surgery and sometimes radiation and the psychological impact of living with cancer. And as discussed earlier, some estrogen advocates also claimed (and still do) that the cancer in estrogen users seemed to be a milder form, and that therefore women had a better prognosis.

Dr. Robert Wilson responded to the news about endometrial cancer by saying that it was "the worst lie in the world, the worst fallacy."(44) He claimed that of 40 doctors working for him all over the world, none had seen a case of cancer.

Dr. John Studd maintained that the results were the product of overdiagnosis of malignancy. "I am convinced," he said, "much of the so-called cancer in the American studies was misdiagnosed. Pseudomalignant hyperplasia can so easily masquerade as cancer."(45)

While it was conceded that the design of the studies was not perfect, the increase in cancer risk—at 500 to 800%—was "too high to be explained away by even major methodological flaws."(46)

In the following year, yet more studies showed that endometrial cancer rates had risen sharply in America, parallel with the expansion in use of estrogen. In the same year, came the first report of a higher breast cancer risk in users of estrogen, an even more alarming prospect than the endometrial cancer risk because of the higher incidence of breast cancer among women and the poor prognosis for even early stage disease.(47) The third possibility raised by researchers during the same period was the possibility of an association of estrogen with coronary heart disease, whether beneficial or harmful. Added to this, in 1974, a report from the Boston Collaborative Drug Surveillance Program had linked estrogen with gallbladder disease.(48) The relative risk of users was two and a half times that of nonusers.

The black marks were accumulating against estrogen. Estrogen had been linked to gall bladder disease and two cancers, and a question mark hung over the issue of coronary heart disease. The wonder hormone was beginning to look not nearly so benign.

The news that use of estrogen was associated with a steeply increased risk of cancer of the endometrium had reverberated among doctors and the public like a bomb blast. If it did not dampen the enthusiasm of some estrogen advocates, it certainly provoked second thoughts among many prescribers and users. The accumulation of evidence against estrogen caused a fall-off in hormone prescriptions in the United Kingdom starting in 1975. A similar pattern was seen in America. Estrogen use declined by 18% from 1975 to 1976, and by another 10% from 1976 to 1977.(49)

One factor in the decline in use in America was the FDA's insistence that every package of estrogen contain an insert warning of the risks of estrogen.(50) This was bitterly opposed by Ayerst, who had contacted clinicians within days of the appearance of the 5 December 1975 issue of *New England Journal of Medicine,* reassuring them that Premarin was safe, in terms the FDA commissioner described as "misleading" and "irresponsible."(51) The American Pharmaceutical Manufacturers' Association joined Ayerst in its opposition to the FDA's plan for a package insert, and took legal action, arguing that "patient information would reduce sales of estrogen drugs and, therefore, reduce profits."(52) Next, the American College of Obstetrics and Gynecology joined the action, with the support of the American College of Internal Medicine and the American Cancer Society. The College maintained that giving patients information violated the physician's right to control how much information to disclose to patients and threatened medicine's professional autonomy. On the other side of the fence, the U.S. National Women's Health Network submitted a brief to the court in support of the FDA's insert.

The estrogen controversy of the mid-1970s constituted a watershed in doctor-patient relationships. There were some physicians who were deeply critical of the *New England Journal of Medicine* for allowing the study results to leak into the mass media where the public could read them, thus denying the medical profession the luxury of deciding about the evidence for themselves. The news that an apparently beneficial drug given to well women could cause cancer led to the troubling idea in women's minds that their doctors could not necessarily be trusted. They had been duped, lulled into a false feeling of security by the promise of professional competence. Doctors may have been duped too, but this didn't alter the fact that they had given the reassurance that the therapy was safe. It seemed that women would have to be more alert and reject blind dependence on the medical profession. There was increasing talk of the need to involve women in decision making about their health, especially when they were well women.

As one commentator explains:

> The information about estrogen introduced the notion of iatrogenesis into the physician-patient relationship and was incompatible with the demand that the physician be trusted.

> The combination of media activity and the FDA-required insert made information on estrogen directly available to the patient, thus breaking the physician's monopoly over the control of information. . . . Once the estrogen was declared potentially

iatrogenic, the old definition of the patient role as essentially passive had to be discarded as no longer appropriate.(53)

New Polemics

Ayerst barely paused in its promotional efforts with Premarin. As well as sending "Dear Doctor" letters to physicians, it continued its pursuit of the public. The public relations firm Hill and Knowlton prepared strategies for Ayerst to counter the adverse news emerging from research programs and to "preserve the identity of estrogen replacement therapy as effective, safe treatment for symptoms of the menopause."(54) As usual, it was proposed that the major focus of attention be magazines read by women. Although Ayerst never implemented this particular plan, Hill and Knowlton advised an intense campaign of articles carefully placed in the mainstream media. *McCall's, Ladies' Home Journal, Redbook,* and *Reader's Digest* were suggested as publications to target, as were 4,500 suburban newspapers. Ayerst was advised to "steer clear of attempting to promote the use of estrogens, and instead concentrate on the menopause." The "estrogen message can be effectively conveyed by discreet references to 'products that your doctor may prescribe.'"

Throughout the period of controversy, estrogen still had staunch medical defenders, undeterred by what they casually called the "cancer scare," as if it had no substance at all. At first they savaged the studies, but when the endometrial cancer association was proven beyond doubt by later research, they moved on to a different strategy.

This involved glibly ignoring the damage done (certainly not taking any responsibility for it), and adopting the "progress of medicine" stance. A New Zealand doctor described the bad news about endometrial cancer this way:

> [HRT] got a slightly bad name in the early years in America because doctors there were giving just one hormone—estrogen. They quickly found out that this was causing a certain amount of cancer—not much—but a little bit of cancer in the womb and of course this was disastrous. . . . This was quickly corrected and the causes were found and now it's catching on in America again because they have found out what the problem is.(55)

In *The Amarant Book of Hormone Replacement Therapy*, women are told that "there were earlier scares about estrogen causing womb cancer. Such scares have been nailed since it was found that what was missing from the therapy was progesterone. Once estrogen and pro-gesterone were combined they make a pretty formidable team and it has been suggested that between them they may actually *protect* women from womb cancer."(56) Clever science could now ensure the endometrium was protected by the addition of another hor-mone—progesterone. By inducing a regular bleed, it was hoped to avoid the dangerous buildup of the uterine lining that occurred un-der the influence of estrogen. This was called "opposed" therapy.

But there were problems with this regime. While postmeno-pausal women continued to produce some estrogen, there is essen-tially no progesterone production in the postmenopause. No one could predict exactly what a progestogen added at this time would do. Also, progesterone has a deserved reputation as a difficult hor-mone. Dr. John Studd calls progesterone "a beastly hormone."(57) Still an enthusiast for postmenopausal hormones, he says: "The only problem about estrogen therapy is progesterone." Progestogens cause premenstrual syndrome in 25% of postmenopausal users of opposed HRT, while the major unwelcome effect of progestogens is a return of menstruation. This is the most common reason women give for discontinuing HRT, especially those who had already passed through menopause and naturally ceased menstruating.

This reluctance on the part of women to resume menstruation has sent doctors in search of methods of delivering hormones that entail less patient "compliance" than swallowing tables. Implants of estrogen, inserted either into the flesh of the stomach, thigh, or but-tock, or sewn into the wound at the time of hysterectomy, remove the ability of women to withdraw from the therapy.

But women were disenchanted with estrogen for other reasons. The debate around HRT had introduced some caution and more careful science into the claims made for estrogen. Fewer doctors were prepared to publicly proclaim that estrogen could keep wrinkles at bay.

It was increasingly recognized that all estrogen could do was help with the recognized signs of menopause—hot flashes and dryness in the vagina. From a woman's point of view, taking a harmless drug for menopause was one thing; taking a possible carcinogen for the sake of hot flashes quite another. There had to be a better reason before women would be convinced it was wise.

There was another reason waiting in the wings and, as we have seen, that was osteoporosis. In the interests of rehabilitating HRT, women have been subjected to "a carefully orchestrated campaign" to advocate estrogen as a prevention for osteoporosis.(58)

Bone Crazy

Prior to the 1960s medical research on the subject of osteoporosis would be found in a medical library under the heading of "other bone diseases."(59) Osteoporosis was seen as a problem of bones, not of women.

This began to change when companies such as Ayerst Laboratories began to market estrogen therapy. The potential of estrogen to retard bone loss had been suspected from the days when scientists were looking for commercially viable sources of estrogen. As far back as the 1930s Dr. Fuller Albright of Harvard Medical School had argued that estrogen might be used to prevent osteoporosis. Dr. Robert Wilson had also made the connection and in one of his papers used an illustration of a woman with a dowager's hump, or, as he put it, "the stigmata of 'Nature's defeminization.'"(60) But 25 years ago the idea of a "youth pill" and a treatment for the emotional distress of menopause had more commercial promise than the strategy of disease prevention.

Nevertheless, Ayerst was alert to the estrogen/osteoporosis link and from its earliest days included treatment of osteoporosis in the indications for using Premarin. There was no proof at this stage that estrogen could retard bone loss, but the statement that it could strengthened estrogen's claim to wonder drug status. Ayerst even devised a special estrogen/androgen/vitamin C preparation called Formatrix, marketed especially for the treatment of bone loss. The symbol for the promotional campaign for Formatrix was, predictably, the woman with the dowager's hump.

The endometrial cancer crisis created a need to find some additional reason to woo women onto hormones. Osteoporosis provided the answer: the condition was prevalent among women, and in serious cases was disfiguring and even deadly. This led to a renewal of interest in the osteoporosis/estrogen connection; in the early 1980s when several timely studies confirmed that estrogen was effective in retarding bone loss, the pharmaceutical promotional juggernaut swung into action. In 1986 estrogen manufacturers obtained permission from the FDA to include prevention of bone loss in the indications for the use of estrogen.

To reorient women's perception of the benefits of estrogen, certain preconditions had to be created: the gravity of osteoporosis needed to be impressed on them, they needed to understand that it was "their" disease, and they had to perceive the cancer risk as trivial when measured against the benefits.

Statements such as these began to appear in the media: "The invalidism which can occur with osteoporosis is far more grave than the putative risk of endometrial cancer," said Dr. Robert Greenblatt, a former student of Dr. Albright.(61) "Even if you took estrogen without progesterone, you are 15 times more likely to die of a hip fracture than of endometrial cancer," said Dr. Howard Judd of UCLA.(62)

Davi Birnbaum of the Menopause Collective of the Boston Women's Health Book Collective commented on the role of osteoporosis in the reselling of HRT: "Osteoporosis is a serious and scary problem, but I'm afraid it's being used to seduce women back to estrogen."(63)

Ayerst's osteoporosis campaign was meticulously planned. In 1985 Ayerst hired the public relations firm Burson-Marsteller to market osteoporosis.(64) Following criticism from women's health groups such as the National Women's Health Network, one of the vice presidents of Burson-Marsteller defended Ayerst. The purpose of the campaign, she said, "is to educate women about the existence of osteoporosis and risk factors associated with it. It is a noble thing. The reality is that there is decreased federal funding for research and public education, resulting in the necessity for corporations to fill the gap."

There were two prongs to the public relations firm's strategy: raise awareness of osteoporosis among the public, and enlist health workers to mediate the message to consumers and providers.

A survey carried out by Burson-Marsteller showed that 77% of the women had never heard of osteoporosis. These women were to be reached by stories on radio, television and in magazines such as *Vogue, McCall's,* and *Reader's Digest.* The thrust of the articles was to be that osteoporosis was a major health problem for which there were remedies and that those at risk should consult a doctor. The patient leaflets developed for this campaign defined osteoporosis as a menopausal disease and used alarming phrases such as "incredible shrinking women" and "little old ladies." They bore Ayerst's name but did not mention estrogen replacement therapy. Instead, talking to your doctor was underscored as the thing to do.

Burson-Marsteller's other strategies ensured that if women did this there was a high degree of likelihood that hormones would be prescribed. Burson-Marsteller used major nursing associations to run seminars on osteoporosis for church groups, women's clubs, and hospital outreach programs. The nurses would also be a useful conduit by which information on osteoporosis would reach doctors.

As part of their media effort, Burson-Marsteller financed a tour of three medical experts who visited 10 major cities with "high risk populations." This tour capitalized on a consensus report on osteoporosis put out by the National Institutes of Health in 1984. The NIH report had warned against widespread use of HRT because of the unknown risks but otherwise had stated that estrogen was the "most effective" way of preventing osteoporosis. On the tour were Dr. William Peck, the NIH panel's chairman; another panel member, Dr. Don Gambrell of the Medical College of Georgia and a known advocate for estrogen; and Dr. Robert Lindsay, a highly regarded researcher of osteoporosis. Dr. Lindsay, said Burson-Marsteller, "has worked a lot with Burson-Marsteller and done extensive work on osteoporosis." Lindsay was also on the board that advised on educational materials for the seminar program.

Meanwhile, doctors were courted in the medical media with a flood of often drug-company-inspired articles promoting the benefits of estrogen for bones, while cautious doctors were castigated for their timidity:

> Their attitude, not necessarily one of benign neglect, is that much can be accomplished by homespun psychology, encouragement, and simple sedatives. Then again, a good proportion of physicians, intimidated by alarming reports dealing with the hazards of estrogen therapy, are reluctant to offer hormone replacement therapy. In avoiding such therapeutic measures, they are relieved of responsibility if a gynecic cancer (breast or uterus) should develop. Brave new world—to do new harm should not be a mandate not to try to do good.(65)

The drug-company-inspired campaign to remarket estrogen with a clean image has been stunningly successful. In the 1990s the reorienting of osteoporosis as a woman's disease is complete. It is now mandatory to include osteoporosis as a major "symptom" in any discussion of menopause. By convincing the public and the medical profession that osteoporosis is a "crippling" and "killing" disorder and estrogen the only cure, HRT has been imbued with a kind of saintliness. HRT offers salvation where otherwise there would be none, rescuing women from an unthinkable fate as deformed old crones. In the face of this, how could anyone be so ungrateful as to raise the question of risks?

An Affair of the Heart

More recently, there has been another twist in the hormone story. Women and doctors are being assailed with stories of yet another reason to use estrogens. This time it is to prevent heart disease. For the advocates of HRT, this is seen as estrogen's final ace. According to one consensus conference "the protective effect of estrogen on cardiovascular disease should be the major indication for ERT."(66)

Heart disease is a major killer of men, the incidence of which increases throughout their lives. A similar pattern is seen in women, but women have far fewer deaths from heart disease than do men. Because the increase in women begins about the same age as menopause, it has been assumed that loss of estrogen is the cause. Estrogen seems to act favorably on the lipids (fatty substances found in the blood), and lipids are involved in the causation of heart disease.

However, the results of studies looking at whether HRT protects against heart disease have been mixed; a clear relationship has not been shown. The studies have almost exclusively been conducted in America where the most used preparation is the estrogen-only Premarin, and many of the women in these studies took estrogen preparations with much higher doses than those used today.

Ayerst was eager to gain approval to cite protection against cardiovascular disease among estrogen's benefits, and in June 1990 the Fertility and Maternal Health Drugs Advisory Committee of the FDA agreed that "the cardiovascular benefits of Premarin may outweigh the risks depending on the individual patient's risk profile for various estrogen-related diseases and conditions."(67) Ayerst is next seeking permission from the FDA to include prevention of coronary heart disease in women who have had hysterectomies as an indication for using Premarin. So far the FDA has withheld its permission. The reason why Ayerst's request is confined to women with hysterectomies is that no one knows what happens when progestogen is added to estrogen. The studies published so far have not adequately addressed the subject of what happens when HRT is opposed. Progestogen may have a negative effect on lipids, so that when it is added to HRT it could undo any positive effect or, worse, cause an increased risk of heart disease.

Although this question is far from resolved, some doctors have begun to argue that HRT should be promoted to women as a prevention for heart disease. They argue that if the protective effect is true, this benefit would outweigh any of the cancer risks attached to hormones. Complicated risk/benefit arguments are put forward, resembling nothing less than an intricate chess game in which bones saved are checked off against malignant tumors in the breast, and canceled heart attacks are measured against cancers in the uterus. Very often, all this amounts to is a sophisticated game playing to put estrogen in a good light. It also involves a subtle fudging of the differing risks between opposed and nonopposed therapy. Women are fed barefaced statements about being saved from heart disease by taking hormones, when this can only be stated for unopposed therapy, and tentatively at that. Women with uteruses need to take opposed therapy with progestogen, so they can't expect this benefit, but these complexities are often hard for laypeople to grasp.

Alternatively, unopposed estrogen is being promoted for all women regardless of whether they have had a hysterectomy or not. A consensus conference on progestogens in menopause held in Florida in 1988 came to this recommendation:

> All postmenopausal women should be made aware of the consequences of untreated menopause and should be "offered" the opportunity to receive estrogen. This statement falls short of the opinion that all postmenopausal women "should" receive estrogen, an attitude that was endorsed by some participants but not by others.(68)

Like faithful brides, the advocates of estrogen appear determined to stay loyal. This has involved considerable contortions of logic and some abandonment of scientific objectivity. The pro-estrogen lobby casts about for new ways to cleanse estrogen of the taint of its past:

its efforts becoming more and more fanciful as the bad news persists. Whether this pro-estrogen mind-set results from feelings of guilt over having caused cancer in healthy women is difficult to know. But doctors and women are still bombarded with messages about the benefits of hormones.

The following optimistic statement is typical of the oversimplification of complex issues that pervades the hormone debate, while the conclusion reached is seriously worrying:

> The fact that estrogen therapy prevents osteoporosis is well established but there is growing evidence that it has a protective role in the development of atherosclerosis [a heart disease]. This, coupled with the evidence that it does not increase the incidence of breast cancer, is adding weight to the argument that HRT should be offered to all menopausal women unless there are contraindications.(69)

Designer Menopauses

The same message is now being put across to the public. "If I don't have any symptoms," a reader asked the medical adviser at the *Australian Women's Weekly*, "why should I take hormones?"(70)

"To protect you against cardiovascular disease, stroke and severe osteoporosis in later life," was the reply. This same article claimed that HRT would "prevent the dread middle-aged spread" and "make women feel psychologically better and have more energy to enjoy life and cope with its ups and downs, less depression and mood disturbances." It went on to state confidently that for most women "the advantages of HRT outweigh the possible disadvantages."

In the *New Zealand Woman's Day*, estrogen was headlined as "the menopause miracle" that ensured "the answer to your change of life nightmares." The article stated that "the majority of women" would need HRT, as it was "necessary for happiness, sexuality and physical well-being." Besides keeping breasts firm, HRT would protect users against serious diseases such as osteoporosis and heart disease.(71)

These promises that HRT can prevent diseases in the future are hard to resist. There is a definite implication that if we don't comply, we are dooming ourselves to disabling, if not killing, illnesses in the future. We almost have an obligation to use it and are depicted as irrationally fearful and old-fashioned if we do not. Modern women should have designer menopauses, not the old sort with hot flashes and night sweats. The side effects and risks are glossed over in this entirely rosy picture of estrogen's benefits.

So too is the meaning of medication in women's lives. HRT was originally proposed for women with symptoms of menopause; it is now being promoted for all women whether they have symptoms or not. When HRT was prescribed for menopausal symptoms, it was for months or one or two years. Now HRT will not be effective for osteoporosis unless it is taken for 10 or 15 years, and the number of years it would need to be taken for the prevention of heart disease has not been established. Presumably it would be lifelong—a matter of some 30 or more years. This would mean a huge cost to the health system and to women in terms of drug-related costs, visits to the doctor, and extra investigatory tests, while for their part the pharmaceutical companies would be laughing all the way to the bank.

HRT's most extreme advocates see nothing the matter with the idea of lifelong use, even though there are no studies of the effects of long-term HRT use. Promoting HRT for the prevention of coronary heart disease also eliminates the problem of selecting "at risk" patients for treatment as proposed for the prevention of osteoporosis. There would be no necessity to push for bone density measurements to determine bone-loss risk before prescribing the drug; HRT could be recommended to all women on the basis of their hypothetical cardiovascular risk. If the story of oral contraceptives was one of a "mass pill experiment," the HRT saga looks set to outstrip it in sheer scale.

What Happened to Medical Ethics?

It sometimes seems that commonsense has permanently fled from the debate surrounding hormone therapy. There is no discussion of the wisdom or ethics of medicating huge numbers of asymptomatic well women with powerful drugs. This is not recommended for any other drug or for the prevention of any other condition. Even with heart disease in men, the major killer of the over-47-year-olds, antihypertensive drugs are only recommended for those with clear indications. The switch from HRT as treatment to HRT as preventive therapy has occurred without debate or justification. It is a shift of the profoundest significance, yet has gone unremarked and undiscussed.

There are over 27 million women in the United States between the ages of 40 and 60. It is hard to grasp that anyone could seriously recommend that this number of women should be offered HRT, but, as we have seen, such suggestions are indeed being made. If large numbers of women were persuaded to take hormones, the public health effect if any serious health risk were to emerge some years later would be catastrophic.

When the FDA Fertility and Maternal Health Drugs Committee looked at the safety of Premarin, committee member Professor James Schlesselman quantified the possible effect of estrogen on breast cancer. He estimated that on the basis of existing data, in a group of 1,000 50-year-old women who used estrogen for 30 years (necessary for cardiovascular protection), there would be 51 additional cases of breast cancer among these women compared to nonusers.(72) Thus, 1 in every 20 long-term estrogen users would be at additional high risk of breast cancer.

There were over one million 50-year-old women in this country in 1991. If 25% of these women took estrogen long-term, there would be 16,498 extra cases of breast cancer within this group. If 80% of them used it, as Dr. Studd suggests, there would be an extra 52,795 cases of breast cancer during the next 30 years.

These figures apply only to women of one age: 50 years old. If we look at all women in their fifties—that is, women between 50 and 59 years (over 11 million)—the corresponding figures for long-term use would be over 144,000 extra cases of breast cancer if 25% of these women were using estrogen, and about 461,000 cases if 80% were using it. The research information so far suggests that estrogen/progestogen preparations would have a similar effect.

These latter figures are hypothetical because many women would die of something else before they had a chance to develop cancer, but it does illustrate the considerable scale of the problem that could be created by widespread long-term hormone use.

The fact that "estrogen drugs are among the most potent drugs in the pharmacopoeia" barely gets stated today.(73) Hormones are depicted as benign, beneficial, and essentially natural. After all, aren't they only putting back what nasty nature took away? Similarly, the principle that "while it may be appropriate to use exceedingly toxic drugs for the treatment of very serious illness, it may not be appropriate to use drugs of minimal toxicity for casual purposes" has gone by the board.(74) The philosophy that a more stringent risk/benefit ratio should apply to drugs used on well people than that applied to people with disease is no longer mentioned, let alone used. To give someone cancer to prevent a heart attack she may never have had, or to stop the thinning of bones that were never going to fracture is a grave responsibility. It is a far different matter from risking leukemia in someone who is having radiation treatment for invasive cancer, a potentially fatal disease. Yet this difference is simply overlooked.

If women do not succumb to the extravagant claims made for HRT in the media and in the plethora of handbooks parading its virtues, the front line in conversion is the general medical practice. Doctors promote HRT to their patients, sometimes without patients' having any symptoms at all, save the attainment of the apparently problematic age of 40.

In Britain there have been two detailed reports on how general practice increases the use of HRT.(75) In the first, a group of general practitioners in Cambridge wrote to their patients aged 50–52 years asking them to complete a survey of their views of menopause and HRT. The major emphasis in the letter was on osteoporosis and HRT's ability to prevent it.

Although nearly 80% of the women said they were not worried about menopause, the same number said the most important problem of menopause was osteoporosis. This could mean either that they have been thoroughly brainwashed by the media or that they took the lead from their physicians! Additionally, three quarters of the women said they would be interested in taking hormones to prevent osteoporosis, although most said they wanted more information.

In the second study Jean Coope, who is a general practitioner in Cheshire, established an osteoporosis prevention clinic for women aged 40–60. All 582 eligible women in the practice were written to, inviting them to attend the clinic, and 43% attended. The aim of the exercise was to "embark on a program of health education and screening, and prescription of hormone replacement therapy for as many women as possible of all social classes, for whom it could be regarded as safe and acceptable."

Women were given a lecture, a history of each woman was taken including risk factors for osteoporosis, and the doctor saw each woman. All women except those with medical contraindications were offered HRT, not just those deemed to be at high risk. Through this strategy, the use of HRT among those women rose from 15% to 45%, although by the end of one year it had fallen to 38%. Dr. Coope said no pressure was put on patients to accept HRT, but she also wrote: "Post-menopausal women were often reluctant to embark on hormone replacement therapy because of a distaste for cyclical bleeding. After an explanation of the benefits of hormone replacement for a limited period (six years' use reducing risk of fractures by 50%) many accepted this."

Who Pulls the Strings?

In addition to such efforts at the primary health level, the pharmaceutical companies are as active as ever, promoting the benefits of their wonder hormones; they have established a key role for themselves in postgraduate medical education on menopause. In Britain, for instance, they promote clinical meetings dealing with menopause and fund hospital menopause clinics and their research programs.(76) The Amarant Trust's newsletter, *Feeling Good* is sponsored by an education grant from two manufacturers of hormones— CIBA-Geigy and Novo Laboratories. (77)

In New Zealand there is a similar involvement by pharmaceutical companies in education on menopause. During 1989 CIBA-Geigy sponsored symposia for general practitioners on the management of menopause. These were conducted by staff from the Family Planning Association's menopause clinics and senior staff from National Women's Hospital. CIBA-Geigy makes Estraderm, an estrogen product that releases hormone through the skin.

The drug companies' strategy to women has continued to be to keep HRT low-key in the patient material. The emphasis is on education about "the problem," whether it is menopause or osteoporosis, rather than on the drug. Doctors are relied on to make the transition from identification of the problem to use of the product. In inviting women to "talk to their doctors," the pharmaceutical industry is confident that the doctors will respond in a way that is in accord with its own commercial interests.

This commercial activity is having an effect. Thirty percent of postmenopausal American women now use HRT, as do 10% of British and Australian women.(78) In Britain, sales for HRT totaled £10 million by 1989, which had doubled over sales figures of two years previously.(79) It was estimated that by the year 2000, a quarter of menopausal British women would be using HRT, amounting to two million women. In Australia, between 1981 and 1987, the sales of estrogens through retail pharmacies increased by nearly 52%. By 1987 there was one prescription unit per year for every 3.7 women aged 45 and over. Over the same period the number of women in this age group increased by slightly under 8%.(80)

The hormone apostles, however, will not be content until substantial numbers of women worldwide are being medicated. They argue that all women must be given "a choice" to use estrogen, as if it were akin to a cosmetic, a new curtain material, or a brand of pet food, not a potent steroidal prescription drug with unknown long-term risks.

Friskies or Whiskas? L'Oreal or Revlon? Premarin or Progynova? The choice, as they say, is yours.

Chapter 9

Mostly Good News About Hormones

Examining the evidence for the effectiveness and safety of HRT is not an easy task because the evidence is so often muddled or of poor quality. The best way of providing reliable evidence would have been to conduct well-designed clinical trials, comparing users of hormones with nonusers. These trials would need to involve large numbers of women carefully followed over a long period of time, decades in fact. Such trials have never been carried out.

Large-scale trials have recently been initiated in several parts of the world. The Postmenopausal Estrogen Progestogen Intervention, or PEPI, study, for instance, is funded by the U.S. government. It is giving similar women estrogen, placebo, or combined therapy and following them for three years to determine the effect of the combinations of hormones on blood lipids, blood pressure, and bone density; but the results of this will not be available for some years. Studies are also needed on the long-term effects of opposed therapy on breast cancer, ovarian cancer, endometrial cancer, liver disease, and fracture rate. All these areas are currently poorly researched.

But it is not possible to wait while trials such as these are conducted. The drug companies and doctors have beaten the gun. Hormones are already in widespread use, so the information we would look to these studies for has to be found in other ways. To discover the facts on HRT we have to rely on epidemiological research.

Unlike clinical medicine, which looks at illness in the individual, epidemiology looks at epidemics of disease. The word epidemiology comes from the Greek *epidemia*, meaning "among the people."

Epidemiology looks at disease incidence or medical or other interventions among the people, among populations.

Epidemiology has only relatively recently been used to look at medical treatments, and research methods have improved as researchers have developed more understanding of how to get reliable results. This means that there are still a lot of unanswered questions about HRT and, in particular, its long-term safety.

As in any medical research, it is possible for unsuspected factors to bias or confound the results unless the researcher controls for them. For example: a researcher might want to compare the incidence of heart disease between users and nonusers of HRT. Unless the researcher makes sure that the groups of users and nonusers are the same in other respects, for instance, weight, age, menopausal status, and smoking, the results could be affected. It could look as if users had less heart disease, but nonsmokers are at less risk of heart disease and it might turn out that HRT users smoke less. Unless the researcher took this into account, she or he might get the wrong result.

There are others ways in which the research into HRT has problems. There is a huge variety of hormonal preparations, using several types of estrogen and several types of progestogens, in differing combinations. Whereas estrogen (Premarin) has dominated in America, the British tended to use opposed therapy from the beginning, although in the early days it was inadequately opposed, the amount of progestogen being low. In most European countries, estradiol valerate and estriol have been used ahead of Premarin, and different progestogens are used in different countries.

In a study of HRT users undertaken by the Department of Community Health and General Practice at Oxford University, the researchers found 175 different treatment combinations among the 4,500 women in the study.(1) In America most of the studies have been carried out on women using Premarin alone, but in the Oxford study only 17% of the women were using Premarin. Similarly, in a Swedish study, 21% of the women were using conjugated estrogens such as Premarin, whereas 30% were using estradiol valerate, and 21% were using an estradiol/norgestrel combination.(2)

The hormone therapy used today generally uses lower doses and different compositions from those used in former years, so that research results from the past are not always totally applicable to women now. In particular, the risks and benefits from studies using estrogen only or inadequately opposed estrogen cannot confidently be applied to women using modern opposed therapy. Since this form of therapy was adopted only after it became clear that unopposed therapy was causing endometrial cancer, there has not been time for much research on the new regimes to be carried out.

In the meantime, many of the claims made for HRT need to be treated with caution because there is not the research to back them up conclusively. There is a tendency for proponents of HRT to gloss over this problem and employ a kind of double-talk when advocating for HRT. For instance, proponents will claim that certain studies show HRT's benefits, but when studies showing risks are pointed out to them, they will dismiss them on the grounds that the hormonal preparations used in these studies are not used today. In other words, they want it both ways. They use studies using old forms of HRT to argue for HRT but will not allow others to use the same kind of studies to highlight the bad news.

We also need to be very careful to name exactly which hormones we are talking about when discussing research. Estrogen used alone will not necessarily have the same effects as estrogen/progestogen combinations. This applies to both beneficial and harmful effects. This is not always clear to the layperson, and doctors sometimes gloss over these differences. They tend to use the generic term "hormone replacement therapy" for estrogen alone and for combined therapy, even when the difference matters. For instance, they will say that HRT is good for blood lipids, whereas the real truth is that while estrogen appears to be good for blood lipids, combined therapy may not be. In this book, the term HRT is used only where the difference in hormonal composition does not matter. Wherever it does, the exact hormone involved will be specified.

Hormone Replacement Therapy Regimens

There are three basic HRT regimens:

- *unopposed therapy* or estrogen alone

- *opposed sequential therapy* where a period of estrogen is followed by a shorter period combined with progestogen

- *opposed continuous combined therapy* using both estrogen and progestogen simultaneously

As noted above, one of the striking things about HRT use is the multiplicity of combinations of hormones used on women. Individual doctors will have their favorite formulas and talk of the need to "tailor" the hormone regimen to the woman. All very well, but then the research on safety and effectiveness, conducted on different regimens, will not necessarily be applicable to the woman getting her own individualized HRT.

Because of the unpleasant side effects and dangers of these hormones, doctors are keen to find the minimum dosages. For instance, the incidence of endometrial cancer in estrogen users was shown to be dose-related—that is, women on high doses of estrogen were more likely to develop cancer than those on lower doses. But there can be a conflict between the desire to give women the smallest possible doses and the need to maintain effectiveness. There would be no point in using estrogen for 15 years to prevent osteoporosis if in fact the dose used was insufficient to prevent bone loss. Doctors perform a balancing act between the need to preserve effectiveness and to minimize risks, but it may not be clear in the short-term whether they are succeeding.

Doctors disagree amongst themselves about what the ideal therapies are. Where one doctor may caution against giving any unopposed estrogen because of the possible risk to the endometrium, liver, and breast (including the possible adverse effect on naturally occurring but as yet undiagnosed cancers), others will argue for as little progestogen as possible because of the effects on blood lipids.(3)

To some extent, a lot of ad hoc experimentation is going on with postmenopausal hormones. It is open season for hormones. By tinkering with dosages, doctors are introducing new methods that have not been properly researched. They try out new methods on individual women in a clinical setting that should really only be attempted in a controlled research environment where the women have given informed consent, the effects are scientifically measured, and the women are given additional tests (such as endometrial biopsies) to protect their health. Women should ask for evidence of safety (chapter and verse) if their doctors want to increase doses beyond standard levels. It is not good enough to be told that the doctor has already "successfully" tried a particular regime on a few of his or her patients. When we are contemplating taking powerful drugs, we deserve *proof* of safety, not speculation.

Unopposed therapy

Far more is known about estrogen-only HRT than any other sort. The research data are clearer because this HRT has been used for longer and there has been the time to conduct research. Because of the link with endometrial cancer, the use of unopposed therapy declined in the 1980s for all but women who had had hysterectomies, and there are firm recommendations that women with a uterus should use opposed therapy. However, in America and other countries, some doctors are beginning to argue in favor of unopposed therapy for all women because the argument for estrogen's effectiveness in preventing cardiovascular disease has come to the forefront.

A recent review of the relative risks of estrogens and progestogens published in *Maturitas* put forward this proposition.(4) The Belgian author favored unopposed therapy because, he argued, the risk of dying from cardiovascular disease from added progestogen outweighed the risks of dying from endometrial cancer. He argued that provided the woman had a sample taken from her endometrium annually to check for hyperplasia, unopposed therapy was quite feasible, although he conceded that this technique "is not always easy, accepted and unharmful. . . " Currently, most doctors reserve unopposed therapy for women who have had hysterectomies.

Opposed therapy: sequential regimens

There are several kinds of opposed sequential regimens. In one, estrogen is taken alone for 11–17 days, then progestogen is added to the estrogen for 10–13 days. Another regimen starts with estrogen and progestogen for 12 days, then continues with estrogen alone. In some regimens, there are table-free days; in others, there are not. The entire cycle takes 28 days. The progestogen usually induces menstrual-like bleeding to prevent a dangerous buildup of endometrium, which can lead to cancer.

Anxiety is sometimes expressed about opposed sequential therapy as it is similar to the sequential oral contraceptives such as Serial C and Sequens which were taken off the market by the FDA in 1976 because they were shown to cause an increased risk of endometrial cancer.(5) This risk, however, appears to be unfounded, and women using sequential forms of HRT do not run the same risk of cancer.

Opposed therapy: Continuous combined estrogen/progestogen therapy

Because the majority of women don't want to retain periods, doctors have been looking for a way of manipulating the drug regimens to protect the endometrium without causing a bleed. Continuous combined estrogen/progestogen medication is being tried to see if this can be achieved. Experience so far shows that while most women will eventually not bleed at all on this regimen and the endometrium will become atrophic, in the first six months of use, breakthrough bleeding is common, especially in women in the early postmenopausal years. This is a frequent reason women give for stopping the therapy, although progestogenic side effects are another common reason for giving up.(6)

Women need to be aware that this type of therapy must be regarded as experimental, for its safety and effectiveness have not been adequately studied. It is a relatively new method and none of the major studies that have looked at the risks of HRT have included it. The results of these trials cannot provide answers about continuous combined hormones.

In an extensive review of the available research on continuous estrogen/progestogen therapy, Dr. Malcolm Whitehead and fellow researchers at King's College School of Medicine in London made some critical points: "[The] published data on this mode of administration are relatively sparse, and many studies have investigated very small numbers of patients for short periods."(7)

The largest study had 265 patients; most were far smaller, some including only 10 or 11 patients. The longest was for 18 months, while most were for less than 12 months. The King's College reviewers said they could not even comment on the studies on lipid and lipoprotein metabolism (important to hearts) because "all of the studies were flawed to some extent, and we believe that their results are largely uninterpretable. For this reason, we have not reviewed the data. This is a most serious criticism." These comments are important because in Europe, America, and Australasia, this form of therapy is increasingly being recommended to general practitioners and prescribed to women, despite its experimental status.

The King's College reviewers expressed concern at this trend: "We believe that the enthusiasm for this new treatment regimen is premature and unjustified on the basis of present studies. We urge caution in the use of this regimen until further, more conclusive, data are available."

They listed four major areas for research:

- control of symptoms

- bleeding patterns

- effect on the endometrium

- effect on lipids and lipoproteins

To this must be added the effect on breast cancer. Several studies so far have pointed to a possible negative effect on the breast when progestogen is added to estrogen. No one has any idea what effect continuous combined therapy will have on the breast.

Similarly, the question of the effect of continuous progestogen on the endometrium is yet to be answered. In a small American study 6.5% of the patients receiving low-dose (2.5 mg) medroxyprogesterone acetate (Provera) along with Premarin were converted from having an atrophic to a proliferative endometrium.(8) The significance of this in relation to endometrial cancer is not known.(9)

Dr. Whitehead says it is probably wise for women undergoing this therapy to have a baseline endometrial biopsy before they start taking it, and then annual biopsies. This is rather an unpleasant prospect for women as the biopsies can be painful. In particular, the pretreatment biopsy could be difficult if not impossible in some women because the cervical canal in women of this age is often contracted and tightly closed.

Some doctors prescribing continuous combined therapy are giving their patients an oral contraceptive called Marvelon, telling the women to take one quarter to half a tablet daily. Marvelon contains a lipid-friendly progestogen—desogestrel—but the estrogen it contains—ethinylestradiol—is considered inappropriate at menopause. In addition, at the dose given, the therapy is likely to be ineffective at protecting bones because it is too low. Women should be aware that using Marvelon in this way is experimental and has not been shown to be either effective or safe.

Different Types of Estrogens

The three major natural female estrogens are *estradiol-17β,* a potent form of estrogen produced primarily in the reproductive years; *estrone,* the estrogen of postmenopause, which is less active; and *estriol,* which is a very weak estrogen. In postmenopause, natural estrone is produced principally by the conversion of androgens in adipose tissue (fat). Most of the hormone preparations used in HRT use one of these forms of estrogen.

Ethinylestradiol, which is used in both oral contraceptives and HRT, is a synthetic hormone with no natural equivalent. It is seen as less suitable for menopause as it breaks down slowly and stimulates the liver.(10)

The estrogens in hormone replacement therapy are often called "natural," but this description is not entirely accurate. As one doctor commented about Premarin, "These estrogenic preparations are natural to horses rather than humans."(11) Although the estrogens are similar to the natural forms, they are all synthetically produced.

Estrogens are inactive when given orally; they all must be modified by the addition of a stabilizer molecule to improve absorption through the intestinal wall and then to stop them being short-circuited as they go through the liver. Two modification processes are used in the commonly prescribed postmenopausal estrogens: *estradiol valerate* is *esterfied* and *estrone sulfate* is *conjugated.* As these estrogens pass through the liver, the stabilizers are removed, leaving the estrogen. Estrogen administered orally is converted primarily to estrone.

Estrogen is usually given orally, but nonoral methods such as skin patches, implants, and creams are also used. Around 30% of the estrogen is deactivated in the intestinal wall and liver when given orally. If nonoral routes of delivery are used, most of the estrogen goes directly into the bloodstream. As only a very small amount of the estrogen passes through the liver, less estrogen is lost. This means that higher doses must be used with oral routes than with the nonoral routes.

As the estrogen directly enters the bloodstream with the nonoral routes, unmodified or natural estradiol can be used. In these methods estradiol levels exceed the estrone levels. There are both advantages and disadvantages to these routes of administration as will be discussed below.

The effect of each preparation will differ with individuals. Each woman will have her own hormone levels onto which the hormones in HRT will be superimposed. Estrogen and progestogen effects can also be synergistic; that is, they can work together to create effects greater than the effects each hormone would cause by itself.

Oral estrogens

Conjugated equine estrogens: The brand names are *Premarin* and *Prempak* when progestogen (norgestrel) is added; they come in estrogen doses of 0.3 mg, 0.625 mg, 0.9 mg, 1.25 mg, and 2.5 mg. These are compounds derived from pregnant mares' urine, comprising 65% estrone sulfate and 35% equine estrogen. They are potent estrogens and because of this can affect the liver. Some doctors recommend that for this reason they should not be used by women with hypertension.(12)

Estradiol valerate: These are *Progynova* or *Progyluton* when progestogen (norgestrel) is added. The estrogen comes in 1 or 2 mg tablets. Although this starts its life as estradiol, some of the estradiol is converted to estrone in the intestines and liver. This estrogen breaks down rapidly and so has less effect on the liver.

Piperazine estrone sulfate: Ogen comes in doses of 1 mg or 2 mg. These types are used in Australia but not in New Zealand.

Micronized estradiol: Estace comes in doses of 1 mg and 2 mg or *Kliogest* when norethisterone acetate is added in a continuous dose, or *Trisequens* in its sequential form. This estrogen has been micronized or reduced to very small particles. It is therefore readily absorbed and passes through the liver without being substantially altered.

Transdermal estrogen patches

Estraderm: Estraderm contains estradiol and is now often administered with supplemental progestogen tablets. It comes in 0.05 mg and 0.1 mg daily dose.

Estraderm contains estradiol in its purest form. A small adhesive patch attached to the skin releases estrogen over a period of three days, after which another patch is applied. Up to one-quarter of women develop a skin irritation at the site of the patch, in which case they are advised to shift the patch around. Nevertheless, some women find the itching annoying enough to stop using this method altogether. The patch can come off in hot humid weather or in a sauna.

With transdermal administration, the estrogen goes straight into the bloodstream, bypassing the intestines and liver, and therefore avoiding any effect on the liver. Women with gallbladder disease or hypertension can take estrogen by this method when they might be advised not to use the oral method. The estrogen is absorbed more slowly and less is converted into estrone, allowing a lower dose of estrogen to be used. Women with a uterus must also take oral progestogen, although research is underway to see if it is possible to deliver progestogen transdermally.(13)

While there have been positive reports of the effects of estrogen delivered this way on menopausal symptoms and vaginal changes, there has been only a small amount of research on its effects on bone loss, and it is not clear what effects it will have on lipids. Research so far suggests it is less beneficial than oral estrogen.(14) It is also possible that nonoral estradiol could have a greater effect than oral estrogens in stimulating the endometrium.(15) Not all women absorb the estrogen at the same rate, and some women may receive insufficient estrogen even at a dose equivalent to the oral dose.

Estraderm was introduced onto the market by CIBA-Geigy in 1988, but it has already quickly achieved a significant share of the hormone market. In Britain it is now the second highest selling brand of HRT.

Subcutaneous estrogen implants

Estradiol: This comes in a dose of 20, 50, or 100 mg, with or without 100 mg testosterone.

Pellets or implants containing estradiol are inserted under the skin of the abdomen or buttock, either surgically or through a cannula. A local anesthetic is used. Alternatively they can be sewn into the skin when a woman has a hysterectomy. The estradiol is slowly released over five to six months, after which time the implant must be replaced, although when it is first put in a high level of estrogens in the body is attained. Women who have not had a hysterectomy must take oral progestogen as well. A study by John Studd showed that 56% of women with implants who did not also take progestogen showed abnormal cell changes in the endometrium.(16) According to Dr. Derek Llewellyn-Jones, implants result in varying amounts of circulating estrogen in individual women.(17) Sometimes this may be too high for safety, sometimes too low to prevent bone loss. He advised women to have a blood test after three months to check their estrogen levels in case they need another implant sooner. There can also be a dosage retention effect where the estrogens build up to very high levels after long-term use.

Implants are controversial and not currently used for menopause in the United States. A disadvantage of this method is that it is difficult to stop it in the short-term if a woman experiences complications. There is also controversy over the effect on the endometrium. This is discussed in the following chapter.

Testosterone is sometimes added to implants for the purpose of increasing sexual desire, but there is considerable debate about whether this is desirable or effective. The way in which medical intervention can lead to further interventions was illustrated by an article advocating the use of testosterone therapy for loss of libido.(18) This hormone, said the doctors, can lead to "slight aggravation of acne, oiliness of skin, and minimal hirsutism [hairiness]." But never mind, they can control these effects "in some patients . . . by adding 50 mg of spironolactone (Aldactone) [a diuretic] once or twice daily."

Vaginal estrogens

Ortho-Dinestrol, Ogen Cream, and *Premarin* creams: Vaginal estrogen creams or pessaries are primarily prescribed for dryness and contraction of the vagina, or urinary problems caused by the thinning of vaginal tissues. Creams are initially used regularly but can be used more occasionally after the vaginal tissue has improved. Creams and pessaries take six to eight weeks to act on vaginal tissue but are also absorbed through the vaginal walls into the bloodstream. In fact, the vaginal walls can absorb hormones more rapidly than the intestines, especially once the treatment has improved the tissue in the vagina. As it is impossible to predict how much estrogen is entering an individual woman's system, vaginal estrogens cannot be relied on for benefits such as preventing bone loss; equally they cannot be regarded as safer than other methods.(19) Doctors variously advise that all women using vaginal estrogens other than for a very short period should also take oral progestogen, or they advise that women who start bleeding on vaginal estrogens must also take oral progestogen.

The policy of the Family Planning Association is to use tiny doses of cream so that there is minimal systemic absorption. They recommend using one-eighth of an applicator to avoid any endometrial buildup.

Vaginal estrogens can be started at any time after menopause, even quite some years after the last period. If treatment does not begin until the vagina has changed markedly, however, it will never be exactly as it was before menopause.

Other forms of estrogen

Estrogen gel containing estradiol is available in some parts of the world, especially France, but is not yet available in America. The woman spreads the gel over a wide area of the abdomen and thighs every second day. This form of administration gives varying levels of absorption. Researchers are also experimenting with nasal sprays and estrogen-releasing silicon vaginal rings. The latter can cause problems with discharge, discomfort, and ulceration.

Progestogen

Progesterone is naturally produced by the ovarian follicles following ovulation and, during pregnancy, by the placenta. It is not naturally present after menopause.

There are several different types of synthetic progesterones, and women have differing tolerances of them. As already mentioned, progestogens have many problems, which will be discussed more fully later. Just as with estrogens, different countries have tended to have their favorite progestogen, which further complicates the applicability of research findings from country to country, especially with regard to breast and endometrial cancer risks and cardiovascular effects.

A common progestogen is *norethindrome acetate,* generally available as *Norlutate* or *Micronor,* in doses of 0.35 mg and 5 mg. This is an androgenic progestogen, meaning it can promote male characteristics. Another progestogen is *medroxyprogesterone acetate* (brand name *Provera*), the same hormone found in Depo Provera. When used orally as part of HRT it is given at a lower dose than its injectable form and, as it goes through the liver, not all the drug enters the bloodstream. Provera is the progestogen most used in America, and some doctors favor it because they argue it is less androgenic and therefore has less effect on blood lipids. But Swedish researchers have said that the different effect on lipids is the result of the use of a larger than necessary dose of norethisterone and levonorgestrel. All progestogens affect lipid metabolism adversely and can lessen or cancel the beneficial effects of estrogen.(20) Even if medroxyprogesterone acetate caused no harm to the blood lipids by itself, it might neutralize any good effect of estrogen.

The primary reason for including progestogen in HRT is to stop the development of endometrial cancer. Some doctors prefer to use norethisterone and levonorgestrel for this purpose because Provera is less effective at preventing endometrial hyperplasia.(21) Researchers are looking for new forms of progestogen that do not have a negative effect on lipids. These newer progestogens such as desogestrel and gestodene may soon be available. Other progestogens that may be used in the future are micronized progestogen and cyproterone acetate. A recent study comparing HRT containing norgestrel and HRT containing cyproterone acetate found that the latter had a more favorable effect on lipoproteins.(22)

Who Uses HRT?

Hormone replacement therapy is predominantly used by white, middle-class women. An FDA assistant commissioner commented at the time the news about estrogen and endometrial cancer was released that "the chronic users [of estrogen] tend to be middle-class and upper-income women, the kind of people who go to doctors . . . It is an interesting example of the poor being spared."(23)

The British study of hormone users at menopausal clinics by the Oxford University researchers is just one of a number that have shown this association between social class and hormone use.(24) They found that 46% of their study subjects were in high social classes—social classes 1 and 2—whereas the corresponding census figure was 23%. These women were also more likely to name the mass media as their source of information about HRT, whereas women in other social classes heard about HRT first from a professional. Reading between the lines, this could mean that women in higher social classes actively sought to go on HRT, influenced by hyped-up claims in the media, while women from other classes were prescribed HRT after complaining of actual menopausal problems to the doctor.

The same pattern of middle-class women being more prone to use estrogen is also seen in Sweden, where higher education led to "a more than twofold increase in the risk of receiving estrogen treatment."(25)

The Oxford study found that 36% of the users had had a hysterectomy, which is 2 to 2.5 times the proportion in the British population, while in Sweden users were four times more likely to have had a hysterectomy. This pattern is consistently seen in all countries. It seems that women who have hysterectomies with or without oophorectomy often have more troubling menopausal symptoms, especially hot flashes. There has been little research to explain why this should be so, although studies have shown that in some women the ovaries do not work as well after a hysterectomy, possibly because of the interruption in the blood supply to the ovaries. This is something women are rarely told about when deciding for or against a hysterectomy.

Studies have also shown that women who have hysterectomies visit the doctor more, so they are possibly more likely to have HRT offered to them. Also, because they have no uterus, they do not run the risk of endometrial cancer, so the doctors may feel more confident about prescribing HRT. The Oxford study also found that a surprising 20% of the users had never had a baby, while the Swedish study found that women with big families (four or more children) were less likely to use HRT.

Most of the studies looking at reasons why women start HRT apply to women who started using it some time ago, so there is not a lot of information about how much women have been affected by the campaign to promote prevention of osteoporosis or how much women are affected by claims that estrogen will protect them against heart disease. A recent study in Iowa showed that the redefinition of menopause as a disease and the inclusion of osteoporosis among its symptoms was having an effect. It found that women using HRT were much more likely than nonusers to see menopause as a medical condition and to believe that women should take HRT if they had distressing menopausal symptoms, even though there was little difference in the actual incidence of menopausal symptoms between the two groups.(26) Women using HRT were likely to have had it recommended by their doctor, and 75% of the women not using HRT said a physician's recommendation would have a positive effect regarding HRT use.

Women taking HRT were far more likely to know about risk factors for osteoporosis and to know that HRT could reduce the risk of developing it (86% of the women taking HRT compared to 28% not taking it). By contrast, only one quarter of the women in either group knew that smoking was a risk factor for osteoporosis. This study suggests that the campaign to raise awareness about osteoporosis and to link it to hormones has been very successful, and that the use of hormones is to some extent doctor-driven.

Benefits of Using HRT

Menopausal symptoms

Some of the research into HRT focuses on objective matters, such as whether it causes endometrial hyperplasia. The proof of this lies in what scientists see when they look at biopsy specimens in the laboratory. But other aspects of the research into HRT are much more subjective. This is particularly true of research that seeks to determine how effective HRT is at alleviating menopausal symptoms. As we have seen, apart from the vasomotor effects and the effects on the vagina, there is no firm proof that psychological symptoms reported by some women are caused first and foremost by menopause. Although the matter is still far from settled, it does seem much more likely that they are coincidental to menopause or alternatively provoked by particularly severe physical symptoms. But as it is widely believed that these symptoms are caused by menopause, in many women's minds, they are. This makes it especially hard to examine just what HRT can do for menopause.

One of the curious findings that has emerged from research into the effectiveness of HRT at relieving menopausal symptoms is what is called "the placebo effect." In studies using hormones and placebos, women can show an improvement in their symptoms, at least initially, even on placebos. British researcher Jean Coope has twice shown this phenomenon in studies of menopausal women, as did two researchers at the Chelsea Hospital in London.(27) In Coope's studies, the women initially showed a distinct improvement in their hot flashes no matter what was in the pills they were taking. The improvement was not lasting however, for women on placebos; when women on estrogen were changed onto placebos, their hot flashes came back. Women on both placebos and estrogen, however, reported the same improvement in depression scores and feelings of well-being.

This effect has not just been shown in menopausal studies but also in studies of other conditions. When people take part in research, they sometimes receive positive benefits such as personal attention to their problems, which help them feel better. Some of us will have had a similar experience in our own lives. A worrying symptom will completely disappear after visiting the doctor, even before we've had a chance to take the prescribed medication or go for any tests.

Unshared problems always feel worse. Once a worry has been taken to the doctor and talked about, and perhaps an explanation has been given or some action taken, the situation will feel more under control. Occasionally, it will disappear. This is not to say that people make things up. Sometimes it means we have exaggerated something in our minds because we don't know what it means. We just needed an explanation. Or we needed a friendly ear to begin to feel on top of the situation and handle it ourselves. There are plenty of reports to suggest that this happens to some women at menopause just as it can happen to men or women at other times. Many women express relief at being able to get together with other women in a support group or at educational sessions such as those run by the Family Planning Association in New Zealand. Knowing that things that are happening to us also happen to other people can be immensely helpful.

In the Oxford study, Kate Hunt commented that "many women felt they had benefited greatly by having their problems treated seriously and sympathetically."(28) She quoted one of these women, who said:

> I found (and I know other ladies I spoke to on HRT felt the same) that the very fact some interest was being shown in the distressing symptoms I was suffering and someone was trying to do something about it was very comforting. It was reassuring to know that not all the medical profession think middle-aged women neurotic idiots with hypochondriac tendencies. This helped a great deal.

This beneficial effect on sympathetic treatment must have an effect on women's perception of the positive benefits of HRT. As Kate Hunt commented:

It is not possible to separate out the positive effects which a referral to a menopause clinic, sympathetic treatment and a prescription for hormone replacement may have apart from any pharmacological effect. This should not be dismissed as further evidence of the triviality of menopausal symptoms; work in other areas suggests that careful explanation of the consequences of a medical procedure or condition can have marked effects on the patient's experience.

Hot flashes and night sweats

Around 80% of women obtain relief from hot flashes and night sweats when they use HRT.(29) If the hot flashes were causing sleeping problems, HRT can also lead to a marked improvement in sleeping patterns, reducing insomnia and wakefulness. Following from this, the Chelsea Hospital researchers found that improved sleep can reduce irritability, worry, headaches, and improve memory, good spirits and optimism. This is called "the domino effect."

When taken for hot flashes, HRT need not be prolonged. A few months up to two years is usually enough to get past the worst of hot flashes. The hormones should then be gradually tapered off by spreading the tablets out, as it is possible for hot flashes to return if the hormones are abruptly withdrawn. This postmenopausal woman has been taking hormones for 10 years, after beginning them for hot flashes. She found that the flashes returned when she tried to stop taking them:

> I went into menopause with a positive attitude. I felt fine, full of energy and with a sense of direction, which had been lacking up to then. Unfortunately, hot flashes went on and on. To say that no one notices hot flashes is rubbish. The sufferer feels terrible even to the point of feeling one is about to die. It was embarrassing and even three showers a day during summer was not enough to eliminate the constant sticky feeling.
>
> I was about the age of 55 when I was first given HRT and it was a marvelous success! Although sometimes I was aware that the hot flashes were occurring approximately once an hour, they no longer bothered me because their effect was diminished to such a degree they no longer caused me distress.

At my last visit to the doctor he asked how long I had been taking this treatment and there was a significant pause when I answered that it must be all of 10 years. The doctor I consulted up until recently has moved away. Over the years I have made attempts to stop taking HRT, each time being full of hope there would no longer be any need to keep on with it, but within a week the hot flashes would return. I have got to the stage I would prefer not to take it, largely because a thrombosis has developed in my leg and I remember reading that HRT is contraindicated if one is prone to clotting.

There are other possible remedies for hot flashes. Some women find regular acupuncture helpful, and clonidine (brand name Dixarit), a drug also used to lower blood pressure, can reduce the dilatation in the blood vessels that precedes a hot flash. It can be used orally or via a skin patch. There have been mixed reports about how effective it is. Clonidine can also cause a range of side effects including a dry mouth, tiredness, dizziness, and constipation. Other hormone treatments are with progestogen drugs such as norethisterone or medroxyprogesterone acetate.

Many women find ways of coping with hot flashes by wearing layered clothing so they can peel them off to cool down quickly. Avoiding situations that provoke hot flashes, such as stress, rushing around, confined spaces, spicy foods, and too much coffee, are all ways of reducing the incidence of flashes. A thermos of cold water beside the bed can help with nighttime sweats. Rosetta Reitz's book *Menopause: A Positive Approach* and Linda Ojeda's *Menopause Without Medicine* both contain many suggestions for ways of helping with hot flashes and other menopausal symptoms.(30)

Vaginal problems and sexual interest

Dryness and fragility of the tissue in the vagina similarly respond well to estrogen treatment in any form, including vaginal creams. Estrogen, taken even some years after the menopause, can improve the vaginal tissues. Bladder problems and increased bacterial infections resulting from thin vaginal walls may also be helped by HRT. If painful intercourse has been caused by vaginal dryness, this should be alleviated by HRT, and if the woman has lost interest in sex because of these difficulties, she will perhaps regain her libido when her physical problems are solved. If her disinterest in sex has other causes, hormones will not help.

The Chelsea Hospital researchers found that while estrogen taken orally did improve vaginal dryness, there was no difference in libido. They commented: "The ability to have sexual intercourse and the desire to have sexual intercourse, of both the patient and her husband, do not seem to be related."(31) Jean Coope's findings were similar. She found that the small group of women who had suffered from dryness of the vagina and painful sex improved greatly on oral HRT, but that none of the women reported an increase in libido and four said it was reduced.(32)

Several studies have shown that women who continue regular sexual activity after menopause usually have less discomfort and less thinning of the vaginal walls. Put crudely, you've got to use it or lose it. Sexual activity can be with a female partner, a male partner, or masturbation. Rosetta Reitz has a very useful discussion of sex after menopause in her book. Women who stop intercourse for some time and then resume it can have special problems. After a period of abstinence, intercourse should be resumed gradually to give the vagina a chance to adjust. KY Jelly and other commercial lubricants such as Sylke can be used to lubricate the vagina, as can plain ordinary saliva.

Psychological symptoms

There is no clear proof that HRT can directly alleviate the psychological symptoms often put down to menopause and discussed in Chapter 4. A number of studies have been carried out to see if HRT improves mood, with differing results, but many of these studies suffer from methodological laws. The selection of subjects and the failure to match for menopausal status, the inclusion of women who have had surgical menopause, and the small size of the studies makes it difficult to take any firm conclusions from them.(33) Because of this lack of proof, drug companies are not allowed to claim psychological or antiaging benefits for hormone replacement therapy in their advertising.

Dr. Wulf Utian summarizes that "Contrary to popular opinion . . . the number and variety of direct, true hormone related effects are fewer than generally assumed."(34) Of these, he lists vasomotor effects, vaginal changes, and vertebral osteoporosis. Psychosociocultural symptoms such as depression, irritability, insomnia, frigidity, headache, and apprehension, he calls nonspecific symptoms. He then goes on to say: "It therefore follows that a case can be made for hormonal treatment of specific symptoms but not for the nonspecific ones."

Jean Coope carried out a double-blind randomized trial of estrogen with 55 clinically depressed menopausal women.(35) She put the women into two matched groups, comparable for depression scores, and each tried both estrogen and placebos without knowing when they were getting which. She found that both groups improved significantly, irrespective of the therapy, as did the patients' own assessment of well-being. Even when they were switched from hormones to placebo, the women maintained their level of improvement. The ineffectiveness of HRT for depression was highlighted by the fact that two women were admitted to hospital for severe depressive illness while they were in the estrogen arm of the trial.

Despite the lack of direct scientific evidence, some doctors talk about estrogen having a "mental tonic effect," and some women say that they "feel better" on it. This woman, who did not have any symptoms before starting HRT, is convinced that HRT enhances her enjoyment of life. She has been part of the research program at Chelsea Hospital in London:

> "It's the change," my mother would say from the time I was about eight, about the migraines, the long stays in bed, and periods of crying. So I cooked regularly and it seems interminably for the seven of us and grew up determined to do all I could to avoid such a debilitating heritage. When I was living in London and approaching 40, I read Wendy Cooper's *No Change* and felt pleased to accept personal responsibility for requesting, administering, and checking any treatment that would prevent osteoporosis, hair on my face, and loss of energy or independence.
>
> My GP seemed alarmed and dismissive, saying she would rather treat my symptoms than mess around with hormones. Finally I went to the menopause clinic at the Chelsea Hospital. Years later I read the notes written by the doctor I first saw there: "This neurotic woman will continue to visit doctor after doctor until she gets what she wants. Prescribed HRT for three months."
>
> The follow-up visit coincided with my return from six weeks' holiday and I remember telling her I felt euphoric. Whether it

was the medication or the holiday, she declared "It obviously suits you" and prescribed six months Premarin.

My mother died at 85 from pneumonia after surgery for a broken bone! It's not only the fears of osteoporosis that concern me now, it is also losing the extra energy that I associate with the original absorption of HRT, particularly the emotional energy of which I seem to have an abundant excess compared to others of my age who often seem to be tired before 10:30 PM. I'll remain a supporter till the indications become more contrary.

Jean Coope reported that 22 of the 30 women in one of her studies said they felt a sense of well-being on HRT and that this often resulted in an improvement in their relationship with their husband.(36) The Chelsea Hospital researchers felt that this improvement in well-being was most likely the domino effect—"the cumulative effect of these small improvements results in an overall enhancement of well-being"; but they too wondered if estrogen could have a "direct tonic effect on the mental state."

Dr. Robert Greenblatt suggests that "Symptoms such as nervousness, depression, insomnia, migrainoid headaches, loss of sexual drive and dyspareunia [painful intercourse] may not be hormone dependent but are frequently hormone responsive."(37) In other words, although these psychological effects may not be caused by loss of estrogen, giving estrogen may help alleviate them. Such a claim is hard to prove. It is generally agreed that depression and nervous symptoms without vasomotor symptoms will not be helped by HRT, whereas these symptoms accompanying hot flashes or vaginal dryness may be.

This 45-year-old woman reported an improvement in her mental state. Her experience provides some support for Dr. John Studd's theory that menopausal mental problems may be a continuation of PMS, or for Dr. Whitehead's view that menopause and PMS are muddled.

I came off the Pill because of high blood pressure and after about 18 months I was bleeding all the time and I had really bad PMS. I was irritable, grumpy, and couldn't get on top of things. At one school I was teaching at, the children would get sent to an "adjustment room" if they were misbehaving. It suddenly dawned on me that one week in every four, my name appeared over and over. During that week, I couldn't handle kids who normally I would manage perfectly all right.

The doctor took a blood test and said I was going through menopause. I was having some hot flashes about every day. He said there was something he could put me onto—he didn't tell me what it was. I went looking in a bookshop and found *The Amarant Book of Hormone Replacement Therapy* which told me something about it.

As soon as I started taking the hormones, all my depression went. I felt like a whole new person. I now feel as if I can cope with life a lot better. When teaching, I stay calm, which means the children don't get upset and everything's much better. The doctor said I could stay on it for 10 years; I just thought if it works, I'll stay on it.

This woman who had had a hysterectomy and so wasn't menstruating has a similar story. She was experiencing headaches and a tightness in her head. It is thought that symptoms such as these may be caused by the withdrawal of estrogen. Women also report this symptom during PMS when estrogen levels fall.

I was tried with antidepressants which did absolutely nothing . . . sleeping tablets were added . . . some weeks later I began getting "overheated" (not the traditional hot flashes). I would be hot during the day for patches, then the same at night. So after a few days of this I decided to go back to the doctor and suggest that it wasn't antidepressants I needed but some hormone replacement. He agreed. This did the trick in a couple of weeks.

Skin and hair

You have only to think about men to realize that thinning hair has little to do with menopause! Thinning hair is primarily a result of aging. If any hormone plays a part, it is the male hormone testosterone that can affect the thickness and quality of hair. One woman who is now in her sixties and who has been on hormones for 10 years wrote: "Recently I read that estrogen prevents hair loss, but I have found this to be untrue, as recently my hair has become noticeably thinner."

As we get older our skin tends to become drier and thinner and to lose its elasticity, causing wrinkles. There are multiple causes of this, including loss of the supporting fiber or collagen in the skin, a decrease in skin thickness, less activity in the sebaceous glands that provide oil to the skin, and lessening of the ability of the skin cells to retain water. These changes begin well before menopause, at about the age of 30.

The evidence about skin and estrogen is mixed, but only extreme enthusiasts for hormones claim that estrogen can halt aging or set the clock back. Despite this, women are frequently told through women's magazines that estrogen will have miraculous effects on their appearance. This is an extremely seductive claim to make to women who may be worried about "losing their looks." In early 1991 a *New Zealand Woman's Day* article contained a statement by Dr. Sandra Cabot, the author of a handbook of women's health, that "many women have found that hormone replacement therapy makes them feel younger and more beautiful."(38) Note that Dr. Cabot does not say that the women actually look younger or more beautiful, only that they "feel" it. Nevertheless, readers will have been given the impression that estrogen is a kind of "youth drug."

Most studies looking at estrogen and skin have not shown a benefit, whether it is used in oral form or as a cream. Those who claim estrogen can benefit skin maintain it may reduce the rate of collagen loss or plump up the skin by increasing fluid retention. This is a double-edged sword because many women say they dislike the bloating that can result from HRT.

Extreme estrogen advocates, such as the Amarant Trust, are adamant that women have improved looks on HRT. Commenting on this, a British writer said:

> Unfortunately, the benefits of HRT are still being oversold, especially by a woman MP who has recently set up a private clinic offering hormone replacement therapy. She is eager to show photographs of herself before and after HRT, for she claims it has transformed her life. It probably has, but one medical newspaper observed sarcastically that HRT also seems to have given her a facelift and a new hairdo and has enabled her to lose several pounds in weight and to throw away her glasses.(39)

In *Women and the Crisis in Sex Hormones*, Barbara and Gideon Seaman noted that women on HRT often imagined they looked younger than they did.(40) The women's own assessment of their youthful appearance did not always coincide with the opinion of a more detached observer. The Seamans went to a local gym and asked to talk to women about using or not using estrogen: "The curious thing was that ERT users imagined they looked young for their ages, but in fact did not. On the other hand, the women who did rely on ERT but instead were very conscientious about exercise and diet were (in our opinion) deceptively young looking."

The Chelsea Hospital researchers found that women believed their skin improved and they looked younger even when they were on placebos! They said that "no reliance should be placed on patient judgment of skin texture and appearance in the evaluation of estrogen therapy."

In the patient insert for Premarin, Ayerst Laboratories had this to say about estrogen's effect on appearance:

> You may have heard that taking estrogens for long periods (years) after the menopause will keep your skin soft and supple and keep you feeling young. There is no evidence that this is so, however, and such long-term treatment carries important risks.

Apart from genetic inheritance, the real culprits in skin deterioration are sun damage, accumulated over a lifetime, and smoking—both self-inflicted. Late nights, air-conditioned and overheated environments, overwork, poor diet, anxiety, and ill health all take their toll on appearance. Attention to these, plus liberal use of skin creams and bath oils, exercise in the fresh air, and an adequate intake of water each day are a woman's best way of looking after her skin.

HRT and Osteoporosis

Estrogen is undeniably effective at preventing bone loss in a significant proportion of women, but this does not mean that most women should be taking it to prevent osteoporosis. First of all, we need to recognize the difference between slowing bone loss and preventing fractures, and then we need to take a hard look at the safety implications of using hormones for decades at a time.

A curious fact emerges when you wade through the medical literature on the relationship between HRT and osteoporosis. The doctors whose work is used to argue for the widespread use of estrogen as a prevention do not recommend it themselves. If you read what they say, you find that they are cautious about the use of estrogen. Nevertheless, despite their own considered views, their work gets used to support the case for estrogen. The same thing has happened with bone density screening: research showing the effectiveness of bone density tests in predicting fractures has been used to argue for screening among the population at large, even though the researchers themselves do not recommend this.

This pattern is not unique to this particular area of medicine. The findings of research scientists often get interpreted differently at the clinical level. In the process, the issues can become oversimplified and depicted as more black and white than they are. Also, findings favorable to particular drugs are often exploited by pharmaceutical companies to encourage the sales of their products.

What the Bone Experts Think

Research scientists maintain that estrogen may be advised for women with definite indications, such as young women who have lost their ovaries; but they disagree on whether it is advisable for larger numbers of women. Dr. Bruce Ettinger, a prominent researcher in this area, agrees that estrogen is effective but also says that the majority of women do not need it: "It definitely works, but you're talking about taking hormones for 10 years—maybe 20 to 30 years—to prevent a largely asymptomatic, self-limited disease. And what are you offering—the risk of endometrial cancer? Lifelong periods? Endometrial biopsies?"(41)

Dr. Lawrence Riggs of the Mayo Clinic says: "Estrogen is a potentially dangerous drug with significant side effects, no matter what anyone says."(42) Joseph Melton, David Eddy, and Conrad Johnston, who wrote what is currently considered to be the definitive paper on screening for osteoporosis, concluded: "Because estrogen replacement therapy entails risks and costs, it should be used only for women who are most likely to benefit."(43)

Dr. Robert Lindsay, one of the foremost researchers of osteoporosis, agrees that "it's dangerous to think of long-term therapy for a large segment of the population." His preferred prevention strategy is exercise and diet.(44) Another proponent of exercise and diet is Dr. Morris Notelovitz, a well-known researcher of estrogen's effect on bone:

If viewed simplistically, postmenopausal osteoporosis is a relatively easy condition to predict and prevent: it is well established that estrogen deficiency per se contributes significantly to bone loss, and that estrogen replacement decreases bone loss and protects against osteoporosis-related fractures. A simple expedient would be to treat all postmenopausal women with estrogen. However, when one considers the physiology of bone formation and loss, it soon becomes apparent that there is much more to postmenopausal osteoporosis than estrogen replacement. For example, consider the fact that black women are relatively immune to osteoporosis, yet they, too, are subject to the same hormonal changes of the senescent ovary. . . . Central to the entire issue is the fact that bone is a living organ and needs to be treated as such.(45)

A group of Danish researchers who showed a beneficial effect of HRT on bone also argued against its widespread use:

Although epidemiological evidence would encourage prophylactic treatment with hormones on a wider scale, considerable skepticism is appropriate. Bone density and bone mass are not the only determinants of crush fractures—for example, many patients with crush fractures have normal vertebral bone mass. Vertebral bone elasticity might also be a factor. The compressive strength of vertebral bodies decreases with age, possibly independently of bone mass. A prerequisite for a more widespread use of hormonal prophylaxis against osteoporosis should be longitudinal studies, of longer duration, of the effects and side effects of different combinations and doses of hormones.(46)

Can hormones halt bone loss . . .

Before starting on this discussion it is important to stress that virtually all the research discussed below looked at unopposed therapy using estrogen by itself rather than estrogen/progestogen combinations. These findings cannot automatically be applied to combined therapy, despite the fact that today this is the most used form of HRT. Firm evidence that modern opposed therapy will prevent fractures is scanty.

Many trials comparing estrogens and placebos have shown that estrogen can halt or slow the loss of bone mass in postmenopause.(47) Some recent studies have also shown that there can be an increase in bone mineral density when HRT is started a number of years after menopause, even where a woman has very low mineral density or vertebral fractures. (48)

. . . and fractures?

The evidence that estrogen can prevent fractures, especially hip fractures, has been obtained indirectly, through epidemiological studies, and is less firm than the data on the prevention of bone loss. Most of these studies were conducted some time ago, and some have methodological flaws. There has been very little recent work on reduction of fractures.

The best way of attaining the proof needed would be to follow matched groups of treated and untreated women from menopause into the age groups when fractures are known to occur. This is possible for vertebral fractures, which occur earlier in the postmenopause, but is not feasible for hip fractures, the peak incidence of which is 30 years or more after menopause. There is also some argument whether such a trial would be ethical, because it would involve doing nothing about women who had been identified as having low bone mass.

Consequently, prospective trials are few and far between. The only randomized controlled trial was carried out by Robert Lindsay in the late 1970s.(49) This showed that oophorectomized women using estrogen were much less likely to suffer vertebral fractures than women in the placebo group. But oophorectomized women are different from women who have had a natural menopause: the former's estrogen is drastically reduced and without hormone therapy these women would be expected to do very badly. Consequently, one could anticipate a big difference between treated and nontreated groups of such women. These results have been widely quoted in support of estrogen, even though the authors themselves caution that oophorectomized women are not representative of all postmenopausal women.

Dr. Bruce Ettinger carried out a retrospective study in an American retirement community which compared the fracture rate in postmenopausal estrogen users identified from prescriptions with matched nonestrogen users.(50) This study suggested that long-term estrogen use could lead to a 50% reduction in fracture incidence in the spine. Estrogen users had 2.5% crush fractures compared to 6.6% in untreated women.

Because of the impossibility of carrying out prospective trials on estrogen's effect on hip fracture, epidemiological work using different study designs has been carried out on this relationship. Case control studies match people who have had hip fractures with similar people who have not. Then the researchers compare the hormone use of the people with fractures with the hormone use of people who have not had fractures.

Many of these studies are far from perfect. There is a persistent failure to differentiate between different types of menopause, whether natural or surgical, which can bias the results, and there can be other problems in design, such as inaccurate recall of estrogen use and the inclusion of few women over 75.(51) Much more is known today about good study design than was known in the 1970s when most of these studies were carried out.

One widely quoted study had only 7 users among the cases and 10 among the controls, which are very small figures from which to come to a firm conclusion.(52) Another much-used study showed a 50–60% reduction.(53) However, this was primarily with continuing or recent long-term use and the study has been criticized for flaws in design, such as the selection of cases.(54) This lack of firmness in the data should lead to some caution about using the results to argue for the widespread long-term use of HRT.

Nevertheless, a number of studies have shown that the women who don't have hip fractures are more likely to have used estrogen. The combined results from 11 observational studies indicated that the risk of hip fracture was about 25% lower among women who had ever used HRT, mainly estrogen therapy. This review also concluded that once women discontinued estrogen they lost any benefit 6 or more years after stopping the therapy.(55) Several studies have shown that estrogen is most beneficial to women who have lost their ovaries and that current use and recent use provide the most protection—the protection dwindles with time after using HRT.(56)

In late 1993 the long-running Massachusetts Framingham Study provided fresh evidence that HRT is not the panacea for fractures it is sometimes claimed to be. This study has been following a group of women who were 30–62 years old when they enrolled in the late 1940s. These women have continued to have regular health checks as part of the study; all their health records are available, the researchers know how many of the women have had hip fractures, and they also know when they had menopause and whether they have used estrogen. This study is important because it is one of the very few to look at the effect of HRT on older women, and it is older women who have hip fractures.(57) The median age for hip fractures in women in America is 80 years.

The researchers found that bone mineral density was definitely higher in women less that 75 years of age who had received long-term estrogen. However, the beneficial effect of estrogen waned with age, so that by the time the women reached the age of greatest fracture risk almost all the benefit had disappeared.

The researchers said that at least seven years of estrogen was needed to have a long-term effect on bone density, but that only one-third of the women in their study who used it stayed on that long. The benefit of seven years or more use persisted until the age of 75 but did not persist beyond that age. In women more than 75 years of age there was little difference in bone density between women who had used estrogen and those who had not.

Reviewing this study, Bruce Ettinger and Dr. Deborah Grady commented that "estrogen treatment for 5–10 years soon after menopause is unlikely to preserve bone density or to prevent fractures in old age." In light of this they said that clinicians might recommend lifelong treatment with hormones after menopause, "but having to take estrogen for the rest of one's life reduces the appeal of this preventive strategy." The other possibility is that estrogen treatment could be started later—at about the age of 70— and continued for life. However, this has not yet been studied.

Another recent large study by Swedish researchers took a cohort of women (over 23,000) all aged over 35, who had been prescribed estrogen in the late 1970s.(58) Over a five-year period the researchers checked the names of all women admitted to hospitals for hip fractures against the names of the women in the study. This ratio was then compared with the known rate of hip fracture among the general population. The results showed that women using potent estrogens (estrone, estradiol) had a 40–60% reduction in hip fracture. The reduction in risk was highest for women who started using hormones before 60 years of age and for current users.

This study was one of several to include women using estrogen/progestogen combinations. A reduction in risk was suggested with these preparations also, although since the numbers were small, the evidence was not as firm. The study showed once again that the reduction in risk diminished as women discontinued using hormone replacement therapy and that women users of HRT were over three times more likely than women in the population at large to have had an oophorectomy and more than twice as likely to have had a hysterectomy.

Impact on individual women

The idea that estrogen can prevent fractures needs to approached with caution, because for individual women a key issue is: what is my risk in the first place? Most of the studies include women at both high and low risk of fracture. The benefit to an individual woman will not be nearly as great if she is not at high risk of fracture to begin with. The lifetime risk of hip fracture for low-risk women is 4%, and of any kind of vertebral fracture, 14%. If there is a 35% reduction in risk for hip fracture and a 50% reduction in risk of vertebral fracture after long-term use of HRT, the risk for a low-risk woman would reduce to 3% and 7% respectively. A reduction in this already low risk is not a lot of gain for years of hormone therapy, with *its* attendant risks. And over 70% of all women are in this category.

A recent analysis looked at how many extra quality years a woman using estrogen could expect to gain. This analysis took into account the benefits of estrogen on bones and hearts, and the risk to the uterus. It calculated that 15 years of estrogen-only therapy in a 50-year-old woman was associated with an additional two-thirds quality-adjusted years of life.(59) In other words, eight months extra life in return for 15 years of hormones. These researchers had proceeded from the assumption that estrogen therapy gave prolonged benefit even after it was stopped, a somewhat arguable proposition. If the benefit of therapy decreases by 50% after treatment stops, the gain is two months; if the benefit of therapy is restricted to the period of use, as some of the studies suggest, the gain would be one month.

This analysis did not take into account the addition of progestogen, which would reduce the endometrial cancer risk but possibly increase the cardiovascular risk. It has to be remembered that extra months of life might not be the only benefits of HRT taken to prevent osteoporosis. For high-risk women, hormones will also reduce the risk of disability arising from the worst effects of osteoporosis.

What happens to bone after HRT stops?

Once hormone therapy is stopped, bone loss commences again. What the hormones have done is effectively delay bone loss rather than stop it forever. The delay buys time—time to die before our bones can go below the fracture threshold, if they were ever destined to do so.

A major unresolved issue is the speed of the bone loss after women stop HRT. There have been conflicting results from studies looking at what happens to bone in women who stop estrogen, which has implications for the amount of time women are urged to stay on HRT. The uncertainty about this point is behind recommendations to women that they stay on HRT indefinitely.

One study by Robert Lindsay showed an accelerated post-treatment bone loss in oophorectomized women, which reached pre-treatment levels in a time interval as short as four years (see the graph below).(60) This study led to some loss of confidence in estrogen's

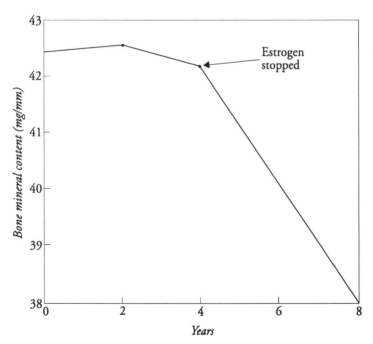

Effect of Withdrawal of Estrogen on Bone Mineral Content after Four Years of Treatment

(Source: Adapted from Lindsay, et al. 1978)

preventive powers. A Leeds group also had similar results.(61) They compared what happened to bone density when they withdrew estrogen from a group of users, and calcium supplements from another group of women. The women using estrogen lost bone density at a much sharper rate than the calcium users. These researchers postulated that estrogen might stimulate the parathyroid glands, leaving them in a prolonged overactive state when the hormone is withdrawn, so that too much bone-resorbing PTH is being secreted.

A Danish crossover study contradicted these findings. Naturally-menopausal women were put on either HRT or placebos, then reversed after two years. The women who had used HRT who were then given placebos did start to lose bone, but they had made a net gain of 8% of bone mass over women who had never had HRT at all, although the follow-up time of 12 months was probably too short to see the full effect of the withdrawal of hormones on bones.(61)

Other unresolved questions

Estrogen may provide a reduction in the likelihood of a fracture; it does not provide a guarantee one will never occur. As we saw in the chapter on osteoporosis, fractures are more than a matter of low bone density. Hormones will not stop us from falling. Added to that, Robert Lindsay says that treatment with estrogen "does not entirely preclude the presence of osteoporosis in some women".(63)

Most of the research in this area has been carried out for estrogens alone. It has been hypothesized that progestogen will not negate the benefit of estrogen to the bone. Some small studies have addressed the issue of the effectiveness of combined therapy in preventing bone loss. Most of this work has been carried out in Northern Europe; a Danish study using both serial and continuous opposed therapy showed a gain in bone in the spine after one year.(64) So far only one observational study and one small randomized control trial using doses of estrogen two to four times higher than those used today have suggested a reduction in hip fractures in women using combined therapy.(65)

The Auckland study that showed loss of bone density in Depo Provera users throws some doubt on the proposition that progestogen will not modify the benefit of estrogen on bones. Depo Provera contains medroxyprogesterone acetate, and it is uncertain whether results from studies using other progestogens can be applied to Provera. It is generally acknowledged that much more work needs to be done to find out what adding progestogen to HRT will do.

It is also not clear what hormones taken transdermally will do for bones. Very short studies have indicated that estrogen taken this way will prevent bone loss, but more work needs to be done.(66)

The need to take HRT long term, if not permanently, is highly controversial. When women take HRT for menopause, they need to take it only for months or at the most one or two years. This will be insufficient to protect against bone loss and coronary heart disease, which will be discussed next. Yet everything we know so far about the risks of HRT points to the fact that the risks increase with duration of use. This is the dilemma faced by women contemplating using HRT. Very little is known about HRT's long-term risks because the studies simply haven't been done. Added to that, the side effects of HRT use, especially periods, may become less tolerable as the years go by.

HRT and Hearts

Headlines such as "estrogen helps to promote longer life" are beginning to sneak their way into newspapers and magazines as coronary heart disease is appropriated as another reason for women to use hormones. Although men are far more likely than women to die of heart disease, it is now being redefined as yet another symptom of menopause, caused by the withdrawal of estrogen.

Because premenopausal women are far less likely than men the same age to suffer from coronary heart disease, some people have assumed women must be protected by their hormones and that this protection will be lost at menopause. This biological cause is disputed by many scientists who point out that sociological factors, such as lifestyle and access to health services, could explain the rise in incidence among women in their older years.

Although heart disease is a leading cause of death in older women, the risk of heart disease does not suddenly increase at menopause. The risk to women only increases rapidly in the third and fourth decades after menopause. About three-quarters of all coronary heart disease deaths and myocardial infarctions (heart attacks) occur after the age of 75 years.

It is largely gynecologists who are promoting the idea of coronary heart disease as a menopausal symptom and arguing for the use of HRT. Many cardiologists—the experts on hearts—are skeptical about the hormonal argument. They say that the drugs proven to benefit hearts should be the first choice of prevention and treatment, not hormones. Other scientists also warn that HRT should not be put into widescale use to prevent coronary heart disease before a benefit has been proven in well-designed prospective studies.

But because some less-than-perfect studies have shown estrogen users to have less heart disease, proponents of HRT see this as compelling reason for women to use it, overshadowing any possible increase in breast cancer or endometrial cancer risk.

The "odd couple" of plasma

To understand how hormones may affect cardiovascular risk, first we need to look at the biological processes at work in heart disease. Saturated animal fat in the diet, and to a lesser extent cholesterol, increase the risk of coronary heart disease. Cholesterol is taken up from the intestine and transported around the body in the bloodstream attached to fatty substances called plasma lipoproteins. There are several classes of lipoprotein. The two important ones for hormones are low density lipoproteins (LDL) and high density lipoproteins (HDL). These two are called the "odd couple" of plasma, as they have an interacting but antagonistic function.

LDL-cholesterol transports serum cholesterol from the liver to body cells, while HDL-cholesterol collects excess cholesterol from body cells and carries it to the liver to be excreted. High levels of serum cholesterol are associated with coronary heart disease, so LDL-cholesterol level is directly associated with increased risk.

On the other hand, HDL-cholesterol is inversely related to coronary heart disease risk: an increased HDL-cholesterol level lessens the chance of heart attack. Women are fortunate to have higher levels of the protective HDL-cholesterol than men.

LDL-cholesterol increases as people age so their coronary heart disease risk increases, although more so in men than in women, and in women who have lost both their ovaries.(68) A low-fat diet, weight reduction, stopping smoking, and exercise can all decrease LDL-cholesterol.

If estrogen has a beneficial effect on coronary heart disease, and as we shall see it is by no means certain that it has, it probably acts by increasing HDL-cholesterol and reducing LDL-cholesterol levels.

The type, strength of dose, and route by which the estrogen is taken may matter here. Ethinylestradiol and conjugated estrogens at their highest dose (1.25 mg) may have more effect than estradiol valerate or conjugated estrogen at lower doses. Some studies have shown no beneficial effect or a weaker effect from estrogen applied through the skin, as patches or gel, or given as implants, but most of these studies have been of very short duration.(69)

There is also the complicating factor of progestogen. Progestogen can decrease HDL-cholesterol and elevate LDL-cholesterol and thus may partly or entirely cancel out any protective effect of estrogen, or, worse, increase the risk of coronary heart disease. Different progestogens could also have varying effects. It is thought that testosterone-derived progestogens (norithisterone and levonorgestrel) may reduce HDL-cholesterol levels, while progesterone types such as medroxyprogesterone acetate may exert a less detrimental effect on lipoproteins. We saw in the previous chapters that several newer types of progestogen may also avoid adversely affecting lipoproteins.

There is also the question of what might be happening to lipoproteins when HRT is given every day as a continuous therapy with estrogen and progestogen. If both HDL-cholesterol and LDL-cholesterol are reduced or are elevated, it is not clear what effect this would have on cardiovascular disease. In one study (using norethisterone) that looked at this question, both LDL-cholesterol and HDL-cholesterol decreased.(70)

Problems in the studies

In any case, this entire scenario is highly speculative. No one is really clear what is going on at a biological level. It has been suggested that estrogen might act directly on artery walls, allowing an increased blood flow.(71) The main argument for the protective effect of estrogen has come from epidemiological studies that have looked at the incidence of coronary heart disease among users of estrogen. Despite the fact that there have been more than 80 of these published in English alone, there is no unequivocal answer to the question of whether estrogen protects hearts. There have been no well-designed large prospective trials to provide answers.

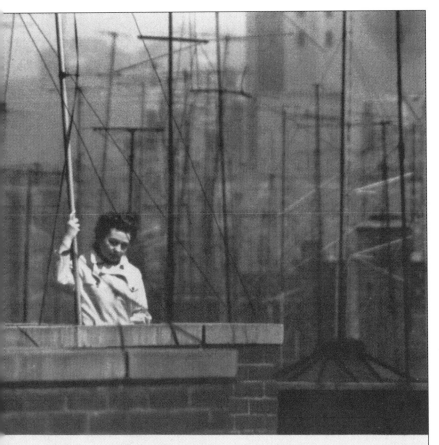

When "change of life" seems the end of life...

With the advancing years, woman's vulnerability to depression often becomes intense. The future looms insecure; menopausal dysfunctions spark somatic concern. And as she faces losing a symbol of femininity, even suicidal panic may supervene.

Menopausal depression has been lifted by Marplan—even when withdrawal and loss of affect were severe.

Episodes of depression can often be controlled by a brief schedule of Marplan treatment, ordinarily 10 mg t.i.d. In some patients, release of new psychic energies may be seen on Marplan in as little as three or four days.

Extensive clinical trials have revealed no hepatitis attributable to Marplan. However, complete dosage information, available on request, should be consulted before administering Marplan.

Supplied: 10-mg tablets in bottles of 100 and 1000.

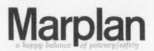

Marplan
a happy balance of potency/safety

MARPLAN®—1-benzyl-2-(5-methyl-3-isoxazolylcarbonyl)hydrazine

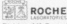 **ROCHE** LABORATORIES
Division of Hoffmann-La Roche Inc.

A cause for suicide: menopause as seen in the medical world in 1960.

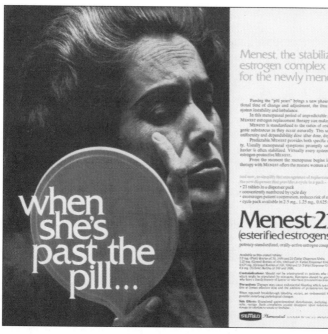

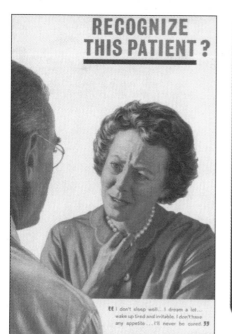
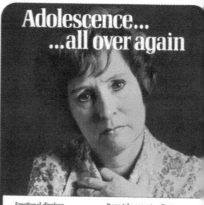

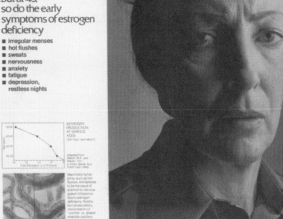

LIFE BEGINS AT FORTY

...but at 45, so do the early symptoms of estrogen deficiency

- irregular menses
- hot flushes
- sweats
- nervousness
- anxiety
- fatigue
- depression, restless nights

Just at the time a woman should be looking forward to one of the most enjoyable periods of her life, her ovarian function begins to wane. And with this waning comes a decreasing supply of estrogen and often the distressing clinical symptoms of estrogen deficiency.

At the age of menopause, primary symptoms are most frequently vasomotor in nature, including the classic flushes and sweats, paresthesias, and palpitations. A number of emotional complaints may also be related to menopausal estrogen deficiency. Usually the appearance of anxiety, nervousness, depression, headache, and insomnia is, at the time of menopause correlates fairly well with declining estrogen levels.

See last page of advertisement for prescribing information.

Here and overleaf: the face of the "untreated" woman, according to the drug companies. These advertisements from the 1950s and 1960s for hormones and tranquilizers depict her as anxious and emotionally out of control. The Premarin advertisement—"Life Begins at Forty"—includes one of Robert Wilson's graphs.

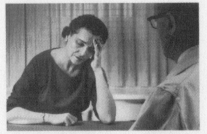

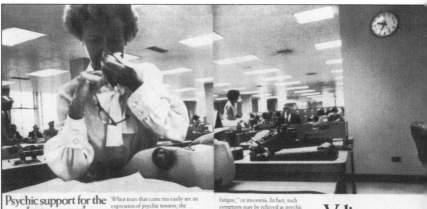
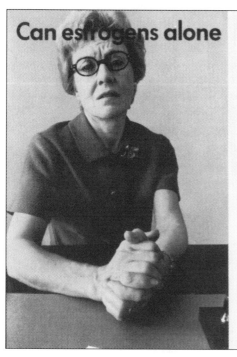

Menrium treats the menopausal symptoms that bother him most.

His wife has a lot of different menopausal symptoms, but only a few really irritate him. Her hot flashes, her vertigo, her palpitations—that's *her* problem. What really bothers him is her nervousness, her irritability and her excessive anxiety, often expressed by endless "book-shuffling, chain-smoking, reading-lamp" insomnia!

Menrium takes care of hot flashes, vertigo, palpitations in most menopausal women. Menrium provides the well-known antianxiety action of chlordiazepoxide (Librium®) and water-soluble esterified estrogens. It therefore relieves more symptoms than either component separately. It takes care of the vasomotor symptoms as well as the emotional symptoms. This means the symptoms that bother his wife most. And the symptoms that irritate him most.

So, to help them both get through *her* menopause, remember Menrium.

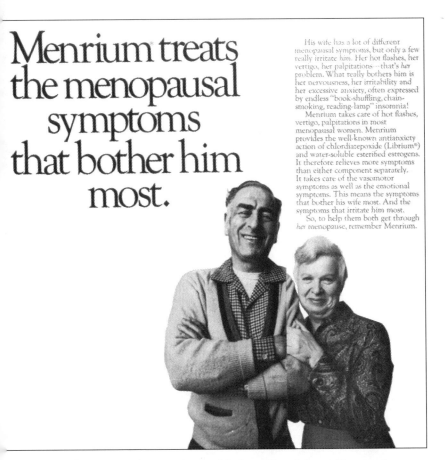

The "treated" menopausal woman is a trouble-free wife and devoted homemaker, unlike the "untreated" woman, who is not only at war with herself but a burden to all around her.

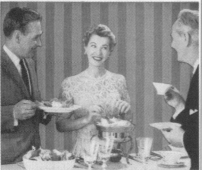
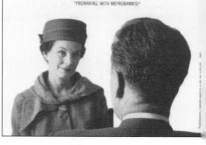
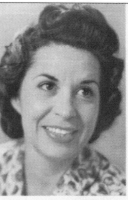
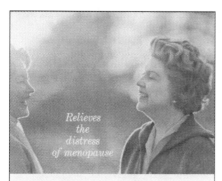

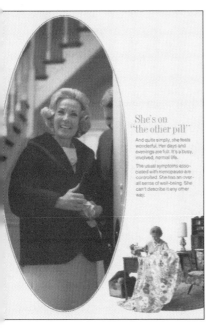

She's on
"the other pill"

And quite simply, she feels
wonderful. Her days and
evenings are full. It's a busy,
involved, normal life.

The usual symptoms asso-
ciated with menopause are
controlled. She has an overall sense of well-being. She
can't describe it any other
way.

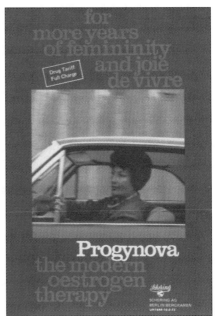

for
more years
of femininity
and joie
de vivre

Progynova

the modern
oestrogen
therapy

Faces of "treated" women from the 1950s
to the 1970s. All these women have been
"cured" by tranquilizers, hormones, or
cocktails of both. The advertisements
make great play of the idea that
hormones give "a sense of well-being,"
make women "feel better," and have a
sense of "joie de vivre."

   "She's on 'the other pill'," enthuses the
Ogen advertisement (above), "and quite
simply, she feels wonderful . . . She has an
overall sense of well-being. She can't
describe it any other way."

   The image of the woman in the car
from the Schering advertisement (above
right), symbolizes freedom and
confidence. The same image was used in
the 1930s to sell cigarettes.

   The happy woman (right) is the
"treated" version of the woman in the
"Life Begins at Forty" advertisement. In
the 1990s the idea that hormones can
induce "a sense of well-being" has been
adopted by the medical profession as a
justification for estrogen's use. The same
slogan could equally be applied to
smoking pot or drinking alcohol.

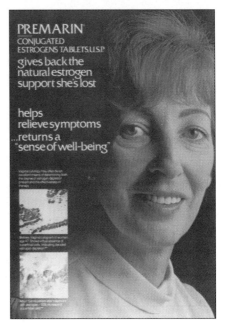

PREMARIN
CONJUGATED
ESTROGENS TABLETS U.S.P
gives back the
natural estrogen
support she's lost

helps
relieve symptoms
...returns a
"sense of well-being"

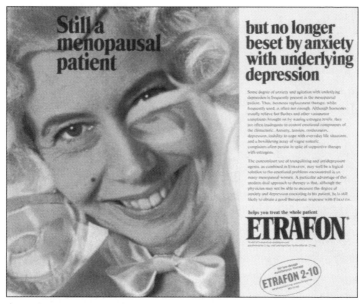

Spot the difference! The face of the menopausal woman (above) cured of anxiety and depression by amitryptiline is indistinguishable from the face of the uncured woman below who gives as indications for treatment (says Merck Sharp & Dohme): dressing "to look too young," nail-biting, and "over-plucked eyebrows."

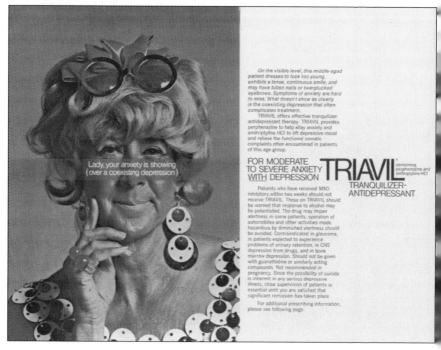

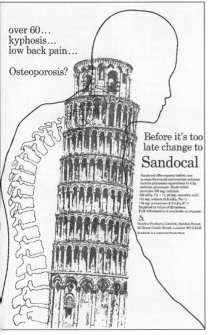

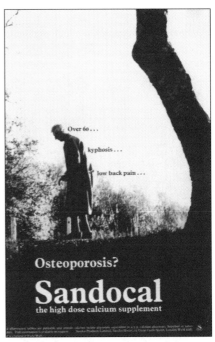

The person with the spinal kyphosis is genderless in these advertisements for calcium supplements from the 1960s (above). The companies marketing hormones, however, have succeeded in redefining the osteoporosis sufferer as a woman. The advertisement by Ayerst for the "littler" old lady marks the beginning of the process.

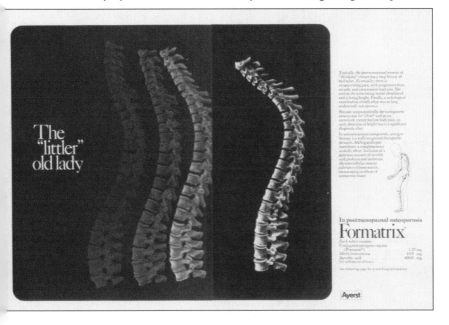

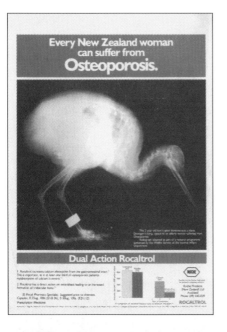

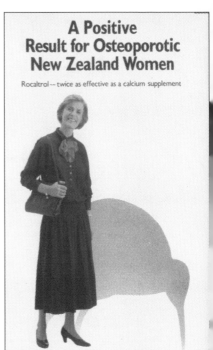

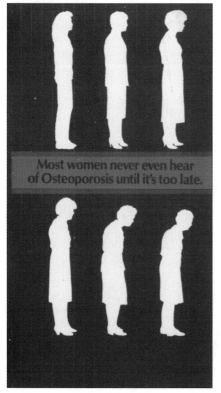

As shown in these advertisements for calcium supplements and vitamin D3, the bent-up old lady has become the key symbol of the New Zealand campaign to encourage people to see osteoporosis as a common health problem.

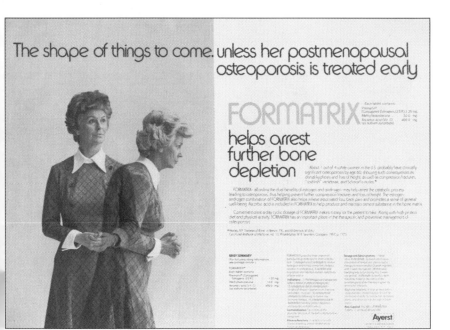

Who took the lead here? The advertisement for the U.S. National Osteoporosis Foundation from 1990 uses the same slogan ("The shape of things to come . . . ") and image as the Ayerst advertisement for estrogen from the 1970s.

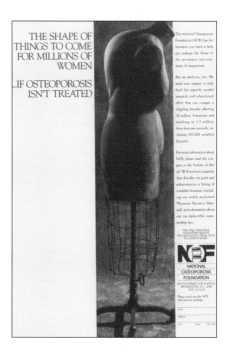

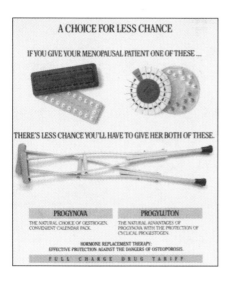

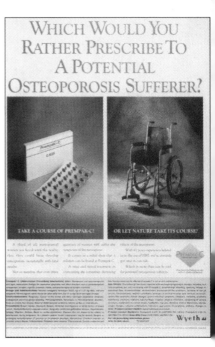

In these advertisements from the 1990s, the wheelchair and crutches are emerging as the new symbol for osteoporosis being used by the makers of hormones, in this case Schering (above) and Ayerst (right). The emphasis is now on hip fracture, allowing the prospect of preventing deaths to be called up on behalf of estrogen. These advertisements encourage long-term use—but ironically, studies indicate that length of use may increase breast cancer risk.

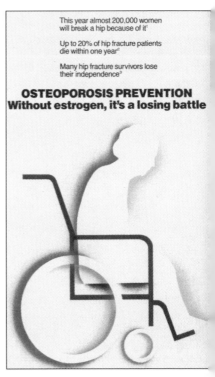

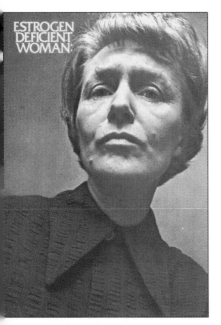

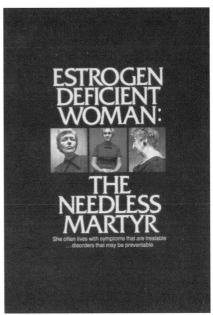

"Classic" pharmaceutical slogans: Ayerst invents the "estrogen deficient woman," a martyr to her own bodily processes, but able to be rescued by the company's wonder hormones.

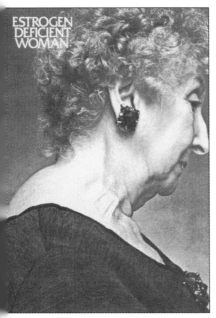

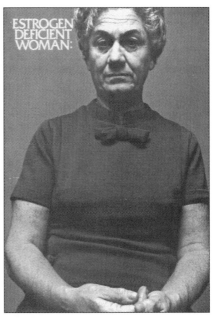

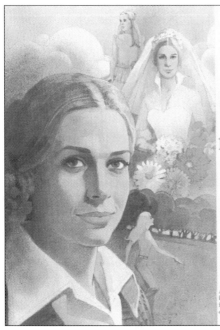

Ogen®
(PIPERAZINE ESTRONE SULFATE)

Estrogen as natural to her body as the estrone it restores.

Ogen is made from pure estrone—chemically and biologically indistinguishable from that produced by the human body.

As in the premenopausal state, the body can freely convert the estrone from Ogen into the other major human estrogens.

Since Ogen is not a hormonal mixture and does not contain unspecified estrogens, you provide the same standardized amount of estrone with every prescription or refill.

See following page for Brief Summary.

The assertion that estrogen replacement is "natural" has persisted as a marketing slogan for HRT, as has the idea that "women outlive their ovaries."

The 1990s advertisement for estrogen patches uses the "new generation" approach to imply both technological advance as well as a long tradition (and therefore by implication, safety) of estrogen use. "New generation" slogans were also used by the makers of the ill-fated Dalkon Shield to distinguish it from older types.

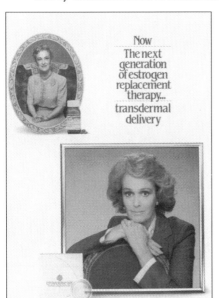

Now
The next generation of estrogen replacement therapy... transdermal delivery

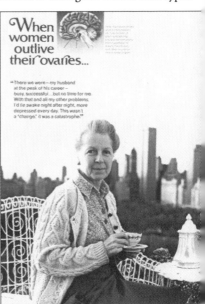

When women outlive their ovaries...

"There we were—my husband at the peak of his career—busy, successful...but no time for me. With that and all my other problems, I'd lie awake night after night, more depressed every day. This wasn't a 'change.' It was a catastrophe."

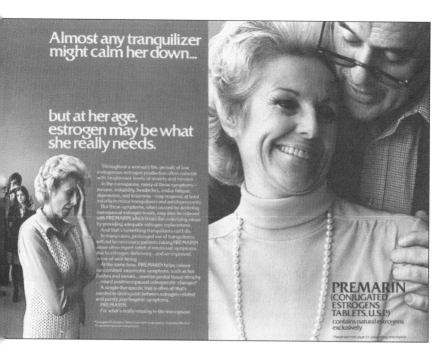

Almost any tranquilizer
might calm her down...

but at her age,
estrogen may be what
she really needs.

PREMARIN
(CONJUGATED
ESTROGENS
TABLETS, U.S.P.)
contains natural estrogens
exclusively

Maintaining markets: Ayerst, the
makers of Premarin, take on the
"psychotropic drug juggernaut" in this
advertisement from 1971 (above).
Ayerst tries a different approach to
counteract the bad news the estrogens
were causing endometrial cancer in
this campaign from 1976.

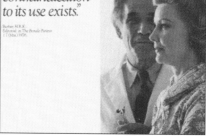

PREMARIN
(CONJUGATED ESTROGENS
TABLETS, U.S.P.)
IN THE
MENOPAUSE
TODAY

*The height of professional integrity
is to prescribe estrogen when needed
and indicated, and to withhold it
if there is no indication or when a
contraindication
to its use exists.*

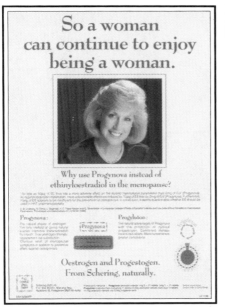

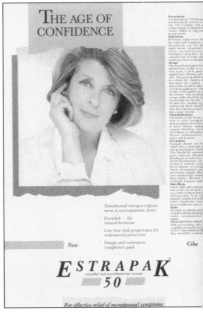

Modern images of the candidate for hormones from Schering, CIBA-Geigy (above) and Ayerst (below): the woman in the Premarin advertisement looks 30 years old, at most.

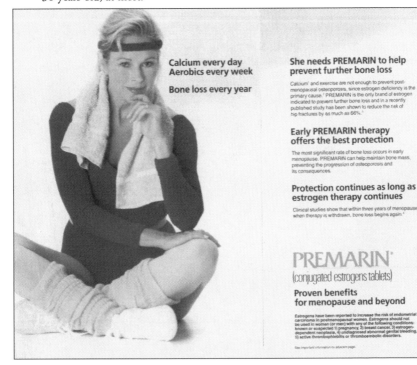

A number of observational studies have shown a reduced incidence of heart attacks among estrogen users. The combined results of 32 studies indicate a 35% lower risk of coronary heart disease in women who had used estrogen. There have not been enough studies to show whether staying on hormones for a long time will further decrease the risk.(72) Only one large study has looked at women on combined treatment. The results of this study suggested that combined treatment also reduced the risk of heart disease but this remains to be confirmed.

Although estrogen users do tend to have a lower incidence of coronary heart disease, it is not clear whether this lower incidence is caused by the estrogen itself or by something else about estrogen users. It has been suggested that the apparent beneficial effect of estrogen on hearts might be the result of differences between women who use HRT and those who don't. "It is entirely possible," said a reviewer in the *Lancet* in 1991, "that a woman who receives a prescription for hormone replacement is subtly healthier, or more determined to stay that way, than a woman who forgoes this therapy."

Overall, women who take HRT are more likely to be white, educated, upper-middle-class, and lean—and therefore at less risk of heart disease than women who do not take HRT.

There is also the issue of compliance. Women who take HRT are compliant women, as up to two-thirds of women continue therapy. Studies of people taking coronary drugs have shown that compliant people have less heart disease than those who do not take their drugs regularly.(74)

Doctors might also be less likely to prescribe HRT to women with existing hypertension or diabetes, or who are overweight. This is called "selection bias." It means that the long-term users of HRT included in the studies may have already been at lower risk of coronary heart disease than the nonusers, which could account for some of the positive results.

There are other considerations to take into account. Most of the studies are American, so the results principally apply to Premarin, not the estrogens used in other countries. Second, doses of estrogen have decreased since these studies were done. The same results might not be gained with weaker doses.

There is also the problem of what HRT might do to women with hypertension. It has been suggested that women with existing arterial problems might increase their risk of myocardial infarction (heart attack) by using estrogens. On the other hand, a recently published study showed a different result. This study compared women with existing mild to moderate coronary heart disease, some of whom were users of estrogen and some of whom were not, with a control group of healthy women who had no disease.(75) The study found that estrogen did provide protection for women with disease, particularly those with severe disease, but made no difference for women who had no disease in the first place. This study did not look at combined therapy with added progestogen.

Progestogen is the wild card, the big unknown. The prediction is that progestogen, or at least some of the most commonly used types, might tip the results in an unfavorable direction. This is a major consideration for the majority of women who use opposed therapy because they still have a uterus. This all adds up to a benefit to the heart that may be more illusory than real.

There are so many ifs and buts in the story of hormones and hearts that it is not possible to claim that using hormone replacement therapy will lower the risk of coronary heart disease. "Perhaps," said the *Lancet* reviewer, "we should demand some colossal well-controlled trials before we let the genie of universal preventive prescription escape from the bottle."(76) The American PEPI study, commenced in 1989, is one such study. In the mean time, the jury is still out.

Chapter 10

The Not-So-Good to Bad News About Hormones

As far as the hormone enthusiasts are concerned, the first problem with HRT is that not enough women take it, and the second problem is that even when women start, not enough women stay on it. There are three main reasons for this:

- The symptoms for which the therapy was started go away.
- Women worry about cancer.
- There are uncomfortable side effects, in particular the return of bleeding.

In the Massachusetts Women's Health Study, Sonja McKinlay reports that by the end of one year, only about half the hormone therapy prescribed is actually being used and that women do not like using it for long periods.(1) Among women receiving HRT for the first time, 20% stopped taking it within nine months, 10% have used it on an intermittent basis only (whenever they remembered), and 20–30% never had the prescription filled because they were not fully convinced of its benefits or safety. This is effectively a 50% discontinuance rate. The main reason women gave for stopping was fear of cancer, even among those using opposed therapy.

As we shall see, women's worries about cancer are well founded, even if some doctors describe them as irrational. In any event, women are right to be cautious. The women in the age group now being targeted for HRT have experience with doctors' promises of the harmlessness of their pharmaceutical offerings. These same women began using oral contraceptives in the 1960s and 1970s as young women, only to learn later that the serial Pill could cause endometrial cancer and that women could die from Pill-induced thrombosis and strokes. It is no use telling them that oral contraceptives used today do not carry the same risks. This may be so, but it does not alter the fact that this generation risked their lives for medicine to make advances, and in some cases they gave their lives for it. There were five hundred Pill-related deaths as late as 1982, over half of them in women 35 years and over.(2)

Then there is Depo Provera. This slipped onto the New Zealand market in 1968. Twenty years later, in 1989, it was suggested that Depo Provera may increase the risk of breast cancer.(3) There is also the IUD. Although it was promoted as safe, easy, and effective, years later it was discovered that particular IUD models had caused dangerous infections, sterility, and even death.

This gulf between the promise and the performance in the medical arena has made many women skeptical. They find hormones worrisome and regard taking them as unnatural. There was a necessity and reason for taking hormones as contraception: to avoid unwanted pregnancy. The woman taking postmenopausal hormones is avoiding what? Old age? Decrepitude? Hypothetical risks? It's hard to accept why it should be necessary, at least for most women. "I don't believe in taking something hormonal unless it is essential. The Pill was hormonal but it was essential or I'd have 10 kids by now."

Even when women have what doctors would consider a clear indication for using hormones, they may decide against it for other reasons:

> It was a fall while hiking last year that alerted me to a bone density problem. The pain in my back next day was quite extreme and my GP requested a bone density scan. I'm 52 and went through my menopause in my mid-forties. These two facts together with his diagnosis of a compression fracture of the spine alerted him to a possible loss of bone density.
>
> So it turned out to be—20% in the spine, 10% in the hip. I was shocked and I grieved for days. Then I went onto "patches" —the least powerful form of HRT—on the advice of the GP (I also have a cholesterol problem). The patches began itching after about a week and I gave up about a month later. I decided

not to proceed with any form of HRT as I suspected it was reactivating a yeast problem I had taken 16 years to overcome.

I went to another doctor who works holistically. He is investigating a form of therapy that uses progesterone only. I will begin this soon. Overseas research has shown positive results— that is, bone density loss can be reversed. I am prepared to try this out. Meanwhile, I have increased the amount of time spent in the sun (gardening mostly) and weight-bearing exercise (walking and hiking). And I get on with my life.

When women consider hormone therapy, they listen to their doctors, but they also have other sources of information—their own experience and the experience of other women. They know what they have observed around them and they do their homework. The medical profession may tell them that menopause is an illness, but their own knowledge does not confirm this. They may be told the world is full of crippled menopausal women, but where are they?

Since I met my birth mother, I asked her how menopause affected her. She said she didn't have any problems, so that was reassuring. I didn't expect any and I haven't had them.

My mother is 80, but she is as straight as a die, and so active she puts the rest of us to shame. She still puts her leather gloves and boots on, takes her slasher and goes out to tackle the cutty grass. She's still in good shape. I can see that keeping active is the way to keep the body going.

Hormones are not for me, but my sister looks better, feels better, runs more, laughs more. Me and my fat probably manufacture as much as she gets given by the chemist. Another sound reason for older women to put on weight. Indeed, maybe that's why we do get fat at middle age.

Another postmenopausal woman who had tried and abandoned HRT in favor of hot flashes because of side effects considered it again for osteoporosis:

I became aware of the use of HRT in the prevention of osteoporosis and decided to read all I could about it because I felt that

I may be confronted with having to make a decision about whether or not to embark on this course of prevention. I have now decided that I will not use this treatment because of what appears to be unknown risks of long-term treatment. I have no family history of osteoporosis and I do not appear to be in the category of women most at risk. I am appalled when I read that it should be offered to *all* women.

Annoying Side Effects

Periods

The medical model of menopause is based on the premise that women are at their most normal in their reproductive years when they have a menstrual cycle. Hormone replacement therapy aims to return women to this state, though without their fertility. Ironically, return of the menses is a major reason women reject hormones. It seems that most women look forward to the end of periods; the idea of periods into the sixties and seventies does not appeal to them.

> I was given hormone cream for a dry vagina and told to use it every other day. After the second time it brought on a period. I hadn't had a period for 18 months and I was mortified I would react so quickly. The doctor hadn't warned me as she didn't think it would bring one on. I never used it again.

It is this factor that has sent doctors and drug companies in search of drug regimes that provide hormones without the bleeding or, failing that, methods that require less "patient compliance," an oblique term doctors use to mean minimizing people's control over their own drug taking.

The 25% of women who have lost their wombs by the time they are 50 will not have periods when they use hormones, but women with wombs must use opposed therapy to protect the endometrium. In 90% of women this results in the return of menstrual-like bleeding, or a "medical curettage" to use the words of one group of researchers. (4) Women can bleed whether their therapy is opposed or not.

There is not a lot of information about the kind of periods women have on hormones. Most women seem to have shorter bleeds of two or four days. In some women, the periods can peter out over the span of about six months, but 60% of women continue to bleed as long as hormones are being used. Pain with the periods is not uncommon.

Spotting and breakthrough bleeding can also occur when women use hormones. This can be worrying as postmenopausal bleeding can be caused by disease. Breakthrough bleeding can occur on all regimens but is a particular problem with continuous combined estrogen/progestogen. When abnormal bleeding occurs, curettes and endometrial biopsies might be needed to check the cause. There is very little in the medical literature about this aspect of HRT so it is hard to know how often this happens and what women think about it.

One study looked at the incidence of dilatation and curettage (D&C) and hysterectomy among hormone users. They were all users of unopposed estrogen therapy only. This study showed that among long-term users of estrogen the incidence of abnormal bleeding was nearly eight times that among women who didn't use estrogen.(5) The users were five times more likely to have a D&C. Over 30% of the users had had a D&C compared to 8.3% of the nonusers, and the prevalence of hysterectomy was 28% among estrogen users compared to 5.3% in nonusers. Users had hysterectomies for endometrial cancer (35%), fibroids (31%), and hyperplasia (21%), whereas the hysterectomies carried out on nonusers were for prolapse (36%), endometrial cancer (27%), and fibroids (18%). The researchers found that 4% of the users had a D&C each year (compared to 0.6% of the nonusers), and every year 2% required a hysterectomy (compared to 0.4% of the nonusers). This means that one woman in five using unopposed estrogen will eventually have a hysterectomy she wouldn't have needed if she hadn't used estrogen.

Other unpleasant effects

Besides periods, the addition of progestogen to HRT can cause other problems:

- premenstrual syndrome-like effects—depression, irritability, bloating, breast tenderness

- uterine cramps and painful periods

- drowsiness (when using micronized progestogen)

Meanwhile, estrogen can cause:

- stomach upsets such as nausea and vomiting (applies to oral and nonoral methods)
- fluid retention and bloating
- swollen, sore breasts, and even mastitis; nipple sensitivity
- weight gain, either because of fluid retention or because estrogen can encourage fat (about 25% of women on HRT put on 2 pounds or more)
- headaches, thought to be caused by fluid retention affecting the brain (migraine headaches can occur because of the estrogen or the progestogen)
- copious vaginal discharge
- acne
- skin pigmentation changes
- enlargement of uterine fibroids
- reactivation of endometriosis
- leg cramps

Transdermal estrogen can cause additional problems:

- itchiness
- allergic reactions

And vaginal creams can cause:

- messiness as the cream leaks out
- estrogen effects on the male partner, if intercourse takes place when cream is in the vagina

These effects are usually passed off in medical texts in a few sentences, although it is acknowledged they are a major reason why women abandon HRT.

In 1985, at the age of 50, I was desperate to find relief from heavy sweating and flushing, especially at night. I tried a course of vitamins which had no effect, so I consulted my GP who prescribed estrogen. It proved a real godsend at first, as for the first time in many months I was able to sleep properly and I felt great. After about two months, I noticed I was gaining weight in spite of the fact that my diet and amount of exercise had not changed, and my breasts became sore. These symptoms gradually became worse, and another month saw my breasts become agonizingly tender and sore, so I abandoned the tablets. In spite of strenuous efforts, I have not yet been able to shed the extra weight I accumulated during that episode. Since then, I have discovered that Dixarit is effective in controlling my problems with hot flashes.

When I was 42 I visited my doctor because I was having many bladder problems related to sexual intercourse. A locum replacing my GP said I should try estrogen cream as my vaginal walls looked "thin" because I was going into menopause. This was a surprise to me, as I had no signs of menopause at all. I lasted for a week. The stuff dripped out everywhere. It was terribly uncomfortable walking around with constantly wet pants. When my GP came back she said there was nothing wrong with my vaginal walls and that they were perfectly healthy. I am now 48 and I have still not gone through menopause.

The significant range of possible negative effects of HRT means that using it is not straight sailing for many women. The following story describes what happened to one woman who took hormones for severe estrogen deficiency, including joint problems, after losing her ovaries because of pelvic inflammatory disease:

I was put on Premarin and my body began to gain weight at an alarming rate, so they tried Progynova, Estraderm TTS 100, and now implants. I am now 2½ stones [35 pounds] heavier than ever before, have constant fluid retention, and they cannot get the balance to the stage where my breasts are comfortable. My breast size ranges from B to DD. As far as the implants are concerned, so far every second one seems to be a dud, and the doctors are very concerned about it. The worst problem is that it takes up to three weeks to get the results of the hormone tests and during that time I get really ill and quite desperate. Mood changes are very severe, depression is very persistent, and I find I have very great difficulty with my vision—my eyesight is very blurry. This time my gynecologist suggests I use patches and top up with Progynova 1 mg on trial for two weeks. I do not see the point of yet another implant when they seem to overdose and then die, all in about two weeks.

Another woman ran into problems after she was given an implant some years after a bilateral oophorectomy:

I am 59 years old and have to have tablets each month to induce "periods," as now, in spite of having no ovaries, I am producing estrogen. My doctor says I am now menopausal even though I already had one lot of menopause in Australia. My specialist thinks that since I am female I am too retarded to know what operations I have had. I have become so angry I have written to the two hospitals overseas where I had my ovaries removed for my records. I have mastitis and still have to take these rotten tablets. My specialist does not tell me anything other than if I don't take these things, I will get cancer. I went to see him last week and he, on being asked if the implant had caused an excess of female hormones, replied "It's too simplistic to say that."

This woman was initially put on oral estrogen for night sweats which came on five years after a hysterectomy with one ovary removed:

The doctor maintained I needed calcium replacement. I then got calcium buildups in my heels and I couldn't walk. I had to have treatment, so they took me off them. They put me on hormone replacement and that made me worse. I mean I got hot flashes in the day then and that wasn't the reason I went. The doctor put me on patches which have not worked and I've got the highest patch you can get. It makes my skin so irritable it sends my body into orbit. It just itches and itches. I leave it off till the itching goes away, then I might put it on the next week. I'm not doing it as a continuous thing because I can't control the itch and it doesn't matter where I put the thing, it brings out a rash.

I feel as if I'm filling up with water till I'm full. And my hands swell. My weight has gone up from 158 pounds which is what I've been for years, to 174 pounds. My dress size has gone from size 14 to 18. I get very irritable, and quick. I fly off the handle for no reason at all, and that's not like me because I have always been quite placid. I've got four children including twins, and nothing's ever fazed me. They maintain that putting you on these patches, things will come right. But it doesn't. Whether I'm an oddball I just don't know.

Even when women experience benefits from HRT and wish to continue it, they may pay a price in annoying side effects:

In the last few months I've been putting on weight and blowing up around the abdomen. Some time ago I went to Jenny Craig and got my weight right down and it's awful to see it going back on. I am cutting down on my food and exercising a lot, but all that has done is make my legs thin and muscly, while my stomach gets fatter and fatter. I was 144 pounds and all of a sudden I leapt up to 149 pounds. The doctor offered diuretics, but I said no. I'm already on beta-blockers for high blood pressure. I have also started to get period pain which I haven't had since I was a teenager, but Ponstan is good for that.

It is hard to know how typical these kinds of problems are because they are considered too trivial to study. Proving something causes or doesn't cause cancer is the stuff of which careers are made; no one reaches the top of the research ladder by studying fluid retention or sore breasts in menopausal women. At least some of these problems might be solved by reducing the dose being used by a woman, but then she may be gaining less of the beneficial effects.

How HRT Medicalizes Women's Lives

These women's experiences illustrate one of the hidden dangers of HRT. Users become locked into constant visits to doctors and become dependent on the health system. Some of these women are worse off because of the therapy, more than they were before they started it. The first intervention—the HRT—has led to more interventions, more drugs, and more tests. The effects of multiple medications are not well known.

There is research to show that exposure to the health system is a health risk because it leads to interventions. Sonja McKinlay has shown that women who visit their doctor regularly are more likely to be given HRT in the first place, and are also more likely to have hysterectomies and breast surgery than matched women who do not.(6)

These are some of the tests and procedures that women on HRT might need to have or have more regularly than women not using HRT:

- blood tests for hormone levels

- diuretics for fluid retention

- Ponstan, aspirin, or other analgesics for uterine cramps

- endometrial biopsies to check the endometrium

- diagnostic curettage for bleeding

- hysterectomy

- blood pressure tests

- blood tests for cholesterol levels

- baseline mammograms before starting therapy and regular mammograms thereafter

- visits for repeat prescriptions of hormones at least every six months

Who should not take HRT

In the early days of HRT a long list of contraindications to using HRT used to be given. As the years have gone by, this list has dwindled considerably. Of the contraindications given below, some doctors now maintain that only breast or endometrial cancer are absolute. This contraction of contraindications is a common process with any drug therapy used by doctors. Sometimes the list shortens because research has shown that fears about a particular risk were unfounded, but at other times there is no firm evidence for striking a particular contraindication off the list. It may simply mean that inadequate research has been carried out and that in the meantime it *appears* there is not a risk.

Definite contraindications:

- women with a history of breast cancer
- women with a history of endometrial cancer

Possible contraindications—should be used only under close medical supervision:

- hypertension
- history of cardiovascular disease
- benign breast disease
- fibroids
- migraine headaches
- endometriosis
- liver and gallbladder disease
- diabetes
- history of thrombosis, pulmonary embolism, or stroke

Risks of HRT

Women who use hormone replacement therapy run the risks of developing endometrial hyperplasia and endometrial cancer, breast cancer, gall bladder and liver disease, and thrombosis—among other risks.

Endometrial hyperplasia and endometrial cancer

Studies have persistently shown that estrogens can cause prolonged overstimulation of the endometrium. This can develop into hyperplasia and abnormal overgrowth in the endometrium. There are two main types of hyperplasia: the most serious is adenomatous hyperplasia, which carries a 30% risk of subsequent endometrial cancer. Cystic hyperplasia has a malignancy risk factor of 1%.(7) Estrogen users have a rate of endometrial cancer two to eight times that of women not using estrogens, and the risk increases the longer a woman uses it. After 10 years, her risk is 10 times that of women not using estrogen; this increased risk in estrogen users persists for at least 10 years after discontinuing therapy.(8)

This is a particularly problematic aspect of hormone use. One study of users of implants showed that stimulation of the endometrium continued for up to 43 months after the women discontinued therapy.(9) Women reported bleeding for a mean period of 35 months. The researchers in this study said that women should be advised to continue taking progestogen after they had discontinued the estrogen until the bleeding stopped; however, they acknowledged that women may not be too enthusiastic about this because of the progestogenic side effects.

Endometrial cancer is not a common cancer; it occurs in about 1 in 1,000 postmenopausal women with a uterus. Using estrogen would increase this risk to between 2 and 10 in 1,000 women. Although most of the research on endometrial cancer has been carried out on conjugated equine estrogen, all types of estrogen carry the risk of endometrial cancer.(10)

Endometrial hyperplasia is more frequent with higher-dose estrogens (over 1 mg conjugated equine estrogen) and with estrogen implants than with lower-dose estrogens. It is not possible to reduce the estrogen dose to a level where the risk is minimal because the therapy will then not be effective in relieving menopausal symptoms or protecting bone. Endometrial hyperplasia can occur whether or not menstruation occurs in women using estrogen.

Progestogen added to estrogen in an adequate dose appears to protect the endometrium, although there is still a need to establish this firmly.(11) Some studies have shown a much lower rate of endometrial cancer—one third or less—among users of opposed therapy than in women who use no hormones at all.(12)

The recommended period for taking progestogen is 13 days each month, although it is frequently given for 10 or 11 days and sometimes for only 7 days. The risk of endometrial hyperplasia increases as the days of progestogen per cycle decrease. In one study a period of seven days was associated with a 5.9–12.5% incidence of hyperplasia.(13) Doctors who recommend 12–13 days of progestogen as the safest regime argue that it is the same number of days of circulating progesterone as occurs naturally during the reproductive years.(14) Approximately 10–11% of women do not bleed at all on opposed therapy. This means that the endometrium has not built up to any appreciable degree.

Different progestogens have differing potencies by weight, so that doses vary. The minimum effective dose of progestogen when prescribed for 12 days is about 0.7 mg of norethisterone and 10 mg of medroxyprogesterone acetate. The dose of levonorgestrel needed to protect the endometrium is not clear.(15)

Some doctors manipulate the regime so that a woman has a bleed only every two, three, or even six months.(16) This practice is experimental and calls for annual endometrial biopsies to check that the endometrium is normal. The safety of continuous combined therapy is also not well researched. When estrogen patches, implants, and creams are used, progestogen must also be taken orally if the woman has not had a hysterectomy.

Until recently it was recommended that endometrial samples be taken annually from women with uteruses taking estrogen, and every two to five years from women on opposed therapy. It is still recommended that any woman with a uterus taking estrogen without progestogen have an annual biopsy, as should women taking continuous therapy, but it is no longer considered necessary for women also taking progestogen, unless there is abnormal bleeding. Abnormal bleeding is considered to be bleeding that occurs at any time other than in the withdrawal bleeding after the tenth day of the progestogen therapy. Any bleeding at any time earlier in the progestogen part of the cycle of very heavy bleeding is considered to be abnormal.

Endometrial biopsies involve taking samples of tissue from the endometrium. They can be performed by a number of different methods, but not all are equally accurate and they have varying degrees of discomfort. The "best" methods are described as being like an IUD insertion, a painful procedure for many women.

Currently the most used methods are,

- the Vabra suction method, which is relatively painful and gives accurate results in 80% of cases(17)

- the Gynoscann method, which seems to give accurate results but still with discomfort, like an IUD insertion(18)

- the Pipelle method, in which a plastic tube is used to take endometrial samples, which can also feel like an IUD insertion

Breast cancer

Breast cancer is the big bogey of hormone replacement therapy. Breast cancer is the most frequent malignant tumor in women and is far more prevalent among women in their midlife and older years than among younger women. The lifetime risk of developing breast cancer is four to five times that of developing endometrial cancer, and the mortality among breast cancer patients is considerable. Even a moderate increase of breast cancer among women using HRT could have catastrophic effects.

Among young American women breast cancer is not a common disease, but for midlife women in the 45–64 age group, the death rate jumps to 76.5 deaths per 100,000 women. The mortality rate for women over 65 is over twice as high. There were over 180,000 new cases of breast cancer diagnosed in the United States in 1992, and there are approximately 46,000 deaths from breast cancer each year. Most of the fatalities are women 45 years of age and older, the very group targeted for hormone replacement therapy.

Because of the biology of breast cancer, there have always been worries that HRT might increase the risk of it occurring. A woman's own natural hormones are implicated in the development of breast cancer in ways that are not yet well understood. Dr. Malcolm Pike, a researcher at the University of Southern California whose field is the Pill and breast cancer, maintains that estrogen stimulates the growth in cells in the breast and that progesterone might potentiate or add to estrogen's effect. Consequently, giving either or both hormones to women at menopause will have an unknown effect on the breasts.

Since 1974 epidemiological studies have been addressing this question. Most of these studies during the 1970s showed no elevation in risk, but beginning in the 1980s several studies started to show small elevations in risk, especially for long-term users. The picture was somewhat confused, but it was reassuring that there was no obvious elevation in risk for women using estrogen.

The U.S. studies published in the 1980s followed this see-sawing pattern. Three showed no increased risk, although in two of them the young age of study subjects was a limitation.(19) One study showed a significant increase in risk for women who had used estrogen for over 20 years but not for others.(20) And one showed an increased risk for all users.(21) In all these studies the women were primarily using unopposed estrogen. Significant numbers of American women did not start using opposed therapy until after the reports on endometrial cancer in the 1970s, so there has been insufficient time for research to demonstrate the effect of opposed hormones on the breast.

In Europe the situation has been different. Other estrogens are commonly used and opposed therapy has had wider use. The study that really set of alarm bells was a Swedish one, published in the *New England Journal of Medicine* in 1989.(22) Leif Bergkvist and other researchers from the University Hospital in Uppsala, Sweden and two American colleagues from the National Cancer Institute, used prescription records to identify 23,000 women living around Uppsala who were using hormones for menopause. The researchers were then able to compare the users' names with those in the Swedish Cancer Registry to see which women with breast cancer had been using hormones. They found that after nine years' use women using hormones had nearly twice the rate of breast cancer compared to women not using hormones.

On top of this bleak news, women using preparations combining both estrogen and progestogen had an even higher rate—over four times the rate of nonusers after they had used opposed therapy for six years. Because the number of cancer cases in women using opposed therapy was small, the researchers were cautious about this finding, but it was the first indication that the progestogen added to HRT to protect the endometrium might be having other, sinister effects.

Bergkvist's study stirred up a hornet's nest among defenders of hormones. Not only were the researchers criticized and their study pulled to pieces, but the *New England Journal of Medicine* was accused of "medical journal sensationalism" for publishing it.(23) One writer in the *Lancet* argued that the results of the Swedish study could not be extrapolated to Britain because different estrogens were used. However, the writer then went on to claim estrogen's benefits to bones and hearts for British women without acknowledging that by the same argument the American studies he cited could not be automatically applied to Britain, where Premarin is hardly used.(24)

Another writer accused the researchers of causing women to stop HRT "which may result in increased osteoporotic fractures and heart attacks" as well as needless suffering from menopausal symptoms.(25) A similar argument—that there will be unwanted pregnancies—is used to criticize anyone who expresses doubts about the safety of various contraceptives.

In late 1992, Bergkvist and his coworkers reported again on a further four years' of follow-up of the women in their study. They found the risks they discovered in 1989 remained, and the risk of combined therapy had increased. This therapy, they said, might be "more hazardous" in terms of breast cancer than estrogen alone.(26)

Other European studies have also shown an increased risk of breast cancer in hormone users. A Danish study showed an increase with duration of use as well as an increase in users of opposed therapy.(27) An Italian study showed an increased risk for any users of HRT, even for a short time, while the results of a British study of hormone users have become more disturbing as time has gone on.(28) When the Oxford researchers of this study first reported, after having followed the women for five years, they had found an increased risk of breast cancer only in those women with a surgical menopause.(29) But by 1990, when they reported again after nearly 10 years' follow-up, the situation had worsened.(30)

This study of 4,544 women is looking at all causes of death in the hormone users, comparing them to the expected rate in the general population. There was no marked change in any of the causes of death from the earlier period (which in general was lower for hormone users), except for breast cancer, its relative risk having almost doubled during the second period. Given the length of time the study has now been going on, this increase could not be explained by a bias caused by the women being more likely to have their cancer found because they are visiting the doctor. This has been suggested by some doctors as an explanation for increased cases of breast cancer among hormone users. The researchers also noted that these findings suggest that the risk is related to duration of use. They called their findings "somewhat worrying."

The sum of these studies is not reassuring, and several epidemiologists have tried to make sense of them. In Australia, Bruce Armstrong, Professor of Epidemiology and Cancer Research at the University of Western Australia, conducted a meta-analysis of 23 of the studies.(31) A meta-analysis involves combining all the study results so that studies with a small number of subjects, or where the statistical result was weak, can contribute to the overall picture. A meta-analysis has more "power" than individual studies and so may achieve a more accurate result. Armstrong's meta-analysis showed that ever having used estrogen did not increase the risk of breast cancer to users. He could find an increased risk only for people using the highest doses and women with a family history of breast cancer, and the increased risk was only slight.

Armstrong's meta-analysis has been widely quoted by those who defend hormones to indicate that HRT does not harm the breast, but reliance on his results should be questioned for two reasons. First, most of the studies included in his meta-analysis were carried out in the U.S. on Premarin users, and it is suspected that if conjugated equine estrogen has an adverse effect on the breast, it is a weak one. Second, Armstrong's results do not include any studies published after 1987, and several of the studies showing the most worrying results appeared after that time, in particular the Swedish, Danish, and Oxford studies. Finally, the studies included in Armstrong's meta-analysis were almost exclusively of estrogen used alone, not of estrogen/progestogen combinations.

Another meta-analysis in 1991 did include the more recent studies (although not the Oxford one). It found a much stronger relationship between HRT and breast cancer. This meta-analysis was carried out by scientists from the Centers for Disease Control, part of the U.S. federal government health system.(32)

The analysts found that an increased risk of breast cancer among HRT users did not begin until after at least five years of use, and applied to women with both surgical and natural menopause. After 15 years' use they found an overall 30% increase in the risk of breast cancer. This increase in risk was largely among women who began using estrogen when they were premenopausal (that is, before periods had ceased) and women using estradiol preparations, with or without progestogen. In these women the risk of breast cancer more than doubled (2.2) compared to nonusers of hormones. In women who had a family history of breast cancer, the risk was even greater (3.4).

Because so many women are using HRT, even a small increase in risk amounts to a large number of preventable breast cancer cases. The authors concluded that, taking a conservative estimate of current levels of hormone use among American women, the added risk of breast cancer would lead to 4,708 preventable cases of breast cancer every year and 1,468 preventable deaths.

Some studies have shown the increased risk is mainly in current users. In 1992 the American Nurses' Health Study—a prospective study with nearly half a million person-years of follow-up—showed an increased risk of one-third in women currently using HRT. There was possibly an even greater risk in women using combined therapy.(33)

This risk in current users in confirmed by a meta-analysis published in 1993. This showed that current users of HRT had a 40% greater risk of breast cancer and that this risk was not related to the duration of therapy. The implication of this is that even short-term use of HRT carries the risk of breast cancer.(34)

These results cast serious doubt on the wisdom of using HRT for more than a very short time. Most of the studies suggest that while five years' of hormone use is safe, a significant risk of cancer appears if the therapy is used for longer. Current users appear to be most at risk and there is a possibility this may apply to even short-term users. A bizarre scenario may emerge whereby women save their bones but get breast cancer in the process. Women with breast cancer are much more likely to die of their disease than are women with thin bones. Eighty percent of women with breast cancer eventually die of their disease.

There is another factor that needs to be remembered. The people who die after fractures are over 80 and are usually not well people. Ironically, the woman who starts taking hormones for bones cannot predict what the general state of her health will be by the time she reaches the fracture age. Her bones might be wonderful, but she may also have Alzheimer's disease or be severely impaired in other ways. Hormones cannot guarantee quality of life. Neither can she know whether she will even live into her eighties; she could die of some unrelated cause before then and so never risk the fracture she thought she was saving herself from. These are tough things to say, but women need to think about them.

By contrast, the woman with breast cancer is a young woman. If the risk of breast cancer in hormone users is confirmed, the woman who starts taking hormones at 50 could develop cancer in her late fifties or early sixties, when she had another quarter-century of her life left. She then faces mutilating surgery, drug treatment, and a question mark hanging over her life forever.

It is important to realize the magnitude of the risk being talked about here. The average midlife woman already has a considerable chance of developing breast cancer; it is a relatively common disease. If hormone replacement therapy increases her risk by 25–40%, she is running a very high chance of developing breast cancer. This is a heavy price to pay for the benefits hormones might give to bones or, less certainly, to hearts. There are other ways of preventing bone loss and other ways of protecting the heart. Stopping smoking and changing lifestyle and diet can minimize the chance of suffering from osteoporosis and cardiovascular disease, without risking any harm at all.

There is another possible problem about HRT and breast cancer. Radiologists have recently reported that it is harder to read mammograms of hormone users compared to those of other postmenopausal women.(35) This was true, they said, of women using estrogen alone or combined therapy. This study in Boston took baseline mammograms of postmenopausal women before they started therapy, then at yearly intervals afterward. The researchers found that in one-fourth of the cases the breast tissue of women became denser while they were on HRT. This dense tissue could obscure a malignant tumor and therefore "the sensitivity of mammographic detection of early breast cancer may be diminished." They said that in such cases the referring doctor and the woman should reevaluate the risks and benefits of HRT and "consider withdrawing therapy."

This is simply another hidden drawback of HRT of which women are unaware. If HRT diminishes the effectiveness of mammography, women will not be obtaining the benefits of mammography discussed in the next chapter. This is a special irony because of the possible elevated cancer risk involved in taking hormones.

Gallbladder and liver

The liver is intimately involved with the metabolization of the hormones given in HRT. Unless hormone therapy is given transdermally, the hormones pass through the liver before entering the bloodstream. This process, called the "hepatic [liver] first pass," can have a number of effects that have implications for cardiovascular disease and for the gallbladder.

The hepatic first pass can result in increased protein and lipid metabolism, and this effect carries potential dangers. The effect on lipoproteins was discussed in the last chapter. Because estrogen affects various liver proteins, it can cause hypertension or worsen it in women who already have raised blood pressure.(36)

Bile, which helps with the digestion of food, is produced by the liver and stored in the gallbladder, just below the liver. The effect of hormones passing through the liver can thicken and concentrate the bile. These concentrations of bile can cause stonelike masses called gallstones to form, which then block the bile ducts, reducing the flow of bile. People with gallstones have indigestion, nausea, and pain, and may require surgery to remove the gallbladder. Studies have shown that women using estrogen are at two-and-a-half times increased risk of gallbladder disease than other women.(37) This is another argument for nonoral methods of HRT.

Thrombosis and other possible risks

Women using estrogen in oral contraceptives are at increased risk for blood clotting, specifically venous thrombosis (a clot in a vein) and pulmonary embolism (a clot in the pulmonary artery), especially if they smoke. This has led to fears that similar events could occur in postmenopausal women. So far this fear has proved unfounded, probably because young women using hormones are receiving a different estrogen—ethinylestradiol—and higher doses of estrogen than postmenopausal women.

At the same time, it has frequently been claimed that HRT will reduce the risk of strokes in users. Some studies have shown a reduced risk, but others have shown an increased risk. In a review of all the evidence, Dr. Deborah Grady and others concluded that there was no convincing evidence that estrogen either increased or decreased the risk of strokes in users, and that there was no information about the effect of combined therapy.(38)

The great concentration of work on risks for users of HRT has gone into researching endometrial cancer, breast cancer, and cardiovascular disease. Other areas have been relatively neglected. Although there seems to be no elevated risk in HRT users, the relationship with ovarian cancer and cervical cancer is not clear. Studies of ovarian cancer have been few and far between: most have shown no increased risk, and one showed a reduced risk for epithelial ovarian cancer.(39) Two, however, showed a slightly increased rate of epidermoid ovarian cancer.(40)

There is still no clear answer as to whether smoking increases any of the risks associated with HRT. If anything, smoking seems to lower estrogen levels, both natural ones, accounting for early menopause in smokers, and artificial estrogens, as in HRT. This may even diminish the effectiveness of HRT, which means there may be less protection to bones in smokers who use HRT. This area is not at all well researched.

Premenopausal Use of HRT

HRT was originally promoted to women who had gone through menopause and had stopped menstruating. The end of periods was a clear sign that production of estrogen by the ovaries had slowed down considerably. The most common indication for prescribing HRT was hot flashes and they usually began late in the climacteric and could continue on after the period had stopped. The second indication for prescribing HRT was vaginal dryness, which is a problem of the postmenopause. Women do not usually complain of vaginal dryness until a few years after bleeding has stopped.

There is an increasing trend to suggest HRT to women in their forties, without any vasomotor symptoms being present and long before periods stop. "Clinicians must bear in mind," writes Robert Wells, Associate Clinical Professor of Obstetrics and Gynecology at the University of California School of Medicine, "that a woman can be a victim of menopausal changes long before her final menstrual curtain goes down. Indeed, women do not have to have stopped menstruating or suffer drenching night sweats to qualify for treatment of menopause . . . . A physician who waits for a patient to complain of terrible hot flashes has missed a golden opportunity to help her."(41) These arguments are possible when menopause is defined as more than the last period and hot flashes. If menopause is viewed as the cause of a plethora of vague emotional symptoms, then it is easy to find something to treat, even in younger women.

It is not possible, however, to describe the practice of giving hormones to premenopausal women as "replacement." The natural hormone system of these women is still active: they are producing their own estrogen. Giving extra hormones to such women is more correctly "supplementation," or "duplication," or even "overdosing." There is very little discussion in the medical literature or anywhere else of how safe this is. Gynecological endocrinologist Dr. Lila Nachtigall is adamant that this practice is unwise and she explains why.

Today we know that, except under special circumstances, taking hormones before menopause, your very last menstrual period, can be dangerous. In fact, it can be especially dangerous during the erratic periods of the perimenopause because that's a time when you may be producing huge amounts of estrogen in response to the frantic activities of the pituitary gland to get your ovaries back in business. If you are still having periods, however irregular, that means you are still making sufficient estrogen to build up your uterine lining.

You do not need estrogen in addition to what you are already producing yourself. You are probably no longer ovulating and so you are not making progesterone. Without the progesterone to clean out the lining, you could develop hyperplasia.(42)

There is also the danger that a woman this age, still fertile, could become pregnant and feed her fetus hormones, with possibly disastrous consequences.

Some doctors recommend a blood test to measure follicle stimulating hormone (FSH) before prescribing HRT. FSH goes up at menopause and so gives an indication that a woman is menopausal. But there are problems with this, for doctors do not agree on the FSH level that indicates menopause has been reached. Also, hormones can fluctuate wildly during the menopausal transition (40–50 years old) and even for some months after the last period.(43) Hormones can be low one month and high the next, therefore, biochemical tests cannot accurately predict whether a woman is menopausal. Thus, these tests are really not much use.

The "Forever" Therapy: Long-Term Use

As noted previously, HRT was originally recommended for short periods at menopause, whereas currently women are told it is quite safe to stay on it for decades, or for life. Dr. John Studd compares it to the wearing of spectacles, which you wear forever!

According to Professor Howard Jacobs of Middlesex Hospital, the definition of "long-term" has stretched with each new study.(44) He considers that five or six years is "reasonably safe," but the prospect of HRT for 15 years causes him "some anxiety."

After discussing his meta-analysis of studies on HRT and breast cancer risk, Professor Bruce Armstrong concluded that until the effects of adding progestogen to HRT were known "the caution that has so far most characterized most use of hormonal replacement therapy at the menopause will continue to be justified."(45)

Dr. Nathan Kase, the Chairman of the Department of Obstetrics and Gynecology at New York's Mt. Sinai School of Medicine, maintains that HRT should only be used for women with the worst menopausal symptoms. He recommends other strategies for the prevention of osteoporosis.(46) Like Professor Armstrong his worry is that there is not enough evidence about the effects of adding progestogen.

These are cautious views. Other gynecologists are encouraging use for decades because of the benefits to bones, even though, as we have seen, the real experts in the osteoporosis area are alarmed at suggestions that women should be using hormones for long periods to prevent bone loss. Recently another medical indication has been summoned on estrogen's behalf: more women should be using HRT, we are told, because it "makes women feel good."(47) Nathan Kase warns against a "numbness of intellect" which would allow "generalized" use of HRT for all menopausal women.(48)

No one can claim that long-term HRT is safe. Most research has been carried out over relatively short periods; doctors then extrapolate evidence for safety into the long term. But this cannot reliably be done.

On the contrary, all the evidence so far points to risks that increase with duration of use, a similar pattern to the one that research has suggested may be occurring in some users of oral contraceptives and Depo Provera. Dr. Klim McPherson of Oxford University, part of the Oxford team conducting long-term research on HRT users in Britain, says that the existing research makes it clear that risks do increase with long-term use: "I would be very surprised if there were not an increased risk of breast cancer associated with the long-term use of HRT."(49)

One writer in a women's magazine called using HRT "a game of hormonal Russian Roulette," which is probably a fairer description of the risks than the promises given by doctors who really don't know.(50)

Part Five

SCREENING PROGRAMS

Chapter 11

The Business of Breasts

Although breast cancer is not the most commonly diagnosed cancer among women (lung cancer is), the American Cancer Society estimates that one in nine American women will develop breast cancer in her lifetime. The disease is uncommon in women in their twenties, becomes more common in their thirties and forties, and increases in incidence with each succeeding decade. Most of the women who develop breast cancer are 50 or older.

In 1992 an estimated 180,000 new cases of breast cancer were diagnosed in America; in 1990 there were approximately 43,700 breast cancer deaths. Although the five-year survival rate for breast cancer has improved to about 70%, the incidence rates and overall death rates have gone up in recent years. It is difficult to know how much of the incidence rate is a real increase in the disease, and how much it reflects increased early detection of the disease by mammography. In other words, mammography might be detecting cancers that otherwise would have appeared in cancer statistics later.

One study suggested that mammography was responsible for some but not all of the apparent increase in breast cancer.(1) This study explained the increase in women 45–64 years old as being totally caused by mammography; but the increase in younger and older women had additional causes. Among young women 25–44 years old, 12% of a 29% increase was attributed to mammography, while the remainder had other causes including, suggested the researchers, oral contraceptive use. Among older women 65–74 years old, 26% of a 57% increase was attributed to mammography; some of the additional increase might be explained by the use of hormone replacement therapy.

Despite improvements in treatment methods for breast cancer, there has been little decrease in the rate at which women die from this disease. Although women now have less mutilating surgery, their chances of survival are little better. Because of the failure of modern treatment methods to improve survival, attention has turned to the possibility of preventing the disease from occurring.

Unfortunately, this is not yet possible because no one knows with any certainty what causes breast cancer. A number of theories have been put forward, but they are only theories rather than known facts around which a prevention program might be built. There are risk factors for breast cancer, but it is not possible for an individual woman to do very much to protect herself from them.

Risk Factors for Breast Cancer

The current estimate that one in nine American women will develop breast cancer is up from 1 in 15 not many years ago. The breast cancer death rate is currently about 17.5 per 1,000 women, up from 14.7 in 1970. These figures are an average for all women, those at high risk and those at low risk. The risk percentage is also a "cumulative" figure obtained by adding a woman's risk of developing cancer between the ages 20 to 30, plus that from 30 to 40, and so on. Thus, a woman with no clear risk factors will have a significantly lower risk that 1 in 9, more like 1 in 20, whereas for the woman with risk factors (blood relative with breast cancer, late first pregnancy, early menarche, etc.), it will be higher. Nevertheless, because women with risk factors are in the minority, approximately 70% of the women who develop breast cancer will actually have no known risk factors.

Environmental factors

There are clues about the possible causes of breast cancer from epidemiology. Breast cancer is very common in countries like the United States, New Zealand, Australia, and in Western Europe, while in other countries the incidence is far smaller. In Japan, for instance, breast cancer is uncommon even though Japan is an industrialized country with a high standard of living like these other countries. The possibility that breast cancer is caused by environmental rather than genetic factors is suggested by the fact that when Japanese women migrate to America their risk of breast cancer increases to reach the American rate within a generation or two, even if they do not inter-marry.

This trend has led to the supposition that fat in the diet increases the risk of breast cancer, but epidemiological studies addressing this question have not confirmed such a breast cancer/fat link. Neverthe-less, there has been widespread publicity claiming fat as a principal cause of breast cancer, leading some women to make major changes in their diet.(2) Reducing fat in the diet is in general a good thing, as fat contributes to coronary heart disease and possibly cancer of the colon, but women should take care not to go to far. Dairy products such as cheese and milk contain some fat, but they also are the best source of calcium, much needed for healthy bones.

The fat hypothesis took a knock when the results of a large study of American nurses became known.(3) The study followed 90,000 nurses for four years, estimating their fat consumption over that pe-riod. During this time, 601 cases of breast cancer were diagnosed among the nurses, but the researchers could find no evidence that the fat consumption of the women who got cancer differed from that of other women. A study of vegetarian nuns that also found no re-duction in breast cancer risk similarly suggests that the fat/breast cancer risk theory may not be correct.(4)

For various reasons, including the possibility that it may be fat consumption during childhood and adolescence that is the problem, the result of the nurses study is not conclusive. Dr. Walter Willett of the Harvard School of Public Health, the principal researcher in the study, points out that if fat consumption in young life is responsible for breast cancer, to stop eating fat in midlife would be an ineffective strategy. In any event, he suggests that the culprit may not be fat at all. Instead, it may be the amount of food eaten in early life, which directly affects body size. Breast cancer may be related to body size. The increase in breast cancer among Japanese women who migrate to Western countries may be related to body size increasing over subsequent generations. If this is the case, it is total calories rather than fat that contributes to breast cancer.

Those who support the fat/breast cancer theory argue that the nurses study did not put the "safe" level of fat low enough. They maintain that if women reduce their fat intake to 20% or less of their diet, they may be at less risk of breast cancer. Support for this theory also comes from the discovery that women on high-fat diets metabolize more estrogen, but whether estrogen is linked to breast cancer is another unknown. Scientists who support this point of view believe that dietary fat could act as a "promoter" of malignancy. The "initiator" may be genetics, radiation, or some other unknown factor. A high-fat diet may provide the conditions in which the abnormal cells flourish. However, all this is currently speculative. There is simply no proof at the moment that this theory is correct.

It is also known that obese postmenopausal women are slightly more at risk of breast cancer, although the cause is still elusive. Increased body size could be the risk factor here but so too could the fact that postmenopausal women produce estrone in fat. Estrogen has also been implicated in the development of breast cancer, although it is not clear how it might be involved. Another possibility is that tumors will be diagnosed late in fat women because they are harder to feel, but this would not explain the fact that fat premenopausal women have lower rates of breast cancer than thin women.

Alcohol consumption, even at moderate levels—a drink or two a day—may be a risk factor. Some studies have shown that moderate to heavy drinkers have higher rates of breast cancer, although it is not clear whether the link is a causal one. It is not known whether it would make any difference to a woman to stop drinking at midlife.

Menstrual and reproductive history

Epidemiology has suggested other possible risk factors for breast cancer. Women whose periods start late have less risk, as do women with early menopause and women who have their first child when young. It seems that the more menstrual periods a woman has during her lifetime, the more she is at risk. The earlier a woman has a baby after starting periods the more protected she is. A woman who has her first child before the age of 18 has about half the risk of breast cancer of a woman who has her first child in her late twenties. It has been speculated that this may be because breast tissue is more sensitive to carcinogens before the first pregnancy.

Women who have no children are at added risk, but those who delay their first pregnancy until they are 35–40 years old have an excess risk of 40% over women who have no children. The trend toward later first pregnancy could possibly explain some of the increase in the number of women developing breast cancer. Breastfeeding may be protective; a woman who breastfeeds for a total of six months over several pregnancies reduces her risk to half.

All these risk factors could be tied to estrogen. It is possible that the more uninterrupted periods of estrogen production a woman has the more she is at risk. This theory has added weight because of the knowledge that women who have both ovaries removed at a young age are at less risk of breast cancer. However, studies that have looked at the relationship between sex hormone levels in blood and urine and the risk of breast cancer have not established consistent findings.

Use of oral contraceptives at a young age, especially long-term use, appears to be associated with an increased risk of breast cancer before the age of 36. Similar risks have been suggested with the use of Depo Provera at a young age, especially with prolonged use.(5) As breast cancer does not commonly occur in these young age groups, the actual statistical chance of an individual woman developing breast cancer from her hormonal contraceptive is small: an increase from approximately 2 in 1,000 among women who do not use hormonal contraception to 3 in 1,000 among users.

Family history

Family history also affects breast cancer risk, suggesting a genetic contribution to the development of the disease. A "first-degree" relative with breast cancer—that is, a mother, daughter, or sister—increases risk markedly, but a "second-degree" relative—a grandmother, aunt, or cousin—only increases risk very slightly. The risk is also greater if the first-degree relative had breast cancer premenopausally or in both breasts, or if two first-degree relatives have had breast cancer.

We have to be cautious about past diagnoses of breast cancer. In years gone by, some women who had mastectomies may not have had breast cancer. It seems that doctors may have been rather quick to remove breasts they would not remove today.

Radiation

Women exposed to high doses of radiation, either environmentally or as treatment for disease, are at added risk of breast cancer, especially if they were exposed in their young adolescent years. This would be very uncommon in the United States.

Early Detection of Breast Cancer

Apart from breastfeeding and choice of contraceptive, there is not a lot women can realistically do to protect themselves from breast cancer. Consequently, attention has turned to early detection of the disease.

The main methods of early detection are

- examination of the breasts by the woman herself
- examination of the breasts by a health professional
- mammographic screening

Breast self-examination (BSE)

For years women have been told that regularly examining their breasts for signs of a thickening, a dimple, or a lump was good for their health. Pamphlets and posters encouraging breast self-examination (BSE) have made dramatic claims, such as "your life is in your hands" and BSE is "a woman's best protection."(6) But the scientific evidence for the effectiveness of BSE is conflicting, to say the least. It is a hard area to research because techniques differ and it is difficult to assess how well a woman is doing it. Still, the fact remains that over 80% of all the breast lumps that can be felt are found by women, not by doctors or mammography.

While there is a good deal of controversy about the effectiveness of BSE in medical circles, others have argued it doesn't matter anyway, the activity is harmless and women may as well do it, whether it is effective or not. But this view is not completely justifiable; besides, it is inherently contradictory to subject mammography to intense scientific scrutiny while neglecting to measure the effectiveness of BSE.

BSE may not be entirely harmless if women rely on it and believe it makes them safe. If a woman is told it is effective, she could decide against mammography thinking that BSE is all she needs and that by performing it she is taking care of herself. Messages given out as part of the promotion of BSE have encouraged women to think that BSE helps a woman "keep in touch with her body."

Overall, the currently available evidence on BSE does not provide support for the claim that the technique will reduce mortality or extend survival. Neither is it known whether BSE leads to less mutilating surgery when a lump is discovered.

A 1990 National Health Interview survey found that while 88.1% of all women know how to do BSE, only 43.1% actually perform it monthly. The survey showed few differences in the profiles of the women who did and did not use BSE: 42.3% of white women versus 50.9% of black women; 43.6% of women with 12 years of education compared to 42.2% of those with more than 12 years. Over 90% of employed women say they know how to perform BSE compared to 83.4% of women who are not in the labor force.(7)

While no research has proved that BSE improves survival rates, it has been fairly consistently shown that women using BSE have smaller and more localized tumors than those who do not.

The American Cancer Society recommends that women begin practicing BSE at age 20. While breast cancer is uncommon in women that young, the longer BSE is performed the more a woman gets to know her breasts, and the more likely she is to spot a change in them. Most public schools teach BSE in girls' health classes now, and instruction can also be obtained from doctors, nurses, a breast cancer health center, American Cancer Society BSE trainers, and most women's health centers.

BSE needs to be carried out regularly and the woman must become familiar with the configuration of her breasts. For women still menstruating, it is recommended that they carry out the examination after their period has finished; after menopause, women need to carry it out by the calendar, on a particular day each month.

Physical examination by a doctor

Many of the studies of mammographic screening programs have noted that a good proportion of the cancers detected were palpable and could have been detected during a clinical examination by a doctor. This was particularly noted among women 40–50 years of age. Despite this, there have been no programs to see if systematic breast examinations of women by their doctors might be an effective way of detecting breast cancer and reducing mortality from the disease. Such a study is under way in Canada, where the National Breast Screening Study is comparing the value of mammography to that of clinical examination, but the results will not be known for some years.

There are no guidelines for doctors on how often they should perform such checks or on whom, and it is not known how well doctors actually perform them. There is little emphasis in medical school training on how to perform breast examination. Consequently, it is done by doctors in a haphazard way, often as an adjunct to taking a cervical smear. Because there are no recommendations for routine breast examination, it is hard for women to raise the issue when it is not offered by the doctor, as evidenced here:

> I discussed self-examination with my doctor and he showed me how to do it. Of course I haven't bothered, I just don't remember. When I've tried it occasionally, I'm always uncertain what to do. When I have my smear I think about asking my doctor to check my breasts, but I'm too embarrassed. I don't mind the smear because it's quite clinical, there's nothing sexual about it. But examining the breasts is not clinical, so I'm a bit shy about initiating it, although I would like him to check me every time I have a smear.

Mammographic screening

Mammography provides an x-ray view of the breast. A skilled operator—a radiographer—takes a picture of the breast while flattened between two plates. The resulting image is read by a radiologist, a doctor who has had special training in this technique.

Mammography does not prevent cancer, so it cannot reduce the incidence of the disease. There would be just as many breast cancers if all women were having mammography as there would be if they were not. The purpose of mammography is to detect tiny cancers when they are impalpable—that is, before the woman or a doctor examining her could feel them. This early diagnosis then allows the cancer to be treated sooner than it otherwise would be. This may improve the woman's chances of cure and survival. The other benefit is that she may need less extensive surgery than if her cancer was detected later.

This is the ideal that mammography hopes to attain. Sadly, the benefits that can actually be achieved with mammography are not that clear-cut—its promise is modified by the behavior of the disease and by limitations of the technology.

The Behavior of Breast Cancer

Breast cancer is a sinister disease. It can grow for a long period without the woman having any idea what is happening in her breast. By the time she finds a lump or other sign of cancer, it has often been silently multiplying for months and usually years. Even when detected by mammography, the cancer will have already been present for some time. Writing about the behavior of breast cancer in the *British Medical Journal,* one doctor pointed out that even the most advanced techniques for detection presently available cannot pick up a breast cancer "early in a biological sense having regard to the overall time scale of the disease."

> If we assume exponential growth of a tumor volume doubling time of two months, a tumor of only 2 mm diameter [the smallest size tumor that can be detected by mammography] will have been resident in the tissues for about three years eight months and will contain about four million cells; by the time it reaches 3 cm diameter it will have been resident for about five years seven months. Thus a tumor diagnosed by screening at the smallest conceivable size detectable will already have gone through 65% of the time taken to reach a size that is easily palpable. Clearly screening is far from being capable of *early* diagnosis.(8)

The vast majority of cancers are poorly differentiated ductal adenocarcinomas. This invasive cancer can be preceded by various precancerous conditions such as atypical hyperplasia or lobular or ductal carcinoma in situ. These conditions increase the risk of breast cancer developing, but progression is by no means certain.

Individual breast cancers can behave differently; some grow rapidly and some are called "indolent" or lazy—they grow more slowly. When cancer is diagnosed, doctors find it very difficult to predict the probable course of an individual woman's disease. Many breast cancers start to metastasize, or spread, early in their biological life, before the tumor can be detected either by mammography or by the woman herself. This means that by the time the tumor is detected, malignant cells may already have silently migrated to the lymph nodes and by way of the lymph or drainage system of the body spread to other parts of the body. The woman may be treated for breast cancer by surgery, radiation, or various kinds of drug therapy, but the malignant cells may have already set up house in some other distant part of the body and be growing there. This lethal biology of breast cancer sets limitations on what any program for early detection can achieve.

Limitations of the Technology

In the words of Heather Mitchell, spokesperson on mammography for the Australasian Epidemiological Association, it is "desperation" induced by the toll from breast cancer that has promoted interest in mammographic screening, despite the many drawbacks.(9)

Mammography cannot detect all cancers. It will miss a proportion of cancers which are already present, even ones that can be seen and felt. Cancers can show up as a white area on a mammogram, but so does breast tissue which has the same density. The breasts of women under 50 are mainly made up of breast tissue, making the mammogram relatively difficult to read. As women age, there is less glandular tissue and more fat in the breasts, so the mammograms become easier to read. This means that mammography is more reliable for over-50-year-olds.

There are also "interval" cancers—cancers that develop rapidly between mammograms. Regular mammography cannot give a woman a guarantee she is free of cancer. Even when cancer is detected, there is no way of being certain that the early treatment she receives will prolong or save the woman's life.

Despite these limitations, there is a tendency to see mammography as holding the key to eliminating the threat of breast cancer in women's lives. Women commonly feel aggrieved that mammography is not more accessible and see it as further evidence of the low priority given to women's needs within the health system. In many health insurance plans, mammography is only covered for diagnostic purposes; women with no symptoms must pay to have a screening mammogram carried out.

Selling Mammography

There is a problem of vested interests in the promotion of mammography. As most mammography screening is done in the private health sector, these units need considerable use to pay for the very expensive technology involved. In the process of recruiting women, the benefits of mammographic screening tend to be somewhat oversold and the drawbacks downplayed or ignored. Women do not understand that mammography cannot protect them against developing breast cancer, and they are usually not told that a cancer detected by mammography could still kill. This limitation of the technology—and it is not the only one—is simply avoided in the promotional literature.

For instance, an advertising leaflet from the Radiology Group in Auckland gives three reasons why women should think about mammography, each one of which is wrong:

- "It's the number one cause of death among women." Not so, heart disease kills five times more women, stroke nearly three times more.

- "One of every 10 women will develop breast cancer sometime during her life." Wrong again. As we have seen, the authoritative figure is 1 in 15.

- "And most cases can now be cured—*if they're detected soon enough.*" Sadly, this is a long way from the truth.

This kind of oversell makes mammography seem absolutely vital and highly effective, but the claims cannot be sustained by any of the scientific evidence.

The National Cancer Institute (NCI) recently released a statement concerning breast cancer screening, updating its recommendation that women have a baseline screening at age 35 and regular mammograms from age 40 on. The statement is a successor to a working guideline formulation drafted in 1987 and will be revised as new information is developed.

NCI convened an International Workshop on Breast Cancer Screening in February 1993. The results from eight randomized clinical trials were reviewed. The workshop conclusions reinforced the advisability of screening for women ages 50 to 69 and stated that the effects of screening in women ages 40 to 49 do not demonstrate a statistically significant reduction in mortality to date.

In America fear is used as a weapon to persuade women to show up for mammography. "All breast cancer needs is a place to hide," says one advertisement. "Have a mammogram, give yourself the

chance of a lifetime." Women are exhorted to have a mammogram
with messages that imply that the woman who does not is stupid: "If
you haven't had a mammogram, you need more than your breast
examined."

None of these promotional messages is really frank about what
mammography can and cannot do, and somewhat extreme claims
have been made in the media. Dr. Laszlo Tabar, principal researcher
in the influential Swedish Two Counties Study, said that breast
screening could save the lives of half of all New Zealand women who
die annually from breast cancer, a claim which is not sustainable on
the evidence from even the most successful trials.(10) As we shall see,
the true figure is probably less than 10%.

A tempering voice in the midst of the pro-mammography enthusiasm has come from the Cancer Society of New Zealand and
from Professor David Skegg, who convened the working party that
drew up guidelines for screening in New Zealand. Professor Skegg
cautions that there has been "too much hype" about mammography:
"I think it's important not to exaggerate the potential benefits of
mammography. This is not a panacea for the problem of breast cancer. There have been some quite unrealistic statements made in the
news media about it."(11)

The Evidence on Mammographic Screening

The purpose of screening programs is to test well people in order to
detect medical conditions at an early stage. Screening is only beneficial if early treatment improves the outcome, in terms of morbidity
and mortality, compared to what would happen if the condition were
not detected until a later stage.

The World Health Organization has established criteria for acceptable mass screening tests (see page 286). While mammographic
screening meets some of these criteria, it does not meet them all. The
critical elements are that

- the disease is not well understood

- an early stage of the disease is hard to recognize

- the test to detect the disease—mammography—is costly and
  imprecise

World Health Organization Principles of Screening

For a screening test to be acceptable it should fulfil the following criteria:

- the condition sought should be an important health problem;

- the natural history of the disease should be well understood;

- there should be a recognisable early stage;

- treatment of the disease at an early stage should be of more benefit than treatment started at a later stage

- there should be a suitable test;

- there should be adequate facilities for the diagnosis and treatment of abnormalities detected;

- for diseases of insidious onset, screening should be repeated at intervals determined by the natural history of the disease

- the chance of physical or psychological harm to those screened should be less than the chance of benefit; and

- the cost of a screening program should be balanced against the benefit it provides.

- acceptability of the test to women is not really known

- there are risks of harm to people who take part in screening

The fact that mammography is a far from perfect screening tool explains the caution with which most countries have approached the idea of using mammography for mass screening programs. One of the few to decide to go ahead is the United Kingdom, although there has also been criticism that the decision to do so was premature.(12) This followed the Forrest Report which decided that although breast screening did not meet all the criteria for successful screening, the benefits of doing so would outweigh the risks.(13)

The final arbiter for the effectiveness of mammography is whether or not it saves lives. There is not a lot of point in detecting cancers unless the woman gains some life by doing so. If mammography does not improve her chances, all that will have been achieved is that she will know she has cancer for longer than she would have otherwise.

Professor Skegg addressed this point at a seminar on breast cancer in Auckland:

> If you talk to any radiologist, they will be able to tell you about breast cancers in women in their 40s that they have been able to detect. The problem is that just because you've detected something, does not prove that you are going to improve that person's survival. A few years ago it was widely recommended that heavy smokers should have regular X-rays in the hope that lung cancers could be picked up early while they were still treatable. It seemed a very logical idea. And when this procedure was used, some heavy smokers were found to have lung cancer before symptoms had developed. But when randomized trials were carried out it was shown that screening actually produced no benefit—the death rate was exactly the same in the people who had regular X-rays and those who didn't. So it is no longer recommended as a screening practice.(14)

The only way to determine if mammography can prevent deaths from cancer is by large-scale studies comparing women who are screened with women who are not. All such studies of mammographic screening use death from breast cancer as their main measuring point. Assessing the effectiveness of screening is potentially complicated by a process called "lead time bias." The screening may have appeared to have given a woman an extra two or more years when these are really only the difference in time between when a mammogram can detect a tumor and when she might have noticed it herself. Most of the studies of mammographic screening have tried to control for this effect.

Arguments in favor of mammographic screening are based primarily on two randomized controlled trials: the New York Health Insurance Plan trial, or HIP study, and the Swedish Two Counties Study. These provide the best evidence for the effectiveness of screening.

The HIP study

The HIP study was the first randomized controlled trial of mammographic screening.(15) In 1963, 62,000 women aged 40–64 who were in an insurance plan were randomly allocated to two groups. One of the groups was offered annual mammography for the next three years. Sixty-five percent of the group took advantage of this offer and had a clinical examination of the breasts and a mammogram. Ten years later (six years after the mammography ended) there were 30% fewer deaths among the screened women, with the major benefit seen in women over 50. By 18 years later, however, the reduction in deaths in the study group had declined to 23%. Critics argue that "catch up" suggests that women who had their breast cancer diagnosed by mammography only had their deaths postponed by screening.(16) It is also possible to say that these women gained some extra years because of screening.

The Swedish Two Counties study

This randomized controlled study in Ostergotland and Kopparbarg in Sweden was similar to the HIP study, although the screening was less frequent: every 24 months for women 40–49, and every 33 months for women over 50, and there was no physical examination.(17) Nearly 90% of the women came to the first screening round. A difference between the screened group and the control group began to emerge after four years. The reduction in deaths among the women having mammographic screening was 31%, although once again this benefit was only marked among women over 50.

These two large studies, indicating a worthwhile reduction in deaths among screened women if they were over 50 years of age, are frequently quoted in support of mammography; but against this has to be set the experience in three further trials which gave rather different results.

The Malmo trial

Another randomized controlled trial was started in Malmo, Sweden, in the same year the Two Counties Study began.(18) This time the women were of a slightly different age, 45–69 years old, and they were offered screening by mammography every 21 months, but no physical examination. Seventy-four percent of the women took part in the first screening round. After 10 years there was no significant difference in breast cancer mortality between the screened and the control group aged over 55 years, and there was a nonsignificant excess of mortality among the younger group of screened women, a result that could have arisen by chance. Problems with this trial arise from the relatively small scale of the study and the fact that nearly one-quarter of the controls had a mammogram of their own accord during the trial period, which could have brought results in the two groups closer together than they otherwise would have been.

The Edinburgh trial

In the Edinburgh study, women aged 45–64 were randomized and the study group was then offered an annual examination: a physical examination one year and a mammographic examination the following year.(19) Sixty-one percent of the eligible women took up the offer; at the end of seven years there was a nonsignificant 17% reduction in deaths in women offered screening, and this was almost entirely confined to the women over 50.

The Canadian trial—the National Breast Screening Study

This Canadian study was the first designed specifically to look at the vexed question of mammography's benefits to under-50-year-olds. None of the previous studies had sufficient numbers in this age group to come up with confident results. This study found that after seven years there were more deaths in the group receiving mammography than the group that did not, a conclusion that shocked many of those who advocated for mammography.(20)

In 1993 the National Cancer Institute held an International Workshop on Screening for Breast Cancer to provide an "objective critical review" of all the study results. It concluded that for women aged 40–49, randomized controlled trials have consistently shown no benefit from screening for the first 5–7 years after study entry. At 10–12 years the benefit is uncertain, but if there is one it is tiny. For women 50–69 years, screening reduces breast cancer mortality by about one-third.(21)

Following this workshop the National Cancer Institute issued a policy statement that it did not support mammographic screening for women under 50.

What Does This Mean for Individuals?

All these studies are of screening programs organized on a population basis and the results are averages across populations. This means that the kind of reductions in mortality achieved in the HIP and Swedish Two Counties studies are worked out over the whole population of women invited to have a mammogram, rather than just the women who actually attended. No study has achieved 100% attendance rates; if this had been achieved, then the reduction in mortality would have been greater. The attendance rate in the Swedish Two Counties study was high, around 90%, so an individual woman could expect to achieve approximately this benefit or slightly more at an abstract statistical level.

There is no way that an individual can be given an accurate personalized prediction of what she can achieve by regular screening for herself. All that can be said for the individual woman over 50 is that she is reducing her chance of dying from breast cancer by 30% or more by having a mammogram every other year.

Professor David Skegg estimates that for a woman over 50 years of age actually having mammograms, the reduction in risk could be as high as 50%. This means a reduction in risk of death from about 3 in 100 to $1\frac{1}{2}$ to 2 in 100. On the other hand, women under 50 need to know that statistically they are probably not achieving anything at all.

The recommended interval between mammograms for asymptomatic women is every two years after the age of 50. The interval for women under 50 must be one year, although it is not recommended in this age group.

Screening Programs

Countries considering mammographic screening programs want to know what can be achieved for the whole population and are looking for significant reductions in total deaths. Screening programs use a large proportion of health resources, so they must be shown to be effective before they are put in place, or money could be squandered for no great benefit. The existence of a particular technology is not an absolute justification for using it. It must be shown to work, without causing undue risks to the users of the services (see below).

Screening programs that fail can do harm. There are always risks and costs involved in screening, both for society and for the individuals involved. This raises ethical considerations, which were summed up by Professor Skegg at a meeting on breast cancer in 1990: "The ethics of someone going to their doctor and saying 'I've got this problem, please help me,' are different from professionals going to the healthy public and saying 'We've got something you need.' In order to do that, we really need to have very clear evidence of the benefits."(22)

The good results achieved in the Swedish Two Counties study resulted from a very high standard of screening. The program was very well designed and organized. Even in Sweden, this experience has not yet been translated into a nationwide program. A lot more than mammography machines are needed to make screening work. Mammography is a specialized technique, and radiologists working in this area need to go through an extensive approved training program to reach a sufficient level of expertise.

Balance Sheet for a National Program of Screening for Breast Cancer in Sweden

Benefits

- One extra survivor
- 1760 women reassured

Losses

- Cost to services and patients of screening 1850 women
- 75 false positive results
- In 15 of the women who were found to have breast cancer the outcome was unchanged.

(Source: Rose, Geoffrey, 1990. Reflections on the changing times, BMJ, 301 683–87.)

There also needs to be a whole extra level of backup to bring into play when an abnormality is suspected from a mammogram. In some countries, such as Britain, there are multidisciplinary assessment teams that specialize in breasts—specially trained clinicians, pathologists, and nurses—who take over the management of cases where a cancer is suspected. In the past, general surgeons have performed breast surgery, but they are not necessarily experienced in handling the tiny cancers that are revealed by mammography. In New Zealand multidisciplinary breast teams are few and far between. The premature commencement of mammographic screening could result in unnecessarily extensive surgery for some women.

Another important consideration in any screening program is how acceptable the screening procedure is for the people expected to use it. If the particular test is so unacceptable to the potential users that they do not avail themselves of it, then it is not a useful screening procedure and will not effectively reduce mortality. Participation rates need to be at least 70% for a screening program to make any appreciable dent in mortality.

In the studies carried out so far, participation rates have been highest in the Swedish studies. It is important to recognize that the Scandinavian countries have highly organized health care systems. In these countries, residents are on population health registers from birth. They are familiar with preventive health care programs, and therefore when they receive an invitation to have a mammogram via the register, they are more likely to respond to it. In countries such as the United States, there are no comprehensive health registers and it is difficult to invite women for screening. People planning the services have to find some other way to reach women, either by using imperfect lists, such as electoral rolls, or through publicity or general practitioners. This is much harder to achieve.

Women in Edinburgh may be more like American women in their response to an approach to take part in mammographic screening, but even there, the Scottish program had the advantage of being able to invite women by using general practitioners' age-sex patient registers. Not many U.S. doctors have such registers. Attendance rates in Edinburgh were best among women in the highest socioeconomic groups—67% for Social Class 1 at the first screen and 54% for Social Class 6.(23)

In all the screening programs it has proven difficult to keep women attending. The dropout rate is high, greater than one-third in some trials. In the Edinburgh study the attendance rate was 61% for the first screen, but 54% by the second screen.(24) The fall was particularly noticeable in older women. It is generally acknowledged that it is easier to get women in their forties to attend for regular tests than women over 50. The younger group are more health conscious and more tuned in to preventive medicine. In the case of mammography, there is no proven benefit to women under 50, while, ironically, the group that would be expected to benefit—the over-50-year-olds—are not so keen on attending. Australian breast clinics report that less than 20% of their clientele are over 50 years of age.(25) This may explain why commercial interests try to appeal to the under-50-year-olds despite the lack of firm evidence for benefit.

Some people argue that screening should be available for women who choose it, without bothering about organizing a program to make it available for all women. But the effect of this would be that women who are better educated and more knowledgeable about mammography would be more likely to have a test, whereas less-educated, poorer women would not. Middle-class women would also be more likely to afford the cost of a mammogram and other costs associated with it, such as unpaid time off work, transport, and childcare costs.

Mammography provided in an unorganized way as part of private health care would mean a privileged service for middle-class women, which other women could not afford. Although in general breast cancer is slightly more common among women in higher socioeconomic groups, it is also prevalent among precisely the group of women who would be unable to take advantage of private screening.

The cervix/breast debate

The statement is frequently heard that less attention should be paid to cervical screening and more to breast screening because breast cancer kills more women than cervical cancer, but there are important differences between the two types of screening programs. A cervical screening program detects precancers and can prevent cancer from ever occurring, whereas the best that mammography can achieve is early detection of existing cancers. In Britain a committee reviewing that country's experience of breast screening worked out that after ten years, Britain's screening program would be expected to be able to prevent 1,250 deaths annually.(26) As 15,000 women die of breast cancer each year in that country, the saved lives amount to 8% of the total breast cancer toll.

Applying these figures in the U.S., this would mean saving the lives of about 3,560 of the 44,500 women who died of breast cancer in 1991. The restricted impact of mammographic screening on total mortality from breast cancer explains why cervical screening can actually prevent a greater number of deaths than regular breast screening.

Is Mammography a Benign Technology?

One of the most poignant commentaries on mammographic screening was written by Dr. Maureen Roberts, who led the Edinburgh Breast Screening Project. The results of this project were published in the *Lancet* in February 1990, but by this time, Dr. Roberts was dead, of breast cancer. Shortly before her death, Dr. Roberts wrote about her reservations about mammography.(27) Before the results of Dr. Roberts' study had been published, Britain had already made the controversial decision to go ahead with a national mammographic screening program at a cost of millions of pounds. Dr. Roberts wrote:

> I am in a reflective mood as I lie here in the sunshine at the end of my life. Breast cancer has caught up with me, after eight good years. It seems a common disease in Britain, and the evidence is strong that it is on the increase. Small wonder that people working with the disease desperately want to do something.

Dr. Roberts then addressed the question: "What can screening actually achieve?"

> We all know that mammography is an unsuitable screening test: it is technologically difficult to perform, the pictures are difficult to interpret, it has a high false positive rate, and we don't know how often to carry it out. We can no longer ignore the possibility that screening may not reduce mortality in women of any age, however disappointing this may be.
>
> I have to go on and ask the next question: If screening does little or no good, could it possibly be doing any harm? We are all reluctant to face this.

Firstly, I'm thinking about the false positive rate. One in 10 women are being asked to come back for further investigations, which is an unacceptably high proportion. It clearly does not cause all women psychological harm, but it is traumatic for many. In most cases it is also unnecessary.

Some 10% to 17% of all cancers will be diagnosed as non-invasive. The screeners are delighted, but non-invasive cancer is a difficult condition for women, and no studies have been done about their thoughts and feelings. We do not know how much it represents an overdiagnosis of cancer, nor do we know its natural course or how to treat it.

For most women who have invasive cancer diagnosed they become "patients" like other women. The difference is that they did not discover their problem, it was discovered for them. There is also an undeniable if subtle pressure on them to be grateful, but no studies have been done to find out what women feel and think. Neither do we know how these women cope with recurrence. After all, they were almost promised (if only by implication) a good outcome if they attended for screening.

Further reservations were expressed in 1991 in an article reviewing preliminary results from the first pilot mammography screening program carried out in Australia.(28) The program had screened 7,000 women in the first 18 months, and 53 cancers had been detected. But 40% of the cancers were palpable; in other words, they could have been detected by a clinical examination without all the expense of a mammographic screening program. The article pointed out that in this program a scrupulous attention to detail had ensured that the negative effects of screening had been kept to a minimum, but the authors were concerned that this might be difficult to translate into a program for the whole community.

In any preventive health program dealing with well persons, an essential feature of the program is the maximization of benefit and the minimization of adverse effects. This is especially true of screening by mammography where the potential for benefit is relatively small (numerically) and the potential for harm considerable. The benefit of screening is the detection of small, clinically occult cancers which can be expected to be treated conservatively with an excellent prognosis. The harm is the intervention into the lives of normal women only to prove they do not have a problem. This harm may be expressed in various ways—anxiety about the possibility of breast cancer, especially if an abnormality is detected at the initial screen; psychological and physical trauma of the investigations necessary to differentiate benign from malignant once an abnormality is found; the experience of open biopsy for a benign screen-detected lesion of which the screenee was oblivious; the disillusionment or anger associated with a missed or interval cancer; the earlier diagnosis of breast cancer for which the outcome may not be altered; and the diagnosis of a breast cancer which may never have become a clinical problem.

These writers stressed the importance of women understanding both the benefits and risks of mammography so they were fully aware when deciding to go ahead with one.

Drawbacks of Mammography

Discomfort and embarrassment of the procedure

To be most effective, mammography has to be uncomfortable. The more the breast can be compressed, the more effectively the mammogram can be "read." It can be more difficult to obtain a good mammogram from a woman with small breasts since it is difficult to compress the breast tissue.

> I have a regular mammogram—it is about as personal as getting a car registration. I learned it was much harder to get a good screen from small breasts. Mine are so small they had difficulty getting them into the "machine."

> Mammography was uncomfortable for me but not painful. The second time, a male did it, which I had not expected would happen. He offered me a choice of exposing one breast at a time from the white coat or both at the same time. No way was I going to have this fella see both my breasts at once. In a hot sweat and blushing I struggled with one sleeve off, one breast out, same sleeve on, next sleeve off, second breast out and back into the

refuge of the little white coat. The comical part was, he was going to see them both anyway. I'm pleased to say my third mammography was at a private x-ray center where all the staff are female and I felt so much more comfortable.

Anxiety

Women can feel anxious about what they might find out or feel anxious when something is discovered that needs further investigation.

Each year when I go for a mammogram, I'm shaking in my shoes as I go through the door thinking this year is going to be the time.

I suggested mammography to my GP five years ago when I was 40 because a couple of women I knew of my age had gotten breast cancer. She was slightly reluctant as she didn't think it was necessary. It was like an insurance: I'd think, oh well, I haven't got breast cancer, I'm fine. Then last time they found something they didn't like and did it again. That freaked me out because I didn't go to be told something was wrong. I went to be told I was fine. I've now persuaded myself there is no evidence that it is useful for women under 50. So I've stopped going.

I was referred for a mammography for a lump which can be felt when lying down and is sore each month the week before my period. The local surgeon could not feel it and insinuated that weight loss would help him find it. I do have some questions unanswered and not even voiced. If the lump is fatty tissue as they say, will it ever go away? Do they have a high chance of becoming malignant? What causes them?

Unnecessary biopsy

Mammography has a false positive rate. This means that a proportion of women who have a mammogram will need further investigation for some apparent abnormality that will subsequently prove to be benign.

In screening programs carried out so far, 5–10% of the women screened required further investigation.(29) In the Australian study, nearly 1,200 of the 7,200 women screened were recalled.(30) In the case of 273 of the women this was because of technical faults, and they needed repeat mammography, while 915 women needed assessment because of suspected abnormality. Of these women, 118 went on to a consultation with a surgeon, 99 had an open biopsy, and 53 were found to have cancer. This 2:1 rate of biopsy per cancer confirmed is very low, although the same rate was recently reported in Britain.(31) This may reflect improvements in technique since the reports from programs of some years ago.

In other overseas programs, 2–4% of the women screened have needed an open biopsy for 0.5% cancers to be detected, a rate of 4:1 or even 8:1. The unnecessary biopsy rate tends to improve with subsequent screens in a screening program, as the first mammogram will have answered many questions about an individual woman's breasts.

Several types of biopsy are used to diagnose breast abnormalities:

- *Fine needle aspiration,* where a fine needle is inserted into the lump and the cells drawn off are sent for cytological appraisal. This is used for lumps that can be felt, although sometimes with a mammographically detected abnormality the needle can be guided into the lump under X-ray. With a palpable lump, if fluid is drawn off when the needle is inserted and the lump collapses, this suggests the lump was probably a harmless cyst. If no fluid is drawn off, the cells removed will provide a provisional diagnosis of the nature of the tissue, but many women proceed to a biopsy after fine needle aspiration. Sampling errors, where no cancer cells are brought up in the syringe, are possible with this technique.

- *Incisional biopsy,* where part of a lump is removed for diagnosis. This is usually only performed for large lumps.

- *Excision biopsy,* where the lump is removed for both diagnosis and treatment.

- *Biopsy by wire localization* is used for abnormal areas detected by mammography that cannot be palpated. In this technique, a fine, hooked wire is guided into the abnormal tissue under mammography. The surgeon then removes the tissue surrounding the wire for examination.

The term "open biopsy" referred to above includes any of the last three types of biopsy.

When it comes to treatment, many women who have a small malignant tumor detected by mammography are able to have a simple lumpectomy followed by radiotherapy. It is wrong to assume, however, that because a tumor is detected by mammography it can always be removed with minimum damage to the breast. If the malignancy is diffuse or badly positioned, such as deep in the breast, against the chest wall, or around the nipple, a mastectomy must still be performed.

Overdiagnosis

In some women mammography will detect a precancer, such as *atypical hyperplasia* or *carcinoma in situ (CIS)*. Left alone, these precancers might or might not progress into a malignancy. *Lobular CIS* has a progression rate of around 16–27% in 30 years, and *ductal CIS* has a progression rate thought to be about 20–25% in 10 years.(32)

If the precancer was not going to progress, without mammography the women would have been oblivious to it. With mammography, the woman is faced with an agonizing choice: to wait or to go ahead and have treatment. She will never know whether or not the treatment was necessary. Mastectomy is sometimes the only treatment available in these cases because the abnormal tissue is spread throughout the breast. This overdiagnosis can be a cause of more cancers apparently occurring in a group of screened women compared to women who are not being screened.

False reassurance

Just as mammograms have a false positive rate, there is also a false negative rate of about the same magnitude, where an actual cancer is missed. A normal mammogram does not exclude malignancy. In the Breast Cancer Detection Demonstration Project carried out by the National Cancer Institute of America and the American Cancer Society, 9% of palpable cancers did not show up on the mammogram.(33) Other studies have shown even higher rates of missed cancers—10–29%.(34) This is more likely to happen in women under 50. When it happens, women are falsely reassured they are safe, and because of this may even ignore actual signs of cancer in the breast, such as a thickening or lump.

Interval cancers are a reason mammography can fail. When this happens, a cancer appears between mammograms, either because it was fast growing or because it was missed on the mammogram. In both the HIP and Swedish Two Counties studies, 30–50% of the cancers in the study groups were interval cancers.

Because the abilities of mammography have been oversold, there is also a tendency to use mammography inappropriately. General practitioners sometimes refer patients for mammography to diagnose palpable lumps. If the mammogram says the lump is harmless, the woman may be left with an untreated cancer that gets bigger and bigger. In the days before mammography, the same lump would have been referred to a surgeon, diagnosed by biopsy, and treatment started if necessary. In this way, mammography, far from ensuring early treatment, can actually cause delays in treatments.

Although mammography can be used as an adjunct to diagnosis, a palpable lump is a matter for a breast specialist. Unless the lump is clearly benign, the specialist would probably need to perform a biopsy to diagnose it.

Disease labeling

Many lumps and masses detected by mammography or by examination turn out to be benign. Doctors and radiologists have various labels for these harmless conditions and know what they mean, but the women who are told they have them can find this quite alarming. Even something as harmless as having one breast bigger than the other may be described as "marked asymmetry"—a potentially alarming term unless you know what it means. Unfortunately, little effort is made to explain the meaning of various terms, leading to unnecessary fear on the part of women.

The classic disease or nondisease label is *fibrocystic disease.* Some women worry that this may mean they are predisposed to develop cancer, but fibrocystic disease simply means lumpy breasts and half of all women have them! Young women who have mammograms that are difficult to read are particularly at risk of being told they have fibrocystic disease.

Dr. Susan Love, director of the Breast Clinic at the Beth Israel Hospital in Boston, writes:

"Fibrocystic disease" is a meaningless umbrella term—a waste-basket into which doctors throw every breast problem that isn't cancerous. The symptoms that it encompasses are so varied and so unrelated to each other that the term is wholly without meaning. Some doctors recognize this and have stopped using the term. Others, unfortunately, have not. Still others will use equally bad terms such as "chronic cystic mastitis" or just "cystic mastitis."(35)

In the U.S. women with this nondisease have even been talked into prophylactic mastectomies and reconstruction by unscrupulous doctors.(36)

Another variation on the dense breasts theme is when women are told they have *mammary dysplasia*. Dysplasia in any other context means abnormal cell changes that can lead to cancer, so to interpret a diagnosis of dysplasia as meaning precancer would seem logical. But such a diagnosis can only be made by a pathologist looking at the cells in the laboratory, not a radiologist looking at an X-ray picture. Mammary dysplasia simply means dense breasts, but to be given this "diagnosis" can be very alarming:

When I was 40 I had a lump and was referred for a mammogram. Now I think the lump was to do with my period as they couldn't find anything, but I came back with a report that said "moderately severe dysplastic changes" in both breasts. They said I would need another mammogram in two years. I took from the report that I was at risk of breast cancer, it wasn't explained. Later I learned that it was just a radiologist's term which simply means density. Now I understand that I have dense breast tissue, which is typical of breasts at 40.

A further worrisome report a woman can be given from a mammogram is to be told she has *microcalcifications*. These are tiny specks of calcium which are sometimes precursors of cancer. However, 80% of microcalcifications are not precursors of cancer and are entirely harmless. Having many microcalcifications usually indicates there is no problem. More worrisome are new microcalcifications or a cluster of them. If there are only one or two, or it is a woman's first mammogram, she may be asked to return for another mammogram in six months' to see what has changed.

Another aspect of disease labeling is when women get caught up in the system, and are told they need frequent mammograms:

I was getting soreness in my left breast premenstrually where I had had mastitis when breastfeeding. The doctor suggested that as I was 43 I should have a mammogram. I knew something was wrong when the nurse came in and didn't make eye contact and said the radiologist wanted another view of the left breast. While I was waiting for the second mammogram I was pretty nervous. I was told there was some shading in the left side, it wasn't specific. They suggested I come back in another six months just to see what was happening. I went back in nine months—I put it off until after Christmas because I thought if I have cancer, at least I'll have had a happy Christmas. After the mammogram the radiologist spoke to me—in language I wouldn't have understood if I hadn't been a medical person. He said the mammogram was all right but to come back in eight months. I asked why, if there was nothing on the mammogram for me to worry about as he had assured me. He said it was routine and it was better to be safe than sorry. He said when you have had a mammogram on which something abnormal has appeared it pays to check it out regularly. I said was there any abnormality on the mammogram, and he said no. It was all so contradictory. I decided in my own mind not to go back, but last week I received a reminder that I was due for a mammogram and to go and get a referral. When the card arrived, I became acutely aware of the pain in my left breast! I threw out the card, but I still have at the back of my mind that maybe I should go to be sure.

Radiation risk

Modern mammography gives extremely low doses of radiation and is generally considered to be safe. However, it is not "no risk" as is commonly claimed, just very low risk, especially when compared to other forms of X-ray. Today, mammography requires only about 0.2 rad exposure to the breast compared to the 2 rad exposure common in the 1960s when mammography was in its infancy. At this low exposure it has been estimated that one woman in a million might develop breast cancer as a result of mammographic screening.(37) The risk is greater in young women, especially women in their thirties. Mammography machines need to be strictly monitored to ensure that women are getting the lowest dose possible.

A Balancing Act

This list of risks of mammography has been full, to counteract the tendency in patient literature to gloss over the drawbacks. Some women will decide that these drawbacks are outweighed by the benefits screening offers in improving the hope of survival if cancer is detected and in offering the chance of less surgery. When weighing up the positive and negative aspects of screening, the factors that will influence each woman will be highly personal and individual:

> My sister has had premenopausal breast cancer, as has a cousin. When my sister got breast cancer, I thought, oh well, I'll definitely have to have a mammogram now. Then I kept on putting it off until I finally realized I was not ready to find out if I had breast cancer. I have seen how utterly my sister's life has been changed, and I do not want to face the possibility myself, yet. She had great difficulty with the idea that the biopsy told her she had cancer when she felt so well. Then she had to undergo terrible treatment for something that seemed unreal. Why cope with all that before you have to? I am not sure the theoretical extra years you gain are worth bringing forward the time when you find out.

> The doctor felt I should have a mammogram because my sister has had a breast removed. I can't feel my breasts well because they are so full of fibrous tissue from breastfeeding my five children. The mammogram stopped me worrying. I was reassured everything was all right.

Jocelyn Chamberlain of the Institute of Cancer Research in the United Kingdom has a similar point of view:

> Screening, like all preventive medicine, can be likened to an insurance policy whereby one pays a certain premium in order to diminish a particular risk. Just as car insurance does not prevent accidents, it merely diminishes the risk of one of their worst

consequences, a write-off of the vehicle, so breast cancer screening does not prevent cancer from developing but it lessens the risk of its worst consequence, death.(38)

Chamberlain argues that screening is not as distressing to women as Dr. Maureen Roberts maintained. She says any anxiety is short-lived. Her interpretation of the evidence led her to make this assessment for herself:

> During the next 20 years, I, in my late 50s, stand a 1 in 40 chance of dying from breast cancer. If screened from age 50 onward I may be able to reduce this risk to 1 in 55. To me this reduction is worth the slight inconvenience of going for mammography every few years; of having a 1 in 14 chance of being referred and a 1 in 170 chance of having a benign biopsy (both of which have happened to me and were more irritating than alarming); and even of artificially increasing my chance of a breast cancer diagnosis . . . . To me it seems a mildly inconvenient but sensible precaution in the same league, albeit at a greater cost, as a cholera or typhoid immunization before a foreign trip.(39)

The ethical issues raised by screening well women can only be resolved by ensuring that women are fully aware of the benefits and risks and are able to make an informed choice. People cope better when they make deliberate decisions rather than enter into a situation "blind" or half-knowledgeable. The more informed women are, the more in control they will feel of the process, whatever it brings them. Conversely, if the facts deter some women, it is their right to decide not to take part.

Chapter 12

All About Cervixes

Of all the disease prevention strategies discussed in this book, cervical screening is the most straightforward, providing significant protection against cervical cancer for individual women. When it is part of a population-based screening program, it also provides the chance of substantially reducing the overall death rate from cervical cancer. Unlike mammography, cervical screening is a method of disease *prevention* because it detects abnormal cell changes before they become malignant. The abnormal cells can then be destroyed or removed, so ensuring that a cancer never occurs.

The aim of cervical screening is not to detect full-blown cancers as women popularly assume. It is to detect earlier nonmalignant stages of the disease called *precancers* or *cancer precursors*. Cervical screening is really an early warning system which can protect women who have regular cervical smears from ever developing invasive disease.

There are some problematic areas in the strategy of cervical screening, as will be discussed later. These relate mainly to the dilemmas raised by detecting large numbers of low-grade abnormalities in women, and then not being sure what to do about them. Many of these low-grade cell changes will disappear of their own accord: should they then be immediately treated, or should a "wait and see" policy be adopted?

When considering the issue of cervical screening, the aim of the exercise needs to be kept in mind. This is "to prevent invasive cervical cancer, not simply to detect preinvasive lesions."(1) The aim is not to obliterate every cell in the cervix that dares to look different, for however brief a time. The overall object of screening is to prevent harm to women, and abnormal cells will only cause harm if they progress. We have to be vigilant that we don't adopt the kind of "search and destroy" mentality which means that in the end the risks of the procedure start to threaten the benefits to women. More treatment is not always the best treatment.

Arguing against overtreatment of mild changes to cervical cells is not the same as failing to treat cells that show more serious changes, as happened at National Women's Hospital over many years in the 1960s and 1970s.(2) The difference is that there is a good chance that viral changes and low grade cell changes will regress of their own accord, while moderate to severe cell changes are quite likely to progress to invasive cancer.

Cervical Cancer in the United States

As cervical cancer can be prevented from occurring, deaths from this disease are an unnecessary tragedy. About 13,500 American women develop cervical cancer each year; in 1990 about three women per thousand died from it. The death rate has been static for some years, but deaths continue.

Although the incidence of cervical cancer is increasing slightly among women under 50 years of age, the actual numbers in this age group are still relatively low. Epidemiologists warn, however, that deaths in this age group could increase without regular smear tests for all women.(3)

As in most countries, it is primarily older women who develop and die from cervical cancer. The incidence rate for women 50 years old or older is over three times that for women under 50; the mortality rate is 8.4 per thousand women compared to 1.3 for women under 50. In 1973 the incidence rate for women under 50 and older was 8.7 per thousand compared to 31 for those 50 and older. The mortality rate has also improved in both groups, from 15 deaths per thousand women 50 and older in 1973 to 8.3 in 1990.

Black women, however, have incidence rates almost twice that of white women (13.3 per thousand for black women compared to 8.3 in white women in 1990). The five-year survival rate for white women has also improved, while for black women it has actually decreased, from 63.2% for 1974–76 to 55.3% for 1983–88.

Cervical Screening

Screening coverage

The different rates of cervical cancer between races and age groups have nothing to do with inherent differences between those groups, rather they are directly related to the prevalence of cervical screening. The rate at which cervical screening occurs in a particular group of women is called *screening coverage*. A high screening coverage equates with a low incidence of cancer, and, conversely, low screening coverage is related to a high incidence of the disease. Cancers occur among groups of women who are not having smear tests at all or who have an outdated *smear history,* meaning they have not had a smear test within the recommended interval of three years.

Statistically, black women are slightly more likely to have had a Pap smear in the last year than are white or Hispanic women. According to the 1990 figures generated by the National Health Interview survey, about half of all women had had a Pap smear in the last year. Figures for most subgroups of women are about the same, although only 37.9% of women with less than 12 years of education had recent Pap tests, compared to 49.6% of women with 12 years of education and 57.2% of those with more than 12 years. Perhaps the most interesting figure was that while 53.5% of currently married woman and 51.5% of those who had never been married had been tested recently, only 39.1% of formerly married women had been tested in the past year.

Opportunistic screening

Cervical screening in America currently occurs spontaneously, either when a woman asks her doctor for a test or the doctor offers her one. This is called *opportunistic screening.* The trouble with this system is that it leads to the uneven screening coverage discussed above. Young women are more likely to ask for or be offered smear tests as they more often see a doctor for matters related to sexuality, such as contraception, pregnancy, and vaginal infections. On the other hand, older women who are not having pelvic examinations do not tend to ask for a smear test or be offered one as frequently.(4) Embarrassment is a factor here. Older women may feel shy about suggesting the test or exposing themselves to the doctor, and research has shown that doctors can also be embarrassed about suggesting it.

The possibility has also been raised that negative attitudes toward older women can come into play here. A writer in the *Lancet* commented that in Britain doctors often did not implement the policy to concentrate on older women: "Clinicians tend to be more excited by the prospects of 'early diagnosis'—which is generally interpreted as diagnosis in 'young' women—than in forestalling disaster in older women with late lesions."(5)

Because of publicity about increases in cervical cancer among young women, there are also doctors who have gotten the impression they should concentrate on young women and that older women do not need smears as much.

This 55-year-old woman reported the following experience of being given the wrong advice:

> My GP tells me that I will need a "menopausal cervical smear" in August, which will be one year from my last period. After that, I will not need any more smears. I have been having regular smears for the past 26 years and nothing abnormal has ever shown up. I am a bit confused as somewhere I have seen that women need to have smears for longer than this, or is this yet another example of the great diversity in medical opinion?

This 44-year-old woman was also given a distorted impression of the relative importance of different health checks:

> In 1990 I went to family planning for a smear. They recommended a mammogram. I was told at my age annual mammogram was more important than a regular smear test. The smear was done but I didn't hear anything about the result.

Screening intervals

Some people argue that it is up to a woman to decide how often she has a smear test. On one level this is true, except that women often have smears on the advice of their doctor rather than as a result of their own informed choice. Most doctors and clinics habitually advise annual tests, especially for younger women. Partly, this stems from a belief that young women can develop a more "aggressive" form of cervical cancer, which could grow rapidly between less frequent smears. It now seems that there is no good evidence for this;

cases of apparently fast-developing cancer were caused by initial smears that were false negatives, leading to the erroneous impression that the disease had developed more quickly than it actually had.(6) Many doctors argue that this makes a yearly smear even more advisable since it lowers the risk of a false negative.

While this is certainly true, the Clinical Laboratory Improvement Amendment of 1988 was passed by the New Zealand Congress to change national standards. Most of the provisions in this amendment took effect in September 1992, and testing conditions have improved since then. There is now a limit to the number of tests a technician may read in a day, and record-keeping and quality control requirements have been tightened. Unfortunately, the last phase probably will not be completed until 1995. This will set up a testing program whereby all technicians will be tested annually to make sure they are sufficiently skilled to interpret difficult Pap smears.

Recommendations of annual smear taking can also simply be the result of ingrained practices, and the commercial aspect cannot be dismissed, at least for GPs. It is simple arithmetic. More money can be earned out of a woman who has three tests in three years than out of a woman who has one test in three years.

From the woman's point of view, she is adding only a little more protection by having a smear test more than every third year. The International Agency for Research on Cancer looked at this question and decided that "there was very little difference in the protection afforded by screening every year compared with every three years."(7) Their Working Group found that three-yearly screening could potentially reduce the incidence of cervical cancer by 91%, whereas annual screening would reduce it by 93%, a difference of only 2%.(8) They also noticed that the protection for a woman increased once she had two or more negative smears compared to only one, and decreased if five or more years had elapsed since the last negative smear. A woman having regular smears once every three years is eight times safer than a woman who has never had a smear test at all.

In light of these recent findings, the American College of Obstetricians and Gynecologists say that some women who have had normal smears three years in a row could reduce their visits to every other year or even every three years. This is certainly good news for women with no health insurance or who are not eligible for subsidized smears at Planned Parenthood and other clinics.

Organized screening programs

In populations with organized cervical screening programs, such as in the Scandinavian countries and British Columbia, the death rate from cervical cancer has been reduced by around 60–70%.(9) Under ideal conditions it should be possible to reduce the incidence of cervical cancer by 90% by screening.(10)

An organized program involves systematically inviting all eligible women to have regular smear tests and making sure they have access to accurate diagnosis and treatment if an abnormality is detected. Cervical screening can fail if screening coverage is poor, but it can also fail if abnormal smears are not followed up and treated. One study showed that among women with CIN 3 (severely abnormal cell changes), 14% had a series of abnormal smears for periods up to five years before being referred for colposcopy.(11)

To organize an effective program, it is necessary to have a management system in place. In most countries that have been successful at reducing the death rate, some basic components have been found to be essential. These include

- a national policy to ensure consistency
- someone in charge who is accountable for the program
- a method of systematically inviting women to take part
- services that are acceptable to women
- quality control at all levels to ensure
    — good standards of taking smears
    — excellent reading of smears in laboratories
    — high standard of treatment facilities for women with abnormalities
- ongoing monitoring and evaluation of the program to see that screening coverage is high in all groups of women and the death rate is falling

In the chapter on mammography we saw the criteria that have been developed to assess the likely effectiveness of any kind of screening program, and it is worth measuring cervical screening against this list. It can be seen that cervical screening meets most of the criteria established by the World Health Organization. Unlike mammography, there is an easily recognizable early stage of the disease which can be detected in women of all age groups, and the available treatment methods are nearly 100% effective. The natural history of cervical cancer is better understood than that of breast cancer, although knowledge is still incomplete.

The Biology of Cervical Cancer

It is well documented that cervical cancer goes through earlier precancerous stages. Cervical cancer usually develops quite slowly, over many years. The precancerous cell changes may disappear or regress at any stage, although the more severe the cell changes, the less likely this becomes.

Unfortunately, doctors have used numerous terminologies for describing cell changes in the cervix, resulting in some confusion on the part of women about what these mean. Attempts are being made to standardize terms, and currently these are the most used:

Low grade	mild dysplasia	CIN 1
High grade	moderate dysplasia	CIN 2
	severe dysplasia	CIN 3 carcinoma in situ (CIS)

CIN stands for *cervical intraepithelial neoplasia* meaning new growth in the epithelium or skinlike tissue covering the cervix. *Dysplasia* has a similar meaning of abnormal development in the cells.

The majority of cases of mild dysplasia do not progress but can disappear after a time without treatment. A large study of cytology records from a laboratory in Toronto showed that in two-thirds of the cases a smear showing mild dysplasia had reverted to normal by the next smear and only 9% had gotten worse.(12) In cases of moderate dysplasia, 22% had reverted to normal, as had 13% of severe dysplasia cases. In 36% of severe dysplasia cases the smear was still severe when it was repeated.

Other studies have had similar findings. In a Belfast study where women with mild dysplasia were followed for two years, there was a 46% regression rate for mild dysplasia, a 29% persistence rate, and in only 15% of the cases did the abnormality get worse.(13) A calculation made as a result of a study in Stockholm was that there was a 23% chance of progression of mild dysplasia over 12–14 years.(14)

This pattern shows that the greater the degree of severity of the smear, the greater the likelihood of progression.

The progression rate for CIS is variously put at anything from 20% to 100%. The reason for the uncertainty is that very few studies have followed untreated women with CIS because it is considered unethical to do so. One of the few was the study at National Women's Hospital in Auckland. When the outcome for these women with inadequately treated CIS was studied, a 20% rate for progression to invasion was found at five years and a 36% invasion rate at 20 years.(15) As all these women had had some kind of biopsy, which might have interfered with the natural progression of the disease, this invasion rate is probably an underestimate.

Taking cervical smears

The place in the cervix where the abnormal cells usually appear is called the *transformation zone* or *squamo-columnar junction*. This is the point where the squamous cells covering the cervix join with the columnar cells that line the cervical canal leading into the interior of the womb.

When a cervical smear is taken, cells need to be obtained from the transformation zone. To achieve this, the smear taker needs to actually look at the cervix and carefully remove cells from the right place. Failure to go to this trouble explains why laboratories are sometimes unable to "read" a smear.

In older women, the transformation zone retreats up the cervical canal, making an adequate smear a little more difficult to obtain. For these women, a cytobrush is sometimes used to take an additional smear. The cytobrush is a tiny brush a bit like a miniature bottle brush which can be inserted in the cervical canal and rotated to obtain some cells. The cytobrush may also be used for women who need repeat smears or who have already had treatment for cervical abnormalities.

For other women, a cytobrush smear does not give any better result than a smear taken with a wooden spatula. Even when a cytobrush smear is taken, it should not replace the spatula smear but be taken in addition to it. A cytobrush can damage or break up the cells if the smear is not taken carefully.(16)

The Causes of Cervical Cancer

Exactly what causes cervical cancer is still something of a mystery. Over the past 30 years, various explanations have been put forward and then discarded. The usual pattern has been that the latest theory is seized upon with great enthusiasm as providing the magical key to explaining the disease. Later, it is modified or abandoned when further research shows it does not stand up. So we have heard in the past that it was uncircumcised men who infected women with some dread organism that caused cancer. The uncircumcised men theory developed because it was noted that Jewish women had low rates of cervical cancer compared to other women. Subsequently, it was discovered that the more probable explanation was not the removal of their foreskins, but the fact that Jewish people were more often monogamous and tended to have only one sexual partner.

The *herpes simplex* virus has also been implicated as being involved somehow in the development of cervical cancer. At first it was hailed as the probable cause of the disease, but this belief has now been modified. Like the circumcised men association, the herpes link could be related to sexual behavior. People who have a number of partners may be more likely to get both cervical cancer and herpes. Alternatively, cervical cancer patients may be more susceptible to herpes infection. It is still possible that herpes simplex may be involved in the development of cervical cancer, but a simple cause-and-effect relationship now looks remote.(17)

In recent years the idea that cervical cancer is tied in some way to sexual behavior has been confirmed in several ways. Nuns, for instance, very rarely develop cervical cancer. It is increasingly suspected that cervical cancer must be caused by a virus that is passed from one person to another during sexual intercourse.

There has been much discussion of what is called the "male factor" in cervical cancer. Although women with cervical cancer may wonder if it is something they have done, in fact, their partner may be involved in the origin of the disease. For instance, cases have been noted where the second wife of a man whose first wife died of cervical cancer also died of the same disease. Studies looking at sexual practices in various societies suggest that the highest rate of cervical cancer occurs in countries with a sexual double standard. In these societies, chastity and fidelity are valued in women, while there is an expectation that men will have many partners, often through prostitution.(18)

Unfortunately, the sexual connection has the potential for a great deal of victim-blaming and feelings of self-blame on the part of women who develop this cancer or even abnormal cells. It can also cause considerable strain between a couple if the woman then thinks her husband has been unfaithful. Cervical cancer is usually a disease that develops slowly, so that if it is caused by something transmitted during sexual intercourse, it may have happened years ago rather than resulting from a current relationship.

In any case, it is really pointless to get into feelings of recrimination and shame about cervical cancer. The number of people—men or women—who are in the position of having a lifelong monogamous relationship with a person who has never had sexual relations with anyone else must be very small indeed. Most Western women have had at least one other sexual partner before they marry, and their husbands probably have, too. Even if they are then faithful to each other for the rest of their lives, the woman could develop cervical cancer as a result of that earlier sexual experience, either hers or her husband's. This does not mean that either has been promiscuous or unfaithful, just normal!

Most cervical cancers are squamous cancers, but there is another sort that occurs in about 10% of cases, called *adenocarcinoma,* which is not related to sexual intercourse at all.

What about warts?

The most recent agent to be implicated in causing cervical cancer is *human papilloma virus,* or *HPV,* also known as *genital warts.* HPV may be visible as genital warts or there may be changes that can only be seen under magnification using a colposcope. The virus can also be detected in a cervical smear.

Viruses are invisible microorganisms that take over control of a normal cell. They have their own genetic structure, or blueprint, coded in their RNA (ribonucleic acid) and DNA (deoxyribonucleic acid). It is RNA and DNA that determine what cells will do. When a virus invades a cell it substitutes its own RNA and DNA structure for the host cell's structure and uses the cell to reproduce itself. The body fights back by trying to mobilize the immune system to form antibodies. Sometimes it is successful, sometimes not. If not, the virus is able to set up permanent home in the host cells.

Wart virus is known to cause cancer in various animals, such as skin cancer in cottontail rabbits and sheep. As wart virus can also infect human beings, scientists began looking to see if it had anything to do with cervical cancer. They found that a high proportion of women with abnormal cell changes on the cervix did indeed have HPV infection in the cervix. This was often detectable in a cervical smear; it was even more obvious when the cervix had been painted with acetic acid and looked at with a colposcope.

With increasingly sophisticated technology that was able to examine the DNA structure of cells, scientists were able to isolate not one but several different types of HPV infection in women. They have also been able to detect these same viral types on the penises of the partners of these women, thus lending weight to the suspicion that HPV may be sexually transmitted. Further work showed that particular types of HPV were associated with abnormal cells that progressed, while other types were associated with abnormal cells that were more inclined to regress or disappear. The low-risk wart viruses were types 6 and 11, while the high-risk types were 16 and 18.

Although it is not possible to tell from a cervical smear or even a biopsy what type of HPV virus a woman has, it is possible through DNA testing. This process is expensive and time-consuming to carry out, but it is hoped that in time cheaper methods will make this technology more widely available. If the viral type causing a woman's abnormal smears is known, then she and the doctors treating her will have a better idea of what her particular disease is likely to do. If it is a low-risk virus, she might decide to delay treatment to see if the cells disappear of their own accord; if it is the high-risk variety, she will know that immediate treatment is necessary.

Even when a woman is shown to have a high-risk type of HPV, she is not automatically marked to get cervical cancer. Statistical estimates are that one cancer may develop for every 300 women with HPV 16, while the risk to women with HPV 6 or 11 is estimated to be one cancer in 2,000 to 3,000 women.(19)

At first, doctors thought that at last they had found the cause of cervical cancer, and this apparent breakthrough was conveyed to women through the media. But subsequent work has thrown this idea into doubt. Some studies have shown that very large numbers of perfectly normal healthy women actually have HPV infection, even HPV of the apparently high-risk variety. Yet most of these women have no abnormal changes in the cells of their cervix. It has been estimated that most HPV infections are transient and will resolve in 80% of women over a two-year period.(20)

The possibility that it may be a relatively common occurrence to have evidence of HPV in the vagina was shown by an intriguing study in Singapore, where 45 virginal and 162 sexually active women going to a hospital clinic were examined under the colposcope for HPV infection.(21) The majority of the sexually active women had been referred for suspected abnormal cells in the cervix, whereas the virginal women were there primarily for menstrual problems. All the virgins had intact hymens.

Astonishingly, it was discovered that 51% of the virginal group had evidence of HPV infection on their cervices, and 86% of these were confirmed histologically by biopsy. In the sexually active group, 69% had evidence of HPV, which was confirmed by biopsy for 86% of the women.

The researchers then went on to look at the husbands of the sexually active women. It was found that 77% of the men whose wives had HPV also showed signs of infection. On the other hand, only 13% of the husbands of women without HPV showed signs of infection. This once again provided confirmation of the idea that men and women can pass the infection to one another.

The researchers speculated that the presence of HPV in the vaginas of the virginal women pointed to some other cause of transmission than sexual contact. They could only speculate about this but mentioned the fact that two of the virginal women with HPV were sisters: "They both shared clothing and towels with their mother who had squamous cell carcinoma of the cervix diagnosed two years previously." They concluded that although transference of the virus by sexual contact was common, so too might be nonsexual transmission: "genital HPV is ubiquitous and should not be considered exclusively a venereal disease." It is now being suggested that HPV can be picked up from shared clothing, towels, incompletely sterilized specula, and bathing suits tried on in shops (keep your panties on!).

This kind of study has thrown the cat among the pigeons as far as theories of HPV go. It is not clear, says Heather Mitchell of the Victorian Cytology Service in Australia, whether HPV is "a major factor in the development of cervical cancer or an innocent passenger."(22) In other words, it could be merely coincidental that women with abnormal cell changes also show HPV infection. It appears increasingly unlikely that the relationship between HPV and cervical cancer is straightforward cause and effect.

It is now being argued that HPV might need a "cofactor" for cervical cancer to develop, meaning "help" from some other source. To use animal examples: wart virus can cause gut cancer in cows, but only if they eat bracken. Sheep with wart virus can develop skin cancer but only in parts of the body directly exposed to sunlight. It is hypothesized that the most likely cofactors would be conditions or substances that weakened the body's immune system. Possible cofactors (and it must be stressed that none of these is proven) are

- smoking
- long-term oral contraceptive use
- vitamin deficiencies
- herpes viruses
- pregnancy
- high parity (many childbirths)

Risk Factors for Cervical Cancer

Despite all the emphasis on the relationship between sexual activity and cervical cancer, the greatest risk factor for cervical cancer is not sex, but not being screened. A woman who is having regular smear tests has only a slim chance of ever developing cervical cancer. Likewise the chance of her dying from it is infinitesimal. If a woman is having regular smears, any abnormality will be picked up and treated. Although a small percentage of women need more than one treatment to eradicate the disease, the chance of complete treatment failure is less than 1%.(23)

Cervical screening is called *secondary prevention* as it prevents cancer but not the precancer stages. *Primary prevention* would consist of measures a woman could take to protect herself. Unfortunately, there is not a lot that can be suggested here. Lifelong celibacy or using condoms for life would be effective but for many women not very practical strategies.

For most adult women such strategies have limited applicability because they have probably already been exposed earlier in their lives to whatever is causing cervical cancer. Women might consider using barrier methods if they start a new relationship, and very young women could be encouraged to protect themselves by always using barrier contraception and being cautious about their sexual behavior, not just because of the risk of cervical cancer, but also to prevent chlamydia, herpes, AIDS, and unwanted pregnancy.

As we have seen, other agents have been implicated in the development of cervical cancer, but the evidence about them is still unclear. A recent study of women with CIS showed that smokers had a relative risk of 4.5 compared to nonsmokers and that women who smoked a lot were more at risk.(24) This study controlled for sexual behavior, previous researchers having suggested that smokers were more likely to have had a number of sexual partners. Smoking may not cause cervical cancer but may act as a "helper" to something else like a virus. It could weaken the immune system or help a virus alter the cervical cells.

Because of the imprecision and uncertainty that still surround risk factors, there is no solid case to be made for more frequent screening of women with risk factors such as smoking or use of oral contraceptives.(25)

Smear Results

Some doctors automatically tell women what their smear results are. If your doctor does not, it is advisable to ask for a copy or to be told the result. Although women are often told to assume if they hear nothing that their smear is normal, this could be a mistake. Administrative slipups do occur. It pays to always check for yourself.

There have been so many systems of reporting smear results that women are often thoroughly confused about what various reports mean. Also some reports that sound alarming are not so at all. The following are some of the reports that can appear on a smear result with an interpretation in plain language.

"Normal"

Normal, of course, means just what it says, and this is the most common smear result by far. *Within normal limits* is another term for normal used in the Bethesda system. The report may also say the smear was *satisfactory,* meaning the laboratory received a good quality smear which it had no difficulty reading.

"Less than optimal" and "unsatisfactory"

These descriptions do not mean there is anything the matter with the cervix; they refer to the quality of the smear sent to the laboratory. The laboratory may describe it as *less than optimal,* meaning it could not be clearly read, or *unsatisfactory,* meaning it could not be read at all.

There are several possible causes of less than optimal or unsatisfactory smears.(26) Sometimes there are insufficient cells. This could be a poorly taken smear, often resulting from the smear taker obtaining a "blind" smear. In other words, the cervix was not properly visualized and therefore the smear did not contain cells from the transformation zone. Menstrual blood can also obscure the cells so that having a smear taken during a menstrual period is not a good idea.

When the smear is taken, it must be quickly spread on a glass slide and sprayed with a fixative. If this process is improperly carried out, the sample may be improperly fixed or air-dried and so not be easily readable.

An unsatisfactory smear result means the smear test should be carried out again. It is basically a dud smear report. A less than optimal smear is usually repeated a year later as there has been enough material on the slide to allow a reading, even if it has been less than perfect.

A survey of 30,000 smears from one large urban laboratory between 1989 and 1990 showed that only 74% of smears were satisfactory, while 26% were less than optimal or unsatisfactory (see page 320).

Benign abnormalities

The smear report might talk about *inflammation* or *infection.* Inflammation is relatively common and might resolve by itself. If it is caused by an infection, such as thrush, gardnerella, or trichomoniasis, it might need to be treated before the smear is repeated. Inflammatory changes in the cervix can make it difficult for the cytopathologist to see if anything else is happening to the cervix. That is why women with a smear report noting inflammation will often be asked to return for another smear in three months' time. If that smear is normal, it should be repeated again in 12 months' time. If it is still abnormal, the woman should be referred for colposcopy.

Smear Quality

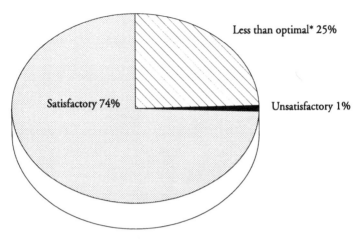

Satisfactory 74%

Less than optimal* 25%

Unsatisfactory 1%

*Includes no endocervical cells

The percentages are based on an analysis of approximately 30,000 cervical smears examined in one New Zealand laboratory in 1989–90.

Wart virus infection

A smear result can show wart virus infection without any kind of dysplastic change. As we have seen, HPV infection is quite common but may disappear of its own accord. In some cases, though, it is not possible for the laboratory to distinguish between HPV changes and dysplasia, which is why the Bethesda system lumps them together as low-grade changes.

This creates a real dilemma for women when the words *wart virus infection without CIN 1* appear on a smear report. There are different medical opinions about what should be done in these cases. Some doctors treat it the same as CIN 1, but other doctors plead for some caution because in many cases the body will deal with the infection itself.(27) It will mobilize its immune defenses and prevent the virus from causing abnormal cell changes. Even if the woman is treated, she may be reinfected by a partner who is also carrying the virus, and there is no known effective treatment for eradicating HPV infection from the genital tract.(28)

For women in this position, there are basically two options:

- Have another smear within three to six months to see if the infection either goes away or progresses to CIN 1. This is the usual advice. This might be a bit nerve-wracking but could avoid unnecessary investigations and treatment. The time for the infection to regress can be two or three years.(29) If it progresses, the woman should be referred for colposcopy. A woman is usually advised that if the infection persists for 12 months she should be referred for colposcopy anyway.

- Proceed to colposcopy to check that the cytology has not missed CIN.

Because of the previous suspicion that HPV "caused" cancer, there has been a certain amount of catastrophizing about HPV, with a tendency to overtreat women who show signs of it. From the individual's point of view, this may lead to unnecessary treatment. From the point of view of the system, this could lead to the treatment services being clogged up with huge numbers of women with the infection, resulting in delays for women with more serious smear reports.

Women who are told they have signs of HPV on their smear need to ensure they are given a clear explanation of the result, in particular whether there is any sign of CIN, before deciding what to do. This situation is complicated by the fact that it may not be possible for the laboratory to distinguish one from the other. Some laboratories make an effort to separate the two wherever possible, while others adhere to the Bethesda reporting system and combine wart virus and CIN 1.

Abnormal cervical smears

This covers dysplastic cell changes from borderline to mild to severe. Some possible reports are

- *Atypical cells,* or *atypical cells of uncertain significance,* or *atypia:* these are borderline cells, meaning cells that are neither completely abnormal or completely normal. These cells could become normal again or could progress.

- *Low-grade squamous intraepithelial lesion:* this category combines wart virus infection and CIN 1, although some laboratories are often able to specify which it is. These cells have a good chance of reverting to normal or they could progress.

The Health Department/Cancer Society working group recommended that women with either of the above should have a repeat smear after three to six months, then further smears annually, possibly for life, unless there are signs that the abnormality has progressed.(30)

- *High-grade squamous intraepithelial lesion:* this combines the categories of moderate and severe dysplasia, CIN 2 and CIN 3, or carcinoma in situ. These cells are more likely to progress.

In addition to these terms, cytopathologists will often spell out the degree of abnormality present using either the *dysplasia* terminology (mild, moderate, and severe) or *cervical intraepithelial neoplasia,* graded 1, 2, or 3, as described earlier.

The laboratory survey quoted above showed that only 1% of satisfactory smears showed high-grade abnormalities, 3% showed low-grade abnormalities, and 5% contained atypia (see page 323).

In an earlier pre-Bethesda study conducted at Lower Hutt laboratory, 5.5% of smears showed some grade of CIN, and only 0.1% showed major abnormalities (suggestive of malignancy). The incidence of CIN was highest among women under 35 years of age, while the major abnormalities were most seen in over-55-year-olds.(31)

For high-grade changes or low-grade changes that persist, referral for colposcopy is usually recommended. A woman with high-grade abnormalities should be seen within a matter of weeks; other women may wait longer, but ideally, for peace of mind if nothing else, no woman should have to wait longer than six weeks to see a colposcopist.

Treatment for CIN is usually by what is called a *locally destructive method,* such as diathermy (burning), cryocautery (freezing), or laser (vaporization). This means that the abnormal cells are destroyed with minimal trauma to the cervix. Some older women may still need a cone biopsy—a cone-shaped piece of tissue cut from the cervix—because the abnormal cells are down the cervical canal and cannot be reached by other methods. Whenever the extent of the abnormal tissue cannot be properly viewed during colposcopy it should be removed by biopsy, either a surgical, laser cone biopsy, or a loop

Smear Abnormality

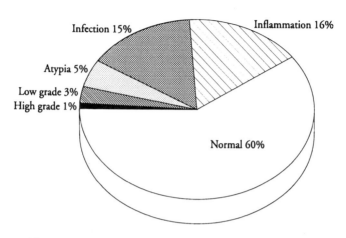

The percentages are based on an analysis of approximately 30,000 cervical smears examined in one New Zealand laboratory in 1989–90.

excision. This provides tissue that can be sent to the laboratory to check that all the abnormal cells have been removed.

Drawbacks of Cervical Screening

There is, according to researchers, "the very real risk that cervical screening could do more harm than good because of over-screening combined with over-diagnosis and over-treatment of minor lesions.(32) Cervical screening is an effective health practice but is not entirely without risks and costs, some of which we have already seen. The smear test itself can be embarrassing and uncomfortable for some women, but the main problems tend to occur when women have other than normal smear results.

Anxiety

Worry is caused by false positive results (about 10% of the cases), which need to be investigated before the woman gets the good news that her cervix is healthy. Uncertain smear results requiring further repeat smears can also lead to an anxious time, as can delays in being referred for colposcopy and periods of waiting to hear the results of biopsies or treatment. There can be a good deal of uncertainty in the process of investigating abnormal smears before the situation is resolved. Even with low-grade abnormalities, the mind does tend to turn to cancer. The whole experience can feel like a brush with a life-threatening disease.

> Three months after I had a smear test I suddenly got a letter through the post from the gynecologist to say my last smear had been abnormal and would I come for a repeat smear. I was absolutely shocked as I had assumed it had been normal. It was as if my whole future suddenly stopped. I was at home alone at the time and I remember thinking what a bombshell to have come in such an innocent-looking white envelope. I felt an enormous threat directed at me, also a feeling of betrayal that the doctor had not told me and also that my body had been tricking me. I had been going on as normal, while all the time I had been harboring something sinister inside me. I felt so angry at the gynecologist I would not return—I went back to my GP for the smear. She explained it was only mildly abnormal, and after a time it went back to normal. I still have all my bits.

The plethora of smear reports for which the meaning is not clear cause unnecessary anxiety. Despite the care taken by her doctor, this woman was still uncertain about what had caused her smear report:

> I have a Pap smear every two years. My last one showed my cervix inflamed. My GP called and explained the possible causes and invited me to call her back for more information. I have heard of a number of mid-30s and 40s women with inflamed cervices. What does it really mean?

Sexual effects

Colposcopy is a diagnostic technique involving extensive exposure of the genital area and invasion of the most intimate part of a woman's body. The vagina is normally private and under the woman's control, but during colposcopy it is invaded by instruments while the colposcopist is seated between the woman's legs. Many women find this embarrassing and even degrading—it can take some adjusting to.

In Britain, 52% of women having outpatient colposcopy in one study reported disturbed feelings about sexual relationships after colposcopy.(33) Another study showed that investigation for CIN had a strong negative effect on sexual feelings and behavior even six months later.(34)

It is also quite common for women to have a profuse vaginal discharge for a month after some treatments, and this can limit interest in sex.

False negative results

A percentage of smears—as high as 30% in some surveys but usually around 20%—are false negatives. This means they appear to give the all clear when there is actually something abnormal happening on the cervix. The main cause of false negatives is a failure by the smear taker to take a good smear.(35) Another cause can be poor-quality smear reading in the laboratory. If there is a great deal of overscreening, smear-reading standards can drop because laboratories cannot cope with the workload and start to cut corners.

False negatives can reassure women they are safe when they are not. False negatives are the reason for the two first smears a woman ever has being one year apart. If the first is a false negative, the chance of the second also being a false negative is remote.(36)

Overdiagnosis and overtreatment

We have already seen that a report of wart virus infection can lead to women having investigations and treatment for something that may never be destined to cause real health problems. The possibility that women with CIN 1 may be getting unnecessary treatment has also been mentioned. This has implications for the individuals who will experience the trauma and disruption caused by the investigation and treatment. Once a woman has an abnormal smear she gets hooked into a system of diagnosis and medical treatment which has the effect of turning her into a patient. What is happening to her cervix will have a major influence on other parts of her life: her sexuality, her relationship with her partner, her work life, her sense of self, and her enjoyment of life. There must be a significant benefit to the person who undergoes this process to risk all this. It is not really justifiable if the benefit is doubtful in the first place.

Most modern methods of treatment for cervical precancers do minimal damage to the cervix, but for some women treatment can result in painful periods caused by stenosis or narrowing of the cervix, and, for young women, there can be a small risk of obstetric problems later.(37)

There are also increasing fears that the health services will be overburdened if large numbers of women are referred for low-grade cell changes.

Many of the negative aspects of cervical screening outlined above are illustrated by the following woman's experience. In 1990, at the age of 41, she was referred for treatment of CIN 1 at a private clinic:

The laser treatment proceeded. After what seemed like 10 to 15 minutes Mr. A said, "I will now do the coning," the first time this had been mentioned. By this time the local anesthetic had worn off and I was finding the procedure extremely uncomfortable. The nurse had said to tell her if I began to find it painful, as she said he can't feel it and the laser tends to become very hot. By now it was very painful. Mr. A then injected more anesthetic, which was actually worse than the laser, and proceeded to finish the coning. The whole operation took about 30 to 40 minutes. When completed, he jumped out of his seat and said, "This treatment doesn't bother most people, you must be one of the few it does," and handed me the specimen jar containing the piece of flesh taken from my cervix.

I was astonished that a biopsy that size would be taken with a local anesthetic. The next day I phoned the GP who had referred me to the clinic to ask her if this operation was usually done under local anesthetic. She said, "No, a coning is usually done under a general anesthetic." I also phoned another gynecologist and was told the same thing.

I felt quite unwell for some time after the operation, and experienced a leaking of clear burning fluid for approximately eight weeks. Having no confidence in Mr. A by this time, I went to see a woman gynecologist, who on examination said all seemed normal and the leaking was part of the healing process.

I feel in spite of much publicity, nothing much has changed for the better. Mr. A did not fully explain what he intended to do, and his attitude and manner I would describe as brutal. If, in fact, the coning should be done under general anesthetic, one would almost conclude that Mr. A and his partners are running a very lucrative cost-saving business.

Toward a Woman-Oriented Screening Service

Many of the drawbacks to screening discussed above can be minimized or eliminated if care is taken in the design of a screening program and the provision of services.

Prerequisites for a service that meets women's needs would include:

- The establishment of national protocols for the management of abnormal smears and for smears showing HPV infection. Consumer representatives must be part of developing these protocols; once they are completed, they should be readily accessible to all women who need them.

- Quality control of laboratory and treatment services so they are of a high standard, uniform throughout the country.

- Adequate information for women on screening, smear results, and treatment options so that they can be fully in control of what happens to them and can make informed choices.

- Ready access to publicly provided diagnostic and treatment facilities without long periods of waiting.

- Support and counseling to be available at treatment services.

Attention to these factors would ensure that screening is not only effective at protecting women from cancer but also achieves its goals at the minimum cost to women.

Chapter 13

Final Thoughts

The "menopause industry" dissected in this book has the potential to damage the quality of life of midlife women. While each individual intervention does hold potential benefit for some women, the combined effect of all the interventions is not benign. Taken together the message is conveyed that

- menopause is not a normal life stage but a disease that affects all women

- women at midlife have the possibility of ill health hanging over them

- medical surveillance of our lives is necessary to ward this off

The ideology of the "menopause industry" poses a threat to the collective well-being of midlife women. Instead of women feeling confident in their abilities and in control of their lives, they are being persuaded to feel anxious, fragile, and prey to a host of unpleasant diseases. "The new danger to our well-being, if we continue to listen to all this talk," noted one doctor, "is in becoming a nation of healthy hypochondriacs, living gingerly, worrying ourselves half to death."(1)

All the interventions discussed in this book are being promoted to women as a population. They are not aimed solely at the individual woman with existing problems but to all women to ward off future ills. Thus, women need to respond on two levels.

Each woman has to make up her own mind for herself, but she also needs to ask: Is this good for my sex? What are the implications for women as a group? Is this where we want resources to go? If we had a choice, would we rather they went somewhere else? For instance, would we rather see money spent on sex education for the young, or support for young mothers, or a mammographic screening program? Do we want information services for women or more technology? How will women benefit most? So far, women have had little input into decision making on such matters; with the move toward population-based screening programs aimed at all women, they must demand a say.

The priorities women have for themselves and their sex may well differ from those of doctors, who tend to bring a mechanistic attitude to bear on the subject. Benefits and risks are weighed by them in purely statistical form, whereas women might take a more subjective view of the matter. "Whether consumers would accept fewer heart attacks for more cancer is unclear," said one doctor in discussing hormone replacement therapy.(2) It is certainly something about which women have never been consulted; instead, the issue is being debated and recommendations and policies made in the absence of any knowledge of women's feelings.

Behind the menopause industry is a belief that mass intervention is acceptable and that drug taking is a normal part of life. Women might see things differently. They are much more likely to be interested in what they can do in their daily lives to preserve their health and enjoy life at the same time. It rarely gets stated that there are other ways of preventing bone loss and other ways of protecting the heart beside taking drugs.

Morris Notelovitz is a voice in the hormone wilderness when he argues for the normality of menopause for most women and that "postmenopausal health can be achieved without the need for hormone therapy":

> Both conditions [osteoporosis and arterial disease] are modulated by the presence or absence of estrogen, but both are also heavily influenced by the individual's genetic makeup, lifestyle, social habits, and physical activity. Women who enter their menopause with adequate bone mass do not develop osteoporosis. Women who are normotensive, have appropriate lipid and lipoprotein profiles, are physically active, and do not smoke are unlikely to experience significant atherogenic disease. Why then should one treat all postmenopausal women with estrogen therapy?(3)

Women need to reject an ideology that leads to a preoccupation with ill health and that inculcates a sense of precarious mortality. Instead of "living gingerly," midlife women should insist on their right to live life with verve, gusto, and spice.

References

1. The Medicalization of Midlife

1. Sontag, Susan. 1974. "Women Grow Old but Men Mature." *Broadsheet* 16: 6–7.

2. Whatley, Marianne. 1988. "Beyond Compliance: Towards a Feminist Health Education." In *Feminism Within the Science and Health Care Professions: Overcoming Resistance*, ed. Sue Rossner. Pergamon Press, Oxford: 131–44.

3. Grace, Victoria. 1990. "Orienting Health Promotion Practice." Paper presented to the First Annual Conference of the Health Promotion Forum of New Zealand, Auckland.

4. O'Hagan, John. 1991. "The Ethics of Informed Consent in Relation to Prevention Screening Programmes." *NZ Med J* 104: 122–25.

5. Taylor, Richard. 1979. *Medicine Out of Control*. Sun Books, Melbourne.

6. Rodgers, Anthony. 1990. "The UK Breast Cancer Screening Programme: An Expensive Mistake." *J Pub Health Med* 12(3/4): 197–204.

7. Illich, Ivan. 1976. *Limits to Medicine*. Marion Boyars, London.

8. Rose, Geoffrey. 1990. "Reflections on the Changing Times." *BMJ* 301: 683–87.

9. Rose, Geoffrey. 1981. "Strategy of Prevention: Lessons from Cardiovascular Disease." *BMJ* 282: 1847–51.

10. Ehrenreich, Barbara, and John Ehrenreich. 1978. "Medicine and Social Control." In *The Cultural Crisis of Modern Medicine*, ed. John Ehrenreich. Monthly Review Press, New York and London: 39–79.

11. Thomas Lewis. 1973. "Notes of a Biology Watcher: The Health-Care System. *N Eng J Med* 293: 1245–47.

12. Rose, Geoffrey. "Reflections on the Changing Times."

13. Guillebaud, John. 1989. "Hormone Replacement Therapy" (letter). *BMJ* 299: 50.

14. Leather, A. T., and J. W. W. Studd. 1990. "Can the Withdrawal Bleed Following Oestrogen Replacement Therapy Be Avoided?" *Br J Obstet Gynaec* 97: 1071–79.

15. Roeber, Johanna. "The Forever Therapy?" *Vogue,* June 1990: 172–73.

16. Armstrong, D. 1983. *The Political Economy of the Body: Medical Knowledge in the Twentieth Century.* Cambridge University Press, Cambridge.

17. Doyal, Lesley. 1979. *The Political Economy of Health*. Pluto Press, London.

18. Taylor, Richard. *Medicine Out of Control*.

19. Ibid.

20. Livingstone, Anna, and David Widgery. 1990. "The New New General Practice: The Changing Philosophies of Primary Care." *BMJ* 301: 708–10.

21. Ibid.
22. Sontag, Susan. 1990. *Illness as Metaphor; Aids and Its Metaphors.* Anchor Books, Doubleday, New York.
23. Slogan of the American Cancer Society.
24. The Radiology Group. 1991. Mammography brochure.
25. McKeown, Thomas. 1976. "An Approach to Screening Policies." *J R Coll Physicians* 10 (2): 1451–52.
26. Rodgers, Anthony. "The UK Breast Cancer Screening Programme."
27. O'Hagan, John. "The Ethics of Informed Consent."
28. Barsky, Arthur. 1988. "The Paradox of Health." *N Eng J Med* 318: 414–18.

2. The Fabulous Midlife Woman

1. Unless otherwise specified, statistical information in this chapter is taken from the following source:

   U.S. Bureau of the Census. 1993. *Statistical Abstract of the United States: 1993* (113th edition) Washington DC.
2. Society for Research on Women in New Zealand. 1988. *The Time of Our Lives: A Study of Mid-Life Women.* Christchurch Branch of SROW, Christchurch.
3. Weideger, Paula. 1978. *Female Cycles.* The Women's Press, London.
4. Housego, Mike. "Battling Father Time: The Winners and Losers." *New Zealand Woman's Weekly,* 12 March 1990: cover and 20–23.
5. Mackenzie, Drew. "Facelifts: Who's Had Them (and Who Hasn't)." *New Zealand Woman's Weekly,* 19 March 1990: 22–23.
6. Shepherd, Rose. "Dieting—Can You Go Too Far? *New Zealand Woman's Day,* 20 Feb. 1991: 12–13.

3. The Construction of the "New" Menopause

1. Kaufert, Patricia, and Penny Gilbert. 1986. "Women, Menopause, and Medicalisation." *Culture, Medicine and Psychiatry* 10: 7–21.
2. Wren, Barry. "Oestrogen Therapy after Menopause: A Viewpoint on Its Rational Use." *Current Therapeutics,* March 1987: 25–36.
3. Gambrell, R. Don. 1987. "The Menopause." *Obstet Gynecol Clin North Am* 14(1).
4. Kaufert and Gilbert. "Women, Menopause and Medicalisation."
5. Greenblatt, Robert (ed.). 1986. *A Modern Approach to the Perimenopausal Years.* De Gruyter, Berlin, New York.
6. Mowat, Wayne. Interview with Dr. Neil McKenzie. National Radio, 28 Feb. 1990.

7. Sauer, M., R. Paulson, and R. Lobo. 1990. "A Preliminary Report on Oocyte Donation Extending Reproductive Potential to Women over 40." *N Eng J Med* 323: 1157–60.

8. Quoted in Kaufert, Patricia. 1982. "Myth and Menopause." *Sociology of Health and Illness* 4(2): 141–66.

9. Greenblatt. *Modern Approach to the Perimenopausal Years.*

10. McCrea, Frances. 1983. "The Politics of Menopause: The 'Discovery' of a Deficiency Disease." *Social Problems* 31(1): 111–23.

11. Ibid.

12. Friedan, Betty. 1965. *The Feminine Mystique.* Norton, New York.

13. McKinlay, John, Sonja McKinlay, and Donald Brambilla. 1987. "The Relative Contributions of Endocrine Changes and Social Circumstances to Depression in Mid-aged Women." *J Health Soc Behav* 28(4 Dec.): 345–63.

14. Deutsch, Helene. 1944, 1945. *The Psychology of Women.* 2 vols. Grune and Stratton, New York.

15. Benedek, Therese. 1950. "Climacterium: A Developmental Phase." *Psychosomatic Quarterly* 19: 1–27.

16. Trethowan, W. 1975. "Pills for Personal Problems." *BMJ* 3: 749–51.

17. Linn, Lawrence, and Milton Davis. 1971. "The Use of Psychotherapeutic Drugs by Middle-aged Women." *J Health Soc Behav* 12(Dec.): 331–40.

18. Parish, Peter. 1971. "The Prescribing of Psychotropic Drugs in General Practice." *J R Coll Gen Pract* 21(92) Suppl. 4: 1–77.

19. Wilson, Robert. 1966. *Fe 3minine Forever.* M. Evans and Company, New York.

20. Judd, Howard, and Wulf Utian. 1987. "Introduction: What We Hope to Learn. Current Perspectives in the Management of the Menopausal and Postmenopausal Patient." *Am J Obstet Gynecol* 156(5): 1279–80.

21. Seaman, Barbara, and Gideon Seaman. 1977. *Women and the Crisis in Sex Hormones.* Bantam Books, New York.

22. Wilson, Robert, and Thelma Wilson. 1963. "The Fate of the Nontreated Postmenopausal Woman: A Plea for the Maintenance of Adequate Estrogen from Puberty to the Grave." *J Am Geriatr Soc* 11: 347–62. All quotes in this chapter from Wilson are from this source, unless otherwise specified.

23. Utian, Wulf. 1987. "The Fate of the Untreated Menopause." *Obstet Gynecol Clin North Am* 14 (1): 1–12. All quotes in this chapter from Utian are from this source, unless otherwise specified.

24. Van Keep, P. 1990. "The History and Rationale of Hormone Replacement Therapy." *Maturitas* 12: 163–70.

25. Ibid.

26. Wilson and Wilson. "The Fate of Nontreated Postmenopausal Women."

27. Utian. "The Fate of the Untreated Menopause."

28. Brown, Karen, and Charles Hammond. 1987. "Urogenital Atrophy." *Obstet Gynecol Clin North Am* 14(1): 13–32.

29. Kahn, Ada, and Linda Holt. 1987. *Menopause: The Best Years of Your Life?* Bloomsbury, London.

30. "Changing Outlook Helps Women with Menopause." *Auckland Star,* 29 Sept. 1986: B4.

31. Utian, Wulf. 1987. "Overview on Menopause." *Am J Obstet Gynecol* 156: 1280–83; Wells, Robert. 1989. "Hormone Replacement before Menopause: Is It a Good Idea?" *Postgrad Med* 86(6): 61–71; Nicosia, Santo. 1987. "The Aging Ovary." *Med Clin North Am* 71(1): 1–10.

32. Llewellyn-Jones, Derek, and Suzanne Abraham. 1988. *Menopause.* Penguin, Ringwood, Victoria.

33. Wells. "Hormone Replacement before Menopause."

34. "How to Treat Menopause." 1990. *New Zealand Doctor,* 2 July: 19–26.

35. Mowat. Interview with McKenzie.

36. Overton, Graeme. 1987. "Hormone Replacement Therapy (HRT) before and after the Menopause: Any Merit?" Unpublished, Auckland.

37. Mowat. Interview with McKenzie.

38. Rae, Bernadette. "Experts Put the Case for Hormone Therapy." *New Zealand Herald,* 28 April 1987, Section 2: 1.

39. McCrea. "Politics of Menopause."

4. Will the Real Menopause Please Stand Up

1. Utian, Wulf. 1986. "Non-hormonal Medication." In *A Modern Approach to the Menopausal Years,* ed. Robert Greenblatt. De Gruyter, Berlin, New York: 117–25.

2. Gorman, Teresa, and Malcolm Whitehead. 1989. *The Amarant Book of Hormone Replacement Therapy.* Pan Books, London.

3. McKinlay, Sonja, and John McKinlay. 1973. "Selected Studies of the Menopause: A Methodological Critique." *J Biosoc Sci* 5: 533–55.

4. Utian, Wulf. 1987. "Overview of Menopause. *Am J Obstet Gynecol* 156: 1280– 83.

5. How to Treat . . . Menopause. *New Zealand Doctor,* 2 July 1990: 19–26.

6. Datan, Nancy. 1986. "Corpses, Lepers, and Menstruating Women: Tradition, Transition, and the Sociology of Knowledge." *Sex Roles* 14: 693–703.

7. Kaufert, Patricia. 1980. "The Perimenopausal Woman and Her Use of Health Services." *Maturitas* 2: 191–205.

8. Avis, N. E., and S. M. McKinlay. 1990. "A Longitudinal Analysis of Women's Attitudes towards Menopause: Results from the Massachusetts Women's Health Study." *Maturitas* (in press).

9. Ballinger, Susan. 1985. "Psychosocial Stress and Symptoms of Menopause: A Comparative Study of Menopause Clinic Patients and Non-patients." *Maturitas* 7: 315–27.

10. Kaufert, Patricia. 1982. "Anthropology and the Menopause: The Development of a Theoretical Framework." *Maturitas* 4: 181–93.

11. *Auckland Star,* 29 Sept. 1987: B4.

12. Tweedie, Jill. "Boning up on the Menopause." *Guardian Weekly,* 22 July 1990.

13. Kaufert. "The Perimenopausal Woman."

14. Gilmore, L., and Judith Madarasz. 1982. "Women's Involvement in Primary Health Care." In *A Report of the National Women's Health Conference.* New Zealand Women's Health Network: 6–11.

15. McKinlay, John, Sonja McKinlay, and Donald Brambilla. 1987: "Health Status and Utilization Behaviour Associated with Menopause." *Am J Epidemiol* 125(1): 110–21.

16. Kaufert, Patricia, et al. 1986. "Menopause Research: The Korpilampi Workshop." *Soc Sci Med* 22: 1285–89.

17. McKinlay, John, Sonja McKinlay, and Donald Brambilla. 1987. "The Relative Contributions of Endocrine Changes and Social Circumstances to Depression in Mid-aged Women." *J Health Soc Behav* 28(4): 345–63.

18. McKinlay, Sonja, and Margot Jefferys. 1974. "The Menopausal Syndrome." *Br J Prev Soc Med* 28: 108–15.

19. Society for Research on Women in New Zealand. 1988. *The Time of Our Lives: A Study of Mid-life Women.* Christchurch Branch of the SROW, Christchurch.

20. Leiblum, Sandra, and Leora Swartzman. 1986. "Women's Attitudes toward the Menopause: An Update." *Maturitas* 8: 47–56.

21. Kaufert, Patricia, and Penny Gilbert. 1986. "Women, Menopause and Medicalization. *Culture, Medicine and Psychiatry* 10: 7–21.

22. McKinlay, John, Christopher Longcope, and Anna Gray. 1989. "The Questionable Physiologic and Epidemiologic Basis for the Male Climacteric: Preliminary Results from the Massachusetts Male Aging Study." *Maturitas* 11: 103–15.

23. Bungay, G., M. Vessey, and C. McPherson. 1980. "Study of Symptoms in Middle Life with Special Reference to the Menopause." *BMJ* 281: 181–84.

24. Kaufert, Patricia, and John Syrotuik. 1981. "Symptom Reporting at Menopause." *Soc Sci Med* 15E: 173–84.

25. Flint, Marcha. 1975. "The Menopause: Reward or Punishment?" *Psychosomatics* 16:161–63.

26. Kaufert and Syrotuik. "Symptom Reporting at Menopause."

27. Lock, Margaret, Patricia Kaufert, and Penny Gilbert. 1988. "Cultural Construction of the Menopausal Syndrome: The Japanese Case." *Maturitas* 10: 317–32.

28. Donovan, John. 1951. "The Menopausal Syndrome: A Study of Case Histories." *Am J Obstet Gynecol* 62(6): 1281–91.

29. Coope, Jean. 1984. "Menopause: Diagnosis and Treatment." *BMJ* 289: 888–90.

30. "Oestrogen Therapy." *New Zealand Herald,* 2 March 1987.

5. Hormones at Menopause

1. Marx, Jean. 1988. "Sexual Responses Are—Almost—All in the Brain." *Science* 241 (4868): 903–04.

2. Hagstad, Anita, and Per Janson. 1986. "The Epidemiology of Climacteric Symptoms." *Acta Obstet Gynecol Scand Suppl* 134: 59–65.

3. McKinlay, Sonja, and Margot Jefferys. 1974. "The Menopausal Syndrome." *Br J Prev Soc Med* 28: 108–15.

4. Hunter, Myra, Rosie Battersby, and Malcolm Whitehead. 1986. "Relationships between Psychological Symptoms, Somatic Complaints and Menopausal Status." *Maturitas* 8: 217–28.

5. Reitz, Rosetta. 1985. *Menopause: A Positive Approach.* Viking Penguin, New York.

6. Schneider, H. 1986. "The Climacteric Syndrome." In *A Modern Approach to the Perimenopausal Years,* ed. Robert Greenblatt. De Gruyter, Berlin, New York: 39–56.

7. Renée. 1983. "Change of Life." *Broadsheet* 114: 8–11.

8. McKinlay and Jefferys. "The Menopausal Syndrome."

9. Hagstad and Janson. "The Epidemiology of Climacteric Symptoms."

10. Hunter et al. "Relationship between Psychological Symptoms, Somatic Complaints, and Menopausal Status."

11. McKinlay and Jefferys. "The Menopausal Syndrome."

12. Kaufert, Patricia. 1980. "The Perimenopausal Woman and Her Use of Health Services." *Maturitas* 2: 191–205.

13. Ibid.

14. Youngs, David. 1990. "Some Misconceptions Concerning the Menopause." *Obstet Gynecol Clin North Am* 75(5): 881–83.

15. Ibid.

16. Bungay, G., M. Vessey, and C. McPherson. 1980. "Study of Symptoms in Middle Life with Special Reference to Menopause." *BMJ* 281: 181–84.

17. Coope, Jean. 1984. "Menopause: Associated Problems." *BMJ* 289: 970–72.

18. Sarrel, Philip. 1987. "Sexuality in the Middle Years." *Obstet Gynecol Clin North Am* 14(1): 49–62.

19. Nachtigall, Lila, and Joan Heilman. 1986. *Estrogen: The Facts Can Change Your Life.* The Body Press, Los Angeles.

20. Society for Research on Women in New Zealand. 1988. *The Time of Our Lives: A Study of Mid-life Women*. Christchurch Branch of SROW, Christchurch.

21. Hagstad and Janson. "The Epidemiology of Climacteric Symptoms."

22. Hunter et al. "Relationship between Psychological Symptoms, Somatic Complaints, and Menopausal Status."

23. O'Connor, Dagmar, 1985. *How to Make Love to the Same Person for the Rest of Your Life—and Still Love It.* Bantam Books, New York.

24. Kaufert, Patricia. 1982. "Myth and Menopause." *Sociology of Health and Illness* 4(2): 141–66.

25. McKinlay, John, Sonja McKinlay, and Donald Brambilla. 1987. "The Relative Contributions of Endocrine Changes and Social Circumstances to Depression in Mid-aged Women." *J Health Soc Behav* 28(4): 345–63.

26. Ibid.

27. Kaufert. "The Perimenopausal Woman."

28. Greene, J. and David Cooke. 1980. "Life Stress and Symptoms at the Climacterium." *Br J Psychiat* 136: 486–91.

29. Cooke, David. 1985. "Social Support and Stressful Life Events During Mid-life." *Maturitas* 7: 303–13.

30. Society for Research on Women in New Zealand. "The Time of Our Lives."

31. McKinlay et al. "The Relative Contributions of Endocrine Changes."

32. McKinlay, Sonja, et al. 1990. "The Relative Contributions of Work and Three Nurturing Roles to the Health of Mid-aged Women: The Experience of the Massachusetts Women's Health Study." In *Gender, Health and Longevity: Multidisciplinary Perspectives.* Springer, New York.

33. Society for Research on Women in New Zealand. "The Time of Our Lives."

34. McKinlay et al. "Relative Contribution of Work."

35. Society for Research on Women in New Zealand. "The Time of Our Lives."

36. Donovan, John. 1951. "The Menopausal Syndrome: A Study of Case Histories." *Am J Obstet Gynecol* 62(6): 1281–91; Ballinger, Barbara. 1976. "Psychiatric Morbidity and the Menopause: Clinical Features." *BMJ* 1: 1183–85; Ballinger, Barbara. 1975. "Psychiatric Morbidity and the Menopause: Screening of General Population Sample." *BMJ* 3: 344–46.

37. Kaufert, Patricia, and John Syrotuik. 1981. "Symptom Reporting at Menopause." *Soc Sci Med* 15E: 173–84.

38. Bungay et al. "Study of Symptoms in Middle Life."

39. Magos, A., and J. Studd. 1986. "Management of the Premenstrual Syndrome." In *A Modern Approach to the Perimenopausal Years,* ed. Robert Greenblatt. De Gruyter, Berlin, New York: 221–32.

40. "Hormone Replacement Therapy: Question Time." 1990. CIBA-Geigy, New Zealand.

41. Flint, Marcha. 1982. "Anthropological Perspectives of the Menopause and Middle Age." *Maturitas* 4: 173–80.

6. The Meaning and Marketing of Osteoporosis

1. Gilchrist, Nigel. 1988. "Bone Density Estimation." *NZ Med J* 101: 259–60.

2. Bonn, Dorothy. "HRT and the Media." Paper given at Women's Health Concern Conference, Cardiff, 31 May 1989.

3. Ibid.

4. Stevenson, John. "Osteoporosis: The Silent Epidemic." *Update*, 1 Aug. 1986: 211–16; Dequeker, J. 1989. "Detection of the Patient at Risk for Osteoporosis at the Time of Menopause." *Maturitas* 11: 85–94; "Osteoporosis–a Matter of Concern for All Women." Arthritis Foundation of New Zealand leaflet.

5. Notelovitz, Morris, and Marsha Ware. 1985. *Stand Tall*. Bantam Books, New York; Cooper, Wendy. 1990. *Understanding Osteoporosis*. Arrow Books, London.

6. Pollner, Fran. "Osteoporosis: Looking at the Whole Picture." *Medical World News,* 14 Jan. 1985: 38–58.

7. Advertisement for Rocatrol. *New Zealand Patient Management,* May 1988.

8. Porter, R., et al. 1990. "Prediction of Hip Fracture in Elderly Women: A Prospective Study." *BMJ* 301: 638–41.

9. Bouillon, R., et al. 1991. "Consensus Development Conference: Prophylaxis and Treatment of Osteoporosis." *Am J Med* 90: 107–10, and abstracts of papers contained in the program for the conference.

10. Riggs, B. Lawrence, and L. Joseph Melton. 1986. "Involutional Osteoporosis." *N Eng J Med* 314(26): 1676–86.

11. Riggs, B. Lawrence. 1987. "Pathogenesis of Osteoporosis." *Am J Obstet Gynecol* 156(5): 1342–51.

12. Ibid.

13. Ibid.

14. Boyle, I. 1989. "Progress in the Understanding and Management of Metabolic Bone Disease." *Scott Med J* 34(5): 515–17.

15. Hui, S., P. Wiske, and J. Norton. 1982. "A Prospective Study of Change in Bone Mass with Age in Postmenopausal Women." *J Chronic Dis* 35: 715–25.

16. Riggs, B. Lawrence, et al. 1982. "Changes in Bone Mineral Density of the Proximal Femur and Spine with Aging: Differences between Postmenopausal and Senile Osteoporosis Syndromes." *J Clin Invest* 70: 716–23.

17. Johnston, C., et al. 1989. "Clinical Indications for Bone Mass Measurements: A Report of the Scientific Advisory Board of the National Osteoporosis Foundation." *J Bone Miner Res* 4, Suppl. 2: 1–28.

18. Bouillon et al. "Prophylaxis and Treatment of Osteoporosis."

19. Cummings, Steven. 1985. "Are Patients with Hip Fractures More Osteoporotic?" *Am J Med* 78: 487–93; Cummings, Steven, et al. 1985. "Epidemiology of Osteoporosis and Osteoporotic Fractures." *Epidemiologic Reviews* 7: 178–208.

20. Elliot, J., et al. 1990. "Effects of Age and Sex on Bone Density at the Hip and Spine in a Normal Caucasian New Zealand Population." *NZ Med J* 103: 33–36.

21. Riggs et al. "Involutional Osteoporosis."

22. Cummings, et al. "Epidemiology of Osteoporosis."

23. Owen, R., L. Melton, and D. Illstrup. 1982. "Incidence of Colles' Fractures in a North American Community." *Am J Public Health* 72: 604–07.

24. Riggs et al. "Involutional Osteoporosis."

25. Cummings, Steven, and D. Black. 1986. "Should Perimenopausal Women Be Screened for Osteoporosis?" *Ann Intern Med* 104: 817.

26. Johnston, et al. "Clinical Indications for Bone Mass Measurements."

27. Resnick, Neil, and Susan Greenspan. 1989. "'Senile' Osteoporosis Reconsidered." *JAMA* 261(7): 1025–29.

28. Cummings, Steven, and Michael Nevitt. 1989. "A Hypothesis: The Causes of Hip Fractures." *J Gerontology* 44: M107–11; Johnson et al. "Clinical Indications for Bone Mass Measurements."

29. Cooper, C. 1989. "Osteoporosis—An Epidemiological Perspective: A Review." *J Roy Soc Med* 82: 753–57.

30. Gibson, M. 1987. "The Prevention of Falls in Later Life: A Report of the Kellogg International Work Group on the Prevention of Falls by the Elderly." *Danish Medical Bulletin* 34, (Gerontology Special Suppl. Series no. 4): 1–24.

31. Campbell, A. John, George Spears, and Michael Borrie. 1991. "Examination by Logistic Regression Modelling of the Variables which Increase the Relative Risk of Elderly Women Falling Compared to Elderly Men." *J Clin Epidemiol* (in press).

32. Porter et al. "Prediction of Hip Fracture in Elderly Women."

33. Gibson. "The Prevention of Falls in Later Life."

34. Gilchrist, Nigel. 1990. Submission to Working Party on Osteoporosis Prevention.

35. Jensen, G., et al. 1982. "Epidemiology of Postmenopausal Spinal and Long Bone Fractures: A Unifying Approach to Postmenopausal Osteoporosis." *Clinical Orthopaedics* 166: 75–81.

36. Ettinger, Bruce, Harry Genant, and Christopher Cann. 1985. "Long-term

Estrogen Replacement Therapy Prevents Bone Loss and Fractures." *Ann Intern Med* 102: 319–24.

37. Johnson et al. "Clinical Indications for Bone Mass Measurements."

38. Van Hemert, Albert, et al. 1990. "Prediction of Osteoporotic Fractures in the General Population by a Fracture Risk Score." *Am J Epidemiol* 132(1): 121–35.

39. Cummings et al. "Epidemiology of Osteoporosis."

40. Hockey, Richard, Michael Hobbs, and Peter Goldswain. 1990. *Femoral Neck Fractures in Western Australia 1971–1988.* University of Western Australia Department of Medicine, Perth: 1–37.

41. Report on the Working Party on Osteoporosis Prevention, 1991. Department of Health, Wellington.

42. Ibid.

43. Hockey et al. "Femoral Neck Fractures."

44. Ibid.

45. Report on the Working Party on Osteoporosis Prevention, 1991. Department of Health, Wellington; Hockey et al. "Femoral Neck Fractures."

46. Sainsbury, Richard, et al. 1986. "An Orthopaedic Geriatric Rehabilitation Unit: The First Two Years' Experience." *NZ Med J* 99: 583–85.

7. Preventing Bone Loss and Fractures

1. Van Hemert, Albert, et al. 1990. "Prediction of Osteoporotic Fractures in the General Population by a Fracture Risk Score." *Am J Epidemiol* 132(1): 121–35.

2. Melton, L. Joseph, David Eddy, and C. Conrad Johnston. 1990. "Screening for Osteoporosis." *Ann Intern Med* 112: 516–28; Slemenda, Charles, et al. 1990. "Predictors of Bone Mass in Perimenopausal Women." *Ann Intern Med* 112(2): 96–101.

3. Melton, et al. "Screening for Osteoporosis."

4. Ibid.

5. Hui, Siu, Charles Slemenda, and C. Conrad Johnston. 1989. "Baseline Measurements of Bone Mass Predicts Fracture in White Women." *Ann Intern Med* 111: 355–61; Hui, Siu, Charles Slemenda, and C. Conrad Johnston. 1988. "Age and Bone Mass as Predictors of Fracture in a Prospective Study." *J Clin Invest* 81: 1804–09; Cummings, Steven. 1990. "Appendicular Bone Density and Age Predict Hip Fracture in Women." *JAMA* 263(5): 665–68.

6. "Osteoporosis is Costly." *New Zealand Doctor,* 23 Oct. 1990; Laracy, Lynne. "Dem Brittle Bones." *More,* Feb. 1991: 122–25; Potter, Leteia. 1991. *Women in Mid Life.* New Women's Press, Auckland.

7. Melton, et al. "Screening for Osteoporosis."

8. Cummings, Steven. 1985. "Are Patients with Hip Fractures More Osteoporotic?" *Am J Med* 78: 487–93.

9. Cummings. "Appendicular Bone Density."

10. Johnston, C., et al. 1989. "Clinical Indications for Bone Mass Measurements: A Report of the Scientific Advisory Board of the National Osteoporosis Foundation." *J Bone Miner Res* 4 Suppl. 2: 1–28; Melton, et al. "Screening for Osteoporosis."

11. Report of the Working Party on Osteoporosis Prevention. 1991. Department of Health, Wellington.

12. Johnston, et al. "Clinical Indications for Bone Mass Measurements."

13. Ibid.

14. Van Hemert, et al. "Prediction of Osteoporosis Fractures."

15. Bouillon, R., et al. 1991. "Consensus Development Conference: Prophylaxis and Treatment of Osteoporosis." *Am J Med* 90: 107–10, and the program for the conference containing abstracts of papers.

16. Cummings, Steven, et al. 1985. "Epidemiology of Osteoporosis and Osteoporotic Fractures." *Epidemiologic Reviews* 7: 178–208.

17. Stevenson, John. 1990. "Pathogenesis, Prevention, and Treatment of Osteoporosis." *Obstet Gynecol Clin North Am* 75(4) Suppl.: 36S– 41S.

18. Reid, I., M. Mackie, and H. Ibbertson. 1986. "Bone Mineral Content in Polynesian and White New Zealand Women." *BMJ* 292: 1547–48.

19. Stott, Susan. 1980. "The Incidence of Femoral Neck Fractures in New Zealand." *NZ Med J* 91: 6–9.

20. Stevenson. "Pathogenesis, Prevention, and Treatment of Osteoporosis."

21. Riggs, B. Lawrence, and L. Joseph Melton. 1986. "Involutional Osteoporosis." *N Eng J Med* 314(26): 1676–86.

22. Reid, Ian. "Determinants of Bone Density in Postmenopausal Women." Paper to a meeting of the Auckland Medical Research Society, 11 Feb. 1991.

23. Cummings. "Epidemiology of Osteoporosis."

24. Seeman, Ego, et al. 1989. "Reduced Bone Mass in Daughters of Women with Osteoporosis." *N Eng J Med* 320: 554–58.

25. Van Hemert, et al. "Prediction of Osteoporosis Fractures."

26. Cummings. "Epidemiology of Osteoporosis."

27. Stevenson. "Pathogenesis, Prevention, and Treatment of Osteoporosis."

28. Riggs and Melton. "Involutional Osteoporosis."

29. Utian, Wulf. 1990. Panel discussion 2. *Obstet Gynecol Clin North Am* 75(4) Suppl.: 31S–35S.

30. Stevenson, John. 1986. "Osteoporosis: The Silent Epidemic." *Update* 33(3): 211–16.

31. Siddle, Nick, Philip Sarrel, and Malcolm Whitehead. 1987. "The Effect of Hysterectomy on the Age of Ovarian Failure: Identification of a Sub-

group of Women with Premature Loss of Ovarian Function," and Literature Review. *Fertil Steril* 47(1): 94–100.

32. Cummings. "Epidemiology of Osteoporosis."

33. Cundy, T., et al. "Reduced Bone Density in Women Using Depot Medroxyprogesterone Acetate for Contraception." *BMJ* (in press).

34. Twomey, Lance. "Physical Activity and Aging Bones." *Patient Management,* March 1989: 29–34.

35. Ibid.

36. Smith, E., et al. 1989. "Deterring Bone Loss by Exercise Intervention in Premenopausal and Postmenopausal Women." *Calcif Tissue Int* 44: 312–21.

37. Krolner, B., et al. 1983. "Physical Exercise as Prophylaxis against Involutional Vertebral Bone Loss: A Controlled Trial." *Clin Sci* 64: 541–46.

38. Sinaki, Mehrsheed. 1989. "Exercise and Osteoporosis." *Arch Phys Med Rehabil* 70: 220–29.

39. Twomey. "Physical Activity and Aging Bones."

40. Orwoll, E., et al. 1989. "The Relationship of Swimming Exercise to Bone Mass in Men and Women." *Arch Intern Med* 149: 2197–200.

41. Sinaki, Mehrsheed, et al. 1986. "Relationship between Bone Mineral Density of Spine and Strength of Back Extensors in Healthy Postmenopausal Women." *Mayo Clin Proc* 61: 116–22.

42. Sinaki, Mehrsheed, and Kenneth Offord. 1988. "Physical Activity in Postmenopausal Women: Effect on Back Muscle Strength and Bone Mineral Density of the Spine." *Arch Phys Med Rehabil* 69: 277–80.

43. Chow, Raphael, and Joan Harrison. 1987. "Relationship of Kyphosis to Physical Fitness and Bone Mass in Postmenopausal Women." *Am J Phys Med Rehabil* 66(5): 219–27.

44. Cooper, C., D. Barker, and C. Wickham, 1988. "Physical Activity, Muscle Strength, and Calcium Intake in Fracture of the Proximal Femur in Britain." *BMJ* 297: 1443–46.

45. Elliot, J., et al. 1991. "A Comparison of Elderly Patients with Proximal Femoral Fractures with a Normal Elderly Population: A Case Controlled Study." *NZ Med J* (in press).

46. Stevenson. "Pathogenesis, Prevention, and Treatment of Osteoporosis."

47. Goulding, Ailsa. 1989. "An Otago Perspective on Osteoporosis." *Proc Nutr Soc NZ* 14: 26–33.

48. Highet, Ruth, 1989. "Athletic Amenorrhoea: An Update on Aetiology, Complications and Management." *Sports Med* 7: 82–108.

49. Ibid.

50. Mellstrom, Dan. 1989. "Epidemiological Aspects." In *Osteoporosis: Pharmacological Treatment and Prophylaxis,* ed. Kjell Strandberg, Bjorn Beermann, and Gudmar Lonnerholm. National Board of Health and Welfare Drug Information Committee, Uppsala, Sweden: 7–21.

51. Cummings. "Epidemiology of Osteoporosis."

52. Resnick, Neil, and Susan Greenspan. 1989. "'Senile' Osteoporosis Reconsid 2ered." *JAMA* 261(7): 1025–29.

53. Cummings. "Epidemiology of Osteoporosis."

54. Resnick and Greenspan. "'Senile' Osteoporosis Reconsidered."

55. Riggs, B. 1990. "Restoration of Skeletal Mass (Fluoride, PTH)." In Consensus Development Conference program: conference report published as reference no. 13.

56. Health Responsibility Systems. 1993. Online reference.

57. Boyle, I. 1989. "Progress in the Understanding and Management of Metabolic Bone Disease." *Scott Med J* 34(5): 515–17.

58. Wallis, Claudia. "A Puzzling Plague." *Time,* 14 Jan. 1991: 40–47.

59. Coope, Jean, and Deborah Roberts. 1990. "A Clinic for the Prevention of Osteoporosis in General Practice." *Br J Gen Prac* 40: 295–99.

60. Goulding, Ailsa. 1990. "Osteoporosis: Why Consuming Less Sodium Chloride Helps to Conserve Bone." *NZ Med J,* 28 March: 120–22.

61. Reid, I. R., et al. 1993. "Effect of Calcium Supplementation on Bone Loss in Postmenopausal Women." *N Eng J Med* 328: 460–4.

62. Stevenson. "Dietary Intake of Calcium."

63. Kiel, Douglas, et al. 1990. "Caffeine and the Risk of Hip Fracture: The Framingham Study." *Am J Epidemiol* 132(4): 675–84.

64. Mellstrom. "Epidemiological Aspects."

65. Notelovitz, Morris. 1986. "Postmenopausal Osteoporosis." *Acta Obstet Gynecol Scand* Suppl. 134: 67–80.

66. Reid, I. R., et al. 1992. "Determinants of Total Body and Regional Bone and Mineral Density in Normal Postmenopausal Women—a Key Role for Fat Mass." *J Clin Endocrinol Metab* 75: 45–51.

67. Kato, Nancy Ton. "Americans Have Fat on the Brain." *American Demographics* 14: March 1992, P. 20, Col. 1.

68. *Report on the Working Party on Osteoporosis Prevention.* 1991. Department of Health, Wellington, New Zealand.

69. Cummings. "Epidemiology of Osteoporosis"; Smith, Roger. 1987. "Osteoporosis: Cause and Management." *BMJ* 294: 329–32.

70. Riggs and Melton. "Involutional Osteoporosis."

71. Cummings. "Epidemiology of Osteoporosis."

72. Bouillon, et al. "Prophylaxis and Treatment of Osteoporosis."

8. All Roads Lead to Hormones

1. Eagan, Andrea. "The Estrogen Fix." *Ms,* April 1989: 38–43.

2. McKinlay, Sonja, and John McKinlay. 1974. "Selected Studies of the Menopause." *J Biosoc Sci* 5: 533–54.

3. Allen, Willard. 1974. "Pros and Cons of Estrogen Therapy for Gynecologic Conditions." In *Controversy in Obstetrics and Gynaecology*, eds. D. Reid and C. D. Christian. Saunders, Philadelphia: 785–93.

4. Sjostrom, Henning, and Robert Nilsson. 1972. *Thalidomide and the Power of the Drug Companies*. Penguin, Harmondsworth, UK.

5. Silverman, Milton, and Philip Lee. 1974. *Pills, Profits and Politics*. University of California Press, Berkeley.

6. Platt, Lord. 1967. "Medical Science: Master or Servant?" *BMJ* 4: 439–44.

7. Silverman and Lee. *Pills, Profits and Politics*.

8. Zola, Ining. 1977. "Healthism and Disabling Medicalization." In *Disabling Professions*. Marion Boyars, London: 41–67; Illich, Ivan. 1976. *Limits to Medicine*. Marion Boyars, London.

9. Platt. "Medical Science."

10. Mintz, Morton. 1985. *At Any Cost: Corporate Greed, Women, and the Dalkon Shield*. Pantheon Books, New York.

11. Van Keep, P. 1990. "The History and Rationale of Hormone Replacement Therapy." *Maturitas* 12: 163–70.

12. McCrea, Frances. 1983. "The Politics of Menopause: The 'Discovery' of a Deficiency Disease." *Social Problems* 31(1): 111–23.

13. Boston Women's Health Book Collective. 1984. *The New Our Bodies Ourselves*. Simon & Schuster, New York.

14. Persson, H-O., et al. 1983. "Practice and Patterns of Estrogen Treatment in Climacteric Women in a Swedish Population." *Acta Obstet Gynecol Scand* 62: 289–96.

15. Seaman, Barbara, and Gideon Seaman. 1977. *Women and the Crisis in Sex Hormones*. Bantam Books, New York.

16. Grant, Ellen. 1985. *The Bitter Pill*. Elm Tree Books, London.

17. Seaman and Seaman. *Women and the Crisis in Sex Hormones*.

18. Sjostrom and Nilsson. *Thalidomide and the Power of the Drug Companies*.

19. Seaman and Seaman. *Women and the Crisis in Sex Hormones*.

20. Silverman and Lee. *Pills, Profits and Politics*.

21. Seaman and Seaman. *Women and the Crisis in Sex Hormones*.

22. *Current Medical Digest*, Nov. 1968.

23. *Current Medical Digest*, Sept. 1968.

24. *Modern Medicine*, Dec. 1976.

25. Seaman and Seaman. *Women and the Crisis in Sex Hormones*.

26. Allen. "Pros and Cons of Estrogen Therapy."

27. Seaman and Seaman. *Women and the Crisis in Sex Hormones*.

28. Ibid.

29. Nachtigall, Lila, and Joan Heilman. 1986. *Estrogen: The Facts Can Change Your Life*. The Body Press, Los Angeles.

30. Gorman, Teresa, and Malcolm Whitehead. 1989. *The Amarant Book of Hormone Replacement Therapy.* Pan Books, London.

31. Whitehead, Malcolm. 1986. "Prevention of Endometrial Abnormalities." In *A Modern Approach to the Perimenopausal Years,* ed. Robert Greenblatt. De Gruyter, Berlin, New York: 189–206.

32. Cooper, Wendy. 1975. *No Change: A Biological Revolution for Women.* Arrow Books, London.

33. Hunt, Kate, and M. Vessey. 1986. "Prospective Study on Long-term Risk of Hormone Replacement Therapy." In *A Modern Approach to the Perimenopausal Years,* ed. Robert Greenblatt. De Gruyter, Berlin, New York; 157–62.

34. Hunt, Kate, 1988. "Perceived Value of Treatment among a Group of Long-term Users of Hormone Replacement Therapy." *J R Coll Gen Pract* 38: 398–401.

35. Cooper. *No Change.*

36. Seaman and Seaman. *Women and the Crisis in Sex Hormones.*

37. Allen. "Pros and Cons of Estrogen Therapy."

38. Ziel, Harry, and William Finkle. 1975. "Increased Risk of Endometrial Carcinoma among Users of Conjugated Estrogens." *N Eng J Med* 293: 1167–70.

39. Allen. "Pros and Cons of Estrogen Therapy."

40. Ziel, Harry, and William Finkle. 1976. "Association of Estrone with the Development of Endometrial Carcinoma." *Am J Obstet Gynecol* 124(7): 735–39.

41. Smith, D. C., et al. 1975. "Association of Exogenous Estrogen and Endometrial Carcinoma. *N Eng J Med* 293: 1164–67.

42. Editorial. 1976. "Oestrogens as a Cause of Endometrial Carcinoma." *BMJ* 1: 791–92.

43. Seaman and Seaman. *Women and the Crisis in Sex Hormones.*

44. Ibid.

45. Cooper, Wendy. "Combined Therapy Makes HRT Safe as Well as Effective." *Modern Medicine,* Jan. 1978: 53–55.

46. Kaufert, Patricia, and Sonja McKinlay. 1985. "Estrogen-replacement Therapy: The Production of Medical Knowledge and the Emergence of Policy." In *Women, Health and Healing,* eds. E. Lewin and V. Olesen. Tavistock Press, London: 113–38.

47. Hoover, R., et al. 1976. "Menopausal Estrogens and Breast Cancer." *N Eng J Med* 295: 401–05.

48. Report from the Boston Collaborative Drug Surveillance Program. 1974. "Surgically Confirmed Gallbladder Disease, Venous Thromboembolism, and Breast Tumors in Relation to Postmenopausal Estrogen Therapy." *N Eng J Med* 290(1): 1519.

49. Kaufert and McKinlay. "Estrogen-replacement Therapy."

50. Ibid.

51. Seaman and Seaman. *Women and the Crisis in Sex Hormones.*

52. Kaufert and McKinlay. "Estrogen-replacement Therapy."

53. Ibid.

54. Lieberman, Sharon. "But You'll Make Such a Feminine Corpse." *Majority Report,* n.d.; "New Discovery: Public Relations Cures Cancer." *Majority Report,* Feb. 1977; Mintz, Morton. "Hawking the Estrogen Fix." *The Progressive,* Sept. 1977: 24–25.

55. Mowat, Wayne. Interview with Dr. Neil McKenzie. National Radio, 28 Feb. 1990.

56. Gorman and Whitehead. *The Amarant Book of Hormone Replacement Therapy.*

57. Studd, John. 1987. "Management of the Menopause." Presentation to Update Conference, New Zealand Obstetrical and Gynaecological Society, February 1987, Auckland.

58. Kaufert and McKinlay. "Estrogen-replacement Therapy."

59. Van Keep. "The History and Rationale of Hormone Replacement Therapy."

60. Wilson, Robert, and Thelma Wilson. 1963. "The Fate of the Nontreated Postmenopausal Woman: A Plea for the Maintenance of Adequate Estrogen from Puberty to the Grave." *J Am Geriatr Soc* 11: 347–62.

61. Neaman, Judith. "Postmenopausal Osteoporosis." *Sexual Medicine Today,* June 1981: 6–12.

62. Heilman, Joan. "The Drug That Made a Comeback." *Parade Magazine,* 20 Oct. 1985: 14.

63. Henig, Robin Marantz. "Estrogen, In and Out of Favor." *Washington Post,* n.d.

64. Dejanikus, Tacie. "Major Drug Manufacturer Funds Osteoporosis Public Education Campaign." *Network News,* May/June 1985: 1–8.

65. Greenblatt, Robert, ed. 1986. *A Modern Approach to the Perimenopausal Years.* De Gruyter, Berlin, New York.

66. Lobo, Rogerio, and Malcolm Whitehead. 1989. "Too Much of a Good Thing? Use of Progestogens in the Menopause: An International Consensus Statement." *Fertil Steril* 51(2): 229–31.

67. Pearson, Cynthia. "FDA Waffles on Premarin Decision." *Network News,* July/Aug. 1990: 1–7.

68. Lobo and Whitehead. "Too Much of a Good Thing?"

69. How to Treat . . . Menopause." *New Zealand Doctor,* 2 July 1990: 19–26.

70. Mackenzie, Frances. "Good health—during and after Menopause." *Australian Women's Weekly,* Nov. 1990: 101.

71. Donaldson, Angela. "Oestrogen—The Menopause Miracle." *New Zealand Woman's Day,* 20 Feb. 1991: 28–29.

72. "Is 1 in 10 Worth It." *Network News,* July/August 1990: 1.

73. Salhanick, Hilton A. 1974. "Pros and Cons of Estrogen Therapy for Gyne-cologic Conditions." In *Controversy in Obstetrics and Gynaecology,* ed. D. Reid and C. D. Christian. Saunders, Philadelphia: 801–08.

74. Ibid.

75. Draper, Juliet, and Martin Roland. 1990. "Perimenopausal Women's Views on Taking Hormone Replacement Therapy to Prevent Osteo-porosis." *BMJ* 300: 786–88; Coope, Jean, and Deborah Roberts. 1990. "A Clinic for the Prevention of Osteoporosis in General Practice." *Br J Gen Prac* 40: 295–99.

76. Bungay, G., M. Vessey, and C. McPherson. "Study of Symptoms in Mid-dle Life with Special Reference to the Menopause." *BMJ,* 281: 181–84.

77. Doress, Paula, Diana Siegal, and Jean Shapiro. 1989. *Ourselves Growing Older.* Simon & Schuster, New York.

78. Roeber, Johanna. "The Forever Therapy?" *Vogue* 1990: 172–73.

79. Roberts, Yvonne. "Fortysomething." *New Statesman and Society,* 12 Jan. 1990: 12–14.

80. Armstrong, Bruce. 1988. "Oestrogen Therapy after the Menopause—Boon or Bane?" *Med J Aust* 148: 213–14.

9. Mostly Good News about Hormones

1. Hunt, Kate, et al. 1987. "Long-term Surveillance of Mortality and Cancer Incidence in Women Receiving Hormone Replacement Therapy." *Br J Ob-stet Gynaecol* 94: 620–35.

2. Persson, H-O., et al. 1983. "Practice and Patterns of Estrogen Treatment in Cli-macteric Women in a Swedish Population." *Acta Obstet Gynecol Scand* 62: 289–96.

3. Overton, G. 1989. "Oestrogens and Progestogens in Clinical Practice." *New Ethicals* 26(6):23–34.

4. L'Hermite, Marc. 1990. "Risks of Estrogens and Progestogens." *Maturitas* 12: 215–46.

5. Overton. "Oestrogens and Progestogens in Clinical Practice."

6. Whitehead, M., T. Hillard, and D. Crook. 1990. "The Role and Use of Progestogens." *Obstet Gynecol Clin North Am* 75: 59S–75S; Weinstein, Louis, Chhanda Bewtra, and J. Chris Gallagher. 1990. "Evaluation of a Continuous Combined Low-dose Regimen of Estrogen-Progestin for Treatment of the Menopausal Patient." *Am J Obstet Gynecol* 162: 1534–39.

7. Whitehead, et al. "The Role and Use of Progetogens."

8. Weinstein, et al. "Evaluation of a Continuous Combined Low-dose Regi-men."

9. Discussion (of paper in above note). *Am J Obstet Gynecol* 162: 1539–42.

10. Studd, John, H. Anderson, and J. Montgomery. 1986. "Selection of Patients
    —Kind and Duration of Treatment." In *A Modern Approach to the Peri-
    meno-pausal Years,* ed. Robert Greenblatt. De Gruyter, Berlin, New York:
    129–40.

11. Noble, Anthony. 1989. "Hormone Replacement Therapy" (letter). *BMJ*
    299: 50.

12. Wren, Barry. 1987. "Oestrogen Therapy after Menopause: A Viewpoint
    on Its Rational Use." *Current Therapeutics,* March: 25–36.

13. Whitehead, M., et al. 1990. "Transdermal Administration of Oestro-
    gen/Progestogen Hormone Replacement Therapy." *lanccet* 335: 310–12.

14. Corson, Stephen. 1990. "Impact of Estrogen Replacement Therapy on
    Cardiovascular Risk." *J Reprod Med* 34(9) Suppl.: 729–43.

15. Cardazo, L. 1986. "Routes of Estrogen Administration." In *A Modern Ap-
    proach to the Perimenopausal Years,* ed. Robert Greenblatt. De Gruyter, Ber-
    lin, New York: 141–48.

16. Studd et al. "Selection of Patients."

17. Llewellyn-Jones, Derek, and Suzanne Abraham. 1988. *Menopause.* Penguin
    Books, Ringwood, Vic.

18. Beard, Mary, and Lindsay Curtis. 1989. "Libido, Menopause, and Estro-
    gen Replacement Therapy." *Postgrad Med* 86(1): 225–28.

19. Cardazo. "Routes of Estrogen Administration."

20. Lobo, Rogerio. 1987. "Absorption and Metabolic Effects of Different
    Types of Estrogens and Progestogens." *Obstet Gynecol Clin North Am*
    14(1): 143–68.

21. Llewellyn-Jones and Abraham. *Menopause.*

22. Hirvonen, E., J. Elliesen, and K. Schmidt-Gollwitzer. 1990. "Comparison
    of Two Hormone Replacement Regimens—Influence on Lipoproteins
    and Bone Mineral Content." *Maturitas* 12: 127–36.

23. "Women and Estrogens." *FDA Consumer,* April 1976: 4–8.

24. Hunt, et al. "Long-term Surveillance of Mortality and Cancer Incidence."

25. Bergkvist, Leif, et al. 1988. "Risk Factors for Breast and Endometrial Can-
    cer in a Cohort of Women Treated with Menopausal Oestrogens." *Int J
    Epidemiol* 17: 732–37.

26. Ferguson, Kristi, Curtis Hoegh, and Susan Johnson. 1989. "Estrogen Re-
    placement Therapy." *Arch Intern* Med 149: 133–36.

27. Coope, Jean. 1981. "Is Oestrogen Therapy Effective in the Treatment of
    Menopausal Depression?" *J R Coll Gen Pract* 31: 134–40; Coope, Jean,
    Jean Thomson, and L. Poller. 1975. "Effect of 'Natural Oestrogen' Re-
    placement Therapy on Menopausal Symptoms and Blood Clotting." *BMJ*
    4: 139–43; Campbell, Stuart, and Malcolm Whitehead. 1977. "Oestro-
    gen Therapy and the Menopausal Syndrome." *Obsta Gynecol* 4(1): 31–47.

28. Hunt, Kate. 1988. "Perceived Value of Treatment among a Group of

Long-term Users of Hormone Replacement Therapy." *J R Coll Gen Pract* 38: 398–401.

29. Campbell and Whitehead. "Oestrogen Therapy and the Menopausal Syndrome"; Coope et al. "Effect of 'Natural Oestrogen'"; Hirvonen et al. "Comparison of Two Hormone Replacement Regimens"; Hunt. "Perceived Value of Treatment."

30. Reitz, Rosetta, 1985. *Menopause: A Positive Approach.* Viking Penguin, New York; Ojeda, Linda. 1992. *Menopause Without Medicine.* Hunter House, Alameda, California.

31. Campbell and Whitehead. "Oestrogen Therapy and the Menopausal Syndrome."

32. Coope et al. "Effect of 'Natural Oestrogen.'"

33. Dennerstein, Lorraine. 1987. "Depression in the Menopause." *Obstet Gynecol Clin North Am* 14(1): 33–48.

34. Utian, Wulf. 1986. "Non-hormonal Medication." In *A Modern Approach to the Perimenopausal Years,* ed. Robert Greenblatt. De Gruyter, Berlin, New York: 117

35. Coope. "Is Oestrogen Therapy Effective?"

36. Coope et al. "Effect of 'Natural Oestrogen.'"

37. Greenblatt, Robert. 1986. "Prologue." In A *Modern Approach to the Perimenopausal Years,* ed. Robert Greenblatt. De Gruyter, Berlin, New York: 3–8.

38. Donaldson, Angela. "Oestrogen: The Menopause Miracle." *New Zealand Woman's Day,* 10 Feb. 1991: 28–29.

39. Bonn, Dorothy. "HRT and the Media." Paper presented to the Women's Health Concern Conference, Cardiff, 31 May 1989.

40. Seaman, Barbara, and Gideon Seaman. 1977. *Women and the Crisis in Sex Hormones.* Bantam Books, New York.

41. Pollner, Fran. "Osteoporosis: Looking at the Whole Picture." *Medical World News,* 14 Jan. 1985: 38–58.

42. Henig, Robin. "Will Estrogen Keep You Young?" *Woman's Day,* April 1985: 64.

43. Melton, L. Joseph, David Eddy, and C. Conrad Johnston. 1990. "Screening for Osteoporosis." *Ann Intern Med* 112: 516–28.

44. Pollner. "Osteoporosis."

45. Notelovitz, Morris. 1986. "Postmenopausal Osteoporosis." *Acta Obstet Gynecol Scand Suppl* 134: 67–80.

46. Munklensen, N., et al. 1988. "Reversal of Postmenopausal Vertebral Bone Loss by Oestrogen and Progestogen: A Double Blind Placebo Controlled Trial." *BMJ* 296: 1150–52.

47. Melton et al. "Screening for Osteoporosis."

48. Lindsay, R. and J.F. Tohme. 1990. "Estrogen Treatment of Patients with Established Postmenopausal Osteoporosis." *Obstet Gynecol* 76: 290;

Lufkin, E. G. et al. 1992. "Treatment of Postmenopausal Osteoporosis with Transdermal Estrogen." *Ann Intern Med* 117: 1–9.

49. Lindsay, R., et al. 1980. "Prevention of Spinal Osteoporosis in Oophorectomised Women." *Lancet* 2: 1151–54.

50. Ettinger, B., H. Genant, and C. Cann. 1985. "Long-term Estrogen Replacement Therapy Prevents Bone Loss and Fractures." *Ann Intern Med* 102: 319–24.

51. Kiel, Douglas, et al. 1987. "Hip Fracture and the Use of Estrogens in Postmenopausal Women: The Framingham Study." *N Eng J Med* 317: 11169–74.

52. Hutchinson, et al. "Postmenopausal Estrogens."

53. Weiss, et al. "Decreased Risk of Fractures."

54. Pitt, Frances, and John Brazier. 1990. "Hormone Replacement Therapy for Osteoporosis" (letter). *lanccet* 335: 978.

55. Grady, D., et al. 1992. "Hormone Replacement Therapy to Prevent Diseases and Prolong Life in Postmenopausal Women." *Ann Intern Med* 117: 1016–1037.

56. Paganini-Hill, et al. "Menopausal Estrogen Therapy and Hip Fractures."

57. Felson, D. T., et al. 1993. "The Effect of Postmenopausal Estrogen Therapy on Bone Density in Elderly Women." *N Eng Med J* 329: 1141–6.

58. Naessen, Tord, et al. 1990. "Hormone Replacement Therapy and the Risk for First Hip Fracture." *Ann Intern Med* 113: 95–103.

59. Hillner, B., J. Hollenberg, and S. Pauker. 1986. "Postmenopausal Estrogens in Prevention of Osteoporosis: Benefit Virtually without Risk if Cardiovascular Effects Are Considered." *Am J Med* 80: 1115–27.

60. Lindsay, R., et al. 1978. "Bone Response to Termination of Oestrogen Treatment." *lanccet* 1: 1325–27.

61. Horsman, A., B. Nordin and R. Crilly. 1979. "Effect on Bone of Withdrawal of Oestrogen Therapy" (letter). *lanccet* 2: 33.

62. Christiansen, Claus, Merete Christiansen, and Ib Transbol. 1981. "Bone Mass in Postmenopausal Women after Withdrawal of Oestrogen/Gestagen Replacement Therapy." *Lancet* 1: 456–61.

63. Lindsay, Robert. 1987. "Estrogen Therapy in the Prevention and Management of Osteoporosis." *Am J Obstet Gynecol* 156: 1347–51.

64. Munktensen, et al. "Reversal of Postmenopausal Vertebral Bone Loss."

65. Nachtigall, Lila, et al. 1979. "Estrogen Replacement Therapy I: A 10-Year Prospective Study in the Relationship to Osteoporosis." *Obstet Gynecol Clin North Am* 53: 277–81; Naessen, et al. "Hormone Replacement Therapy."

66. Stevenson, John, et al. 1990. "Effects of Transdermal Versus Oral Hormone Replacement Therapy on Bone Density in Spine and Proximal Femur in Postmenopausal Women." *Lancet* 335: 265–69; Whitehead, et al. "Transdermal Administration of Oestrogen/Progestogen."

67. "Oestrogen Helps to Promote Longer Life." *New Zealand Herald,* 15 Jan. 1991.

68. Colditz, Graham, et al. 1987. "Menopause and the Risk of Coronary Heart Disease in Women." *N Eng J Med* 316: 1105–10.

69. Larsson-Cohn, V., and L. Wallentin. 1986. "Sex Steroids and Lipoproteins." In *A Modern Approach to the Perimenopausal Years,* ed. Robert Greenblatt. De Gruyter, Berlin, New York: 153–56; Teran, Ana-Zully, Robert Greenblatt, and Jaswant Chaddha. 1987. "Changes in Lipoproteins with Various Sex Steroids." *Obstet Gynecol Clin North Am* 14(1):107–20; Sitruk-Ware, R., and P. Ibarra de Palacios. 1989. "Oestrogen Replacement Therapy and Cardiovascular Disease in Postmenopausal Women: A Review." *Maturitas* 11: 259–74.

70. Mattson, L., G. Cullberg, and G. Samsoie. 1982. "Evaluation of a Continuous Oestrogen-Progestogen Regimen for Climacteric Complaints." *Maturitas* 4: 95–102.

71. Lobo, Rogerio. 1990. "Cardiovascular Implications of Estrogen Replacement Therapy." *Obstet Gynecol Clin North Am* 75: 18S–25S; Bourne, T., et al. 1990. "Oestrogens, Arterial Status, and Postmenopausal Women." *lanccet* 335: 1470–71.

72. Grady, D., et al. "Hormone Therapy to Prevent Disease and Prolong Life."

73. Vanderbroucke, Jan P. 1991. "Postmenopausal Oestrogen and Cardioprotection." *Lancet* 337: 833–34.

74. Barrett-Connor, E. and T. L. Bush. 1991. "Estrogen and Coronary Heart Disease in Women." *JAMA* 265: 1861–67.

75. Sullivan, Jay, et al. 1990. "Estrogen Replacement and Coronary Artery Disease." *Arch Intern Med* 150: 2557–62.

76. Vanderbroucke. 1991. "Postmenopausal Oestrogen and Cardioprotection."

10. The Not-So-Good to Bad News About Hormones

1. Ravnikar, Veronica, 1987. "Compliance with Hormone Therapy." *Am J Obstet Gynecol* 156: 1332–34.

2. Douress, Paula Brown and Diana Laskin Siegal. 1987, 1994. *Ourselves Growing Older.* New York: Simon & Schuster.

3. Paul, C., D. Skegg, and G. Spears. 1989. "Depot-medroxyprogesterone (Depo Provera) and Risk of Breast Cancer." *BMJ* 299: 759–62.

4. Baber, R., and John Studd. 1980. "Hormone Replacement Therapy and Cancer." *Br J Hosp Med* 41: 142–49.

5. Ettinger, B., I. Golditch, and G. Friedman. 1988. "Gynecologic Consequences of Long-term Unopposed Estrogen Replacement Therapy." *Maturitas* 10: 271–82.

6. McKinlay, Sonja. Presentation at Auckland Medical School, 10 Sept. 1989.

7. Whitehead, Malcolm. 1986. "Prevention of Endometrial Abnormalities."

In *A Modern Approach to the Perimenopausal Years,* ed. Robert Greenblatt. De Gruyter, Berlin, New York: 189–206.

8. Shapiro, Samuel, et al. 1985. "Risk of Localized and Widespread Endometrial Cancer in Relation to Recent and Discontinued Use of Conjugated Estrogens." *N Eng J Med* 313: 969–72.

9. Gangar, Kevin, et al. 1990. "Prolonged Endometrial Stimulation Associated with Oestradiol Implants." *BMJ* 300: 436–38.

10. Whitehead, et al. "Prevention of Endometrial Abnormalities."

11. Persson, Ingemar, et al. 1989. "Risk of Endometrial Cancer after Treatment with Oestrogens Alone or in Conjunction with Progestogens: Results of a Prospective Study." *BMJ* 298: 147–51; Armstrong, Bruce. 1988. "Oestrogen Therapy after Menopause—Boon or Bane?" *Med J Aust* 148: 213–14.

12. Gambrell, R. Don. 1987. "Use of Progestogen Therapy." *Am Obstet Gynecol* 156: 1304–13; Whitehead. "Prevention of Endometrial Abnormalities."

13. Studd, John. 1986. "Selection of Patients—Kind and Duration of Treatment." In *A Modern Approach to the Perimenopausal Years,* ed. Robert Greenblatt. De Gruyter, Berlin, New York: 129–40.

14. Ibid.; Gambrell. "Use of Progestogen Therapy."

15. Whitehead. "Prevention of Endometrial Abnormalities."

16. Kemp, John, Judith Fryer, and Rodney Baber. 1989. "An Alternative Regimen of Hormone Replacement Therapy to Improve Patient Compliance." *Aust NZ Obstet Gynaecol* 29: 66–69.

17. Studd, John, et al. 1979. "Value of Cytology for Detecting Endometrial Abnormalities in Climacteric Women Receiving Hormone Replacement Therapy. *BMJ* 1: 846–48.

18. Kovacs, G., and H. Burger. 1988. "Endometrial Sampling for Women on Perimenopausal Hormone Replacement Therapy." *Maturitas* 10: 259–62.

19. Wingo, P., et al. 1987. "The Risk of Breast Cancer in Postmenopausal Women Who Have Used Estrogen Replacement Therapy." *JAMA* 257: 209–15; Buring, J., et al. 1987. "A Prospective Cohort Study of Postmenopausal Hormone Use and Risk of Breast Cancer in U.S. Women." *Am J Epidemiol* 125: 939–47; McDonald, J., et al. 1986. "Menopausal Estrogen Use and the Risk of Breast Cancer." *Breast Cancer Res Treat* 7: 193–99.

20. Brinton, L., R. Hoover, and J. Fraumeni. 1986. "Menopausal Oestrogens and Breast Cancer Risk: An Expanded Case-Control Study." *Br J Cancer* 54: 825–32.

21. Mills, Paul K., et al. 1989. "Prospective Study of Exogenous Hormone Use and Breast Cancer in Seventh Day Adventists." *Cancer* 64: 591–97.

22. Bergkvist, L., et al. 1989. "The Risk of Breast Cancer after Estrogens and Estrogen-Progestin Replacement." *N Eng J Med* 321: 293–97.

23. Gambrell, R. Don. 1990. "Estrogen Therapy and Breast Cancer." *Int J Fertil* 35(4): 202–04.

24. Editorial. 1989. "Hormone Replacement Therapy and Cancer: Is There Cause for Concern?" *lanccet* 2: 368.

25. Gambrell. "Estrogen Therapy and Breast Cancer."

26. Persson, I., et al. 1992. "Combined Oestrogen-Progestogen Replacement and Breast Cancer Risk" (letter). *lanccet* 340: 1044.

27. Ewertz, Marianne. 1988. "Influence of Non-contraceptive Exogenous and Endogenous Sex Hormones on Breast Cancer Risk in Denmark." *Int J Cancer* 42: 832–38.

28. La Vecchia, C., et al. 1986. "Non-contraceptive Oestrogens and the Risk of Breast Cancer in Women." *Int J Cancer* 38: 853–58.

29. Hunt, Kate, et al. 1987. "Long-term Surveillance of Mortality and Cancer Incidence in Women Receiving Hormone Replacement Therapy." *Br J Obstet and Gynaecol* 94: 620–35.

30. Hunt, Kate, Martin Vessey, and Klim McPherson. 1990. "Mortality in a Cohort of Long-term Users of Hormone Replacement Therapy: An Updated Analysis." *Br J Obstet Gynaecol* 97: 1080–86.

31. Armstrong. "Oestrogen Therapy after Menopause."

32. Steinberg, Karen K., et al. 1991. "A Meta-analysis of the Effect of Estrogen Replacement Therapy on the Risk of Breast Cancer." *JAMA* 265: 1985–90.

33. Colditz, G. A., et al. 1992. "Type of Postmenopausal Hormone Use and Risk of Breast Cancer: 12-Year Follow-up from the Nurses' Health Study." *Cancer Causes and Control* 3: 433–439.

34. Colditz, G. A., K. M. Egan, and M. J. Stampfer. 1993. "Hormone Replacement Therapy and Risk of Breast Cancer: Results from Epidemiologic Studies." *Am J Obstet Gynecol* 168: 1473–80.

35. Stomper, Paul, et al. 1990. "Mammographic Changes Associated with Postmenopausal Hormone Replacement Therapy: A Longitudinal Study." *Radiology* 175: 487–90.

36. Cedars, Marcell, and Howard Judd. 1987. "Non-oral Routes of Estrogen Administration." *Obstet Gynecol Clin North Am* 14: 269–99.

37. Boston Collaborative Drug Surveillance Program. 1974. "Surgically Confirmed Gallbladder Disease, Venous Thromboembolism, and Breast Tumors in Relation to Postmenopausal Estrogen Therapy." *N Eng J Med* 290: 15–19.

38. Grady, D., et al. 1992. "Hormone Therapy to Prevent Disease and Prolong Life in Postmenopausal Women." *Ann Intern Med* 117: 1016–37.

39. Hartge, P., et al. 1988. "Menopause and Ovarian Cancer." *Am J Epidemiol* 127(5): 990–98.

40. Baber, R., and John Studd. 1989. "Hormone Replacement Therapy and Cancer." *Br J Hosp Med* 41: 142–49.

41. Wells, Robert. 1989. "Hormone Replacement before Menopause." *Postgrad Med* 86: 61–71.

42. Natchtigall, Lila, and Joan Heilman. 1986. *Estrogen: The Facts Can Change Your Life*. The Body Press, Los Angeles.

43. Metcalf, M. G. 1988. "The Approach of Menopause: A New Zealand Study." *NZ Med J* 101: 103–06.

44. Roeber, Johanna. "The Forever Therapy." *Vogue*, 1990: 172–73.

45. Gambrell. "Use of Progestogen Therapy."

46. Roeber. "The Forever Therapy."

47. Burgher, Harry. National Radio. 10 Aug. 1990.

48. "Ob-Gyn Urges Prudence in Prescribing ERT, Proposes Alternatives." *Medical World News*, 1984: 31–36.

49. Roeber. "The Forever Therapy."

50. Ibid.

11. The Business of Breasts

1. White, Emily, Chung Yul Lee, and Alar Kristal. 1990. "Evaluation of the Increase in Breast Cancer Incidence in Relation to Mammographic Use." *J Natl Cancer Inst* 82(19): 1546–52.

2. Wallis, Claudia. "A Puzzling Plague." *Time*, 14 Jan. 1991: 40–46.

3. Willett, Walter, et al. 1987. "Dietary Fat and the Risk of Breast Cancer." *N Eng J Med* 316: 22–28.

4. Kinlen, L. 1982. "Meat and Fat Consumption and Mortality: A Study of Strict Religious Orders in Britain." *Lancet* 1: 946–49.

5. Paul, Charlotte, D. Skegg, and G. Spears. 1989. "Depot-medrodroxyprogesterone (Depo Provera) and Risk of Breast Cancer." *BMJ* 299: 759–62.

6. Marshall, Betsy. 1987. "Breast Self-examination: Why the Debate?" Paper presented at the Cancer Early Detection Workshop, Public Health Association of Australia and the Cancer Society of New Zealand, Christchurch.

7. U.S. National Center for Health Statistics. 1991. *Health Promotion and Disease Prevention, United States 1990, Vital and Health Statistics*. Series 10, No. 185.

8. Hewitt, Harold. 1989. "Breast Screening: A Response to Dr. Maureen Roberts" (letter). *BMJ* 299: 1337.

9. Mitchell, Heather. 1987. "Organized Mammographic Screening Programmes, A Benign or Malignant Neglect." *Med J Aust* 146: 87–90.

10. Sands, Sarah. "Breast Screening Could Save 250 Lives a Year." *Christchurch Press*, 10 Oct. 1988.

11. Skegg, David. 1990. "Screening for Breast Cancer—Should We Be Using Mammography?" Presentation to Breast Cancer Seminar: Options for Mammography, Detection and Treatment. Fertility Action, Auckland.

12. Rodgers, Anthony. 1990. "The UK Breast Cancer Screening Programme: An Expensive Mistake." *J Pub Health Med* 12(3/4): 197–204.

13. Forrest, O. 1986. *Breast Cancer Screening*. Report to the health ministers of England, Wales, Scotland, and Northern Ireland, DHSS. HMSO, London.

14. Skegg. "Screening for Breast Cancer."

15. Shapiro, S. 1977. "Evidence on Breast Screening from a Randomised Trial." *Cancer* 39: 2772–82; Shapiro, S., et al. 1982. "Ten to Fourteen-Year Effect of Screening on Breast Cancer Mortality." *J Natl Cancer Inst* 69: 349–55.

16. Rodgers. "The UK Breast Cancer Screening Programme."

17. Tabar, L., and A. Gad. 1981. "Screening for Breast Cancer: The Swedish Trial." *Radiology* 138: 219–22; Tabar, L., et al. 1985. "Reduction in Mortality from Breast Cancer after Mass Screening with Mammography." *Lancet* 1: 829–32.

18. Andersson, I., et al. 1988. "Mammographic Screening and Mortality from Breast Cancer: The Malmo Mammographic Screening Trial." *BMJ* 297: 943–48.

19. Roberts, Maureen, et al. 1990. "Edinburgh Trial of Screening for Breast Cancer: Mortality at Seven Years." *lanccet* 335: 241–46.

20. Miller, A. B., et al. 1992. Canadian National Breast Screening Study, 1. "Breast Cancer Detection and Death Rates among Women Aged 40 to 49 Years." *Can Med Assoc J* 147: 1459–76.

21. Fletcher, S. W., et al. 1993. "Report of the International Workshop on Screening for Breast Cancer." *Journal of the National Cancer Institute* 85: 1644–56.

22. Skegg. "Screening for Breast Cancer."

23. Roberts. "Edinburgh Trial."

24. Ibid.

25. Bell, Glenys. "Breast Cancer: A Medical Scandal." *The Bulletin,* 30 May 1989: 44–54.

26. Vessey, Martin and Muir Gray. 1991. *Breast Cancer Screening 1991: Evidence and Experience since the Forrest Report.* NHS Breast Cancer Screening Programme, Sheffield.

27. Roberts, Maureen. 1989. "Breast Screening: Time for a Rethink?" *BMJ* 299: 1153–55.

28. Hirst, Cherrell, and John Kearsley. 1991. "Breast Cancer Screening: 'One Swallow Doth Not a Summer Make.'" *Med J Aust* 154: 76–78.

29. Richardson, Ann, Terence Doyle, and Mark Elwood. 1990. "Mammographic Screening for Breast Cancer: Beneficial for Women over 50." *Professional Bulletin,* Cancer Society of New Zealand, No. 3.

30. Rickard, Mary, et al. 1991. "Breast Cancer Diagnosis by Screening Mam-

mography: Early Results of the Central Sydney Area Health Service Breast X-ray Programme." *Med J Aust* 154: 126–31.

31. Chamberlain, Jocelyn. 1989. "An Insurance Policy to Reduce the Risk of Dying from Breast Cancer." *Clin Radiol* 40: 1–3.

32. Love, Susan M. 1990. *Dr. Susan Love's Breast Book*. Addison-Wesley, Reading, Mass.

33. Baker, L. 1982. "Breast Cancer Detection Demonstration Project: Five-Year Summary Report." *CA* 32(4): 194.

34. Day, Peter, and Michael O'Rourke. 1990. "The Diagnosis of Breast Cancer: A Clinical and Mammographic Comparison." *Med J Aust* 152: 635–39.

35. Love. *Dr. Susan Love's Breast Book.*

36. Alderson, Jeremy. "An Indecent Proposal." *Mother Jones,* May 1985: 52–56.

37. Kopans, D. B. 1989. *Breast Imaging.* Lippincott, Philadelphia.

38. Chamberlain. "An Insurance Policy."

39. Chamberlain, Jocelyn, 1989. "Breast Screening: A Response to Dr. Maureen Roberts" (letter). *BMJ* 299: 1336–37.

12. All About Cervixes

1. ARC Working Group on Evaluation of Cervical Cancer Screening Programmes. 1986. "Screening for Squamous Cervical Cancer: Duration of Low Risk after Negative Results of Cervical Cytology and Its Implications for Screening Policies." *BMJ* 293: 659–64.

2. Cartwright, Silvia. 1988. *The Report of the Cervical Cancer Inquiry.* Committee of Inquiry into Allegations Concerning the Treatment of Cervical Cancer at National Women's Hospital and into Other Related Matters, Auckland.

3. Cox, Brian. 1989. "The Epidemiology and Control of Cervical Cancer." Ph.D. thesis, University of Otago.

4. Grace, Victoria. 1985. "Factors Affecting the Response of Women to Cervical Screening." *NZ Family Physician* 12: 139–42.

5. Anonymous, 1985. "Cancer of the Cervix: Death by Incompetence." *lancet* 2: 363–64.

6. ARC Working Group. "Screening for Squamous Cervical Cancer"; Hakama, M. 1986. "Cervical Cancer: Risk Groups for Screening." In *Screening for Cancer of the Uterine Cervix,* ed. M. Hakama, A. Miller, and N. Day. International Agency for Research on Cancer, Lyon: 213–16; Silcocks, P. 1988. "Rapidly Progressing Cervical Cancer: Is It a Real Problem?" *Br J Obstet Gynaecol* 95: 1111–16.

7. ARC Working Group. "Screening for Squamos Cervical Cancer."

8. Ibid.

9. Hakama, M., and K. Louhivuori. 1988. "A Screening Programme for Cervical Cancer That Worked." *Cancer Surveys* 7(3): 403–16.

10. ARC Working Group. "Screening for Squamous Cervical Cancer."

11. Maclean, Allan, et al. 1985. "Cytology, Colposcopy and Cervical Neoplasia." *NZ Med J* 98: 756–58.

12. Miller, A. 1990. "Natural History of Cancer of the Cervix." Paper presented to UICC International Workshop on Cancer Screening, Cambridge, UK.

13. Ellman, R. 1990. "Indications for Colposcopy from a UK Viewpoint." Paper presented to UICC International Workshop on Cancer Screening, Cambridge, UK.

14. Ibid.

15. McIndoe, W., et al. 1984. "The Invasive Potential of Carcinoma In Situ of the Cervix." *Obstet Gynecol* 64: 451–58.

16. Fitzgerald, Norman. 1988. "Endocervical Cells, Adequate Smears and the Cytobrush." *NZ Family Physician* 15: 3–4.

17. Singer, Albert, and Anne Szarewski. 1988. *Cervical Smear Test: What Every Woman Should Know.* Macdonald Optima, London; Hakama. "Cervical Cancer."

18. Skegg, D., et al. 1982. "Importance of the Male Factor in Cancer of the Cervix." *Lancet* 2: 581–83.

19. Mitchell, Heather. 1990. "An Update on Human Papillomavirus Infection of the Cervix." *Aust Family Physician* 19(6): 887–93.

20. Ibid.

21. Sun-Kuie, Tay, Ho Tew-Hong, and Lim-Tan Soo-Kim. 1990. "Is Genital Human Papillomavirus Infection Always Sexually Transmitted?" *Aust NZ J Obstet Gynaecol* 30: 240–42.

22. Mitchell. "Update on Papillomavirus."

23. Chamberlain, J. 1986. "Reasons That Some Screening Programmes Fail to Control Cervical Cancer." In *Screening for Cancer of the Uterine Cervix,* ed. M. Hakama, A. Miller, and N. Day. International Agency for Research on Cancer, Lyon: 161–68.

24. Brock, K., et al. 1980. "Smoking and Infectious Agents and Risk of In Situ Cervical Cancer in Sydney, Australia." *Cancer Research* 49: 4925–28.

25. Hakama. "Cervical Cancer."

26. Chang, A. 1988. "How to Obtain an Optimal Cervical Smear." *Professional Bulletin,* Cancer Society of New Zealand, No. 2, 1988.

27. Singer, Albert, and David Jenkins. 1991. "Viruses and Cervical Cancer." *BMJ* 302: 251–52.

28. Mitchell. "Update on Papillomavirus."

29. Ibid.

30. Paul, Charlotte, et al. 1991. "1991 Cervical Screening Recommendations: A Working Group Report." *NZ Med J* (in press).

31. McCafferty, John, Carol Green, and Chris Miller. 1989. "Cervical Cytology in a Community Laboratory." *NZ Med J* 102: 316–17.

32. Paul. "1991 Cervical Screening Recommendations."

33. Posner, T., and M. Vessey. 1988. *Prevention of Cervical Cancer: The Patient's View.* King Edward's Hospital Fund for London, King's Fund Publishing Office, London.

34. Campion, M. J., et. al. 1988. "Psychosexual Trauma of an Abnormal Cervical Smear." *Br J Obstet and Gynaecol* 95: 175–81.

35. Chang. "How to Obtain an Optimal Cervical Smear."

36. Chamberlain. "Reasons Some Screening Programmes Fail."

37. Ellman. "Indications for Colposcopy."

13. Final Thoughts

1. Thomas, Lewis. 1975. "Notes of a Biology-Watcher: The Health-Care System." *N Eng J Med* 293(24): 1245–47.

2. Burkman, Ronald. 1990. "Discussion, Following "Evaluation of a Continuous Combined Low-dose Regimen of Estrogen-Progestin for Treatment of the Menopausal Patient, by Louis Weinstein, Chhandra Bewtra and J. Chris Gallagher." *Am J Obstet Gynecol* 162: 1534–42.

3. Notelovitz, Morris. 1989. "Estrogen in Postmenopausal Women: An Opposing View." *J Fam Prac* 29(4): 410–15.

Selected Bibliography

This bibliography contains a selection of the most useful texts under subject headings. The works listed here primarily provide an overview or review of the topic. Other works consulted are listed under the references given for each chapter.

Ethical and Political Issues

Doyal, Lesley. 1979. *The Political Economy of Health.* Pluto Press, London.

Ehrenreich, John (ed.). 1978. *The Cultural Crisis of Modern Medicine.* Monthly Review Press, New York.

Illich, Ivan. 1976. *Limits to Medicine.* Marion Boyars, London.

Kawachi, Ichiro. 1990. *Pharmaceutical Advertising and Promotion—Options for Action.* Public Health Association of New Zealand, Wellington.

Kennedy, Ian. 1981. *The Unmasking of Medicine.* Allen and Unwin, London.

Silverman, Milton, and Philip Lee. 1974. *Pills, Profits and Politics.* University of California Press, Berkeley.

Taylor, Richard. 1979. *Medicine Out of Control.* Sun Books, Melbourne.

World Health Organisation. 1988. *The World Drug Situation.* World Health Organization, Geneva.

Papers

Adams, Stanley. 1985. "World Drugs and Profit Addiction." *New Scientist,* 23 May: 34–37.

Barsky, Arthur. 1988. "The Paradox of Health." *New Eng J Med* 318: 414–18.

O'Hagan, John. 1991. "The Ethics of Informed Consent in Relation to Prevention Screening Programmes." *NZ Med J* 104: 122–25.

Robertson, Ann. 1990. "The Politics of Alzheimer's Disease: A Case Study in Apocalyptic Demography." *Int Health Sciences* 20(3): 429–42.

Rose, Geoffrey, 1990. "Reflections on Changing Times." *BMJ* 301: 683–87.

Thomas, Lewis. 1975. "The Health-Care System." *New Eng J Med* 293(24): 1245–47.

Osteoporosis

Notelovitz, Morris, and Marsha Wane. 1985. *Stand Tall! Every Woman's Guide to Preventing Osteoporosis.* Bantam Books, Toronto.

Working Party on Osteoporosis Prevention. 1991. *Report of the Working Party on Osteoporosis Prevention.* Department of Health, Wellington.

Papers

Campbell, A. J. 1989. "Epidemiology and Prevention of Proximal Femur Fractures." *Patient Management,* March: 13–26.

Campbell, A. J. 1990. "Falls, Fractures and Drugs." *NZ Med J* 103: 580–81.

Cummings, Steven, et al. 1985. "Epidemiology of Osteoporosis and Osteoporotic Fractures." *Epidemiologic Reviews* 7: 178–208.

Johnston, C. Conrad, et al. 1989. "Clinical Indications for Bone Mass Measurements: A Report of the Scientific Advisory Board of the National Osteoporosis Foundation." *Bone Miner Res* 4 (Suppl. 2): 1–28.

Melton, L. Joseph, David Eddy, and C. Conrad Johnston. 1990. "Screening for Osteoporosis." *Ann Int Med* 112: 516–28.

Rutherford, Olga, 1990. "The Role of Exercise in Prevention of Osteoporosis." *Physiotherapy* 76(9): 522–26.

Sinaki, Mehrsheed. 1989. "Exercise and Osteoporosis." *Arch Phys Med Rehabil* 70: 22–29.

Stevenson, John. 1990. "Pathogenesis, Prevention and Treatment of Osteoporosis." *Obstet Gynecol* 75: 36S–41S.

Menopause and Aging

Doress-Worters, Paula, and Diana Siegal. 1994. *The New Ourselves Growing Older.* Simon & Schuster, New York.

Llewellyn-Jones, Derek, and Suzanne Abraham. 1988. *Menopause.* Penguin, Ringwood, Victoria.

Ojeda, Linda. 1992. Menopause Without Medicine. Hunter House, Alameda, Calif.

Potter, Leteia.1991. *Women in Mid-Life.* New Women's Press, Auckland.

Reitz, Rosetta. 1985. *Menopause: A Positive Approach.* Viking Penguin, New York.

Society for Research on Women in New Zealand. 1988. *The Time of Our Lives: A Study of Mid-Life Women.* Christchurch Branch of the Society for Research on Women, Christchurch.

Weideger, Paula. 1978. *Female Cycles.* The Women's Press, London.

Papers

Bungay, G., M. Vessey, and C. McPherson. 1980. "Study of Symptoms in Middle Life with Special Reference to the Menopause." *BMJ* 181: 181–84.

Flint, Marcha. 1975. "The Menopause: Reward or Punishment?" *Psychosomatics* 16: 161–63.

Gath, Dennis, and Susan Iles. 1990. "Depression and the Menopause." *BMJ* 300: 1287–88.

Hunter, Myra, Rosie Batterby, and Malcolm Whitehead. 1986. "Relationship between Psychological Symptoms, Somatic Complaints and Menopausal Status." *Maturitas* 8: 217–28.

Kaufert, Patricia. 1982. "Anthropology and the Menopause: The Development of a Theoretical Framework." *Maturitas* 4: 181–93.

Kaufert, Patricia. 1982. "Myth and the Menopause." *Sociology of Health and Illness* 4(2): 141–66.

Kaufert, Patricia, and John Syrotiuk. 1981. "Symptom Reporting at the Menopause." *Soc Sci Med* 15E: 173–84.

Kaufert, Patricia, and Penny Gilbert. 1986. "Women, Menopause and Medicalisation." *Culture, Medicine and Psychiatry* 10: 7–21.

Leiblum, Sandra, and Leora Swartzman. 1986. "Women's Attitudes towards Menopause." *Maturitas* 8: 47–56.

McCrea, Frances. 1983. "The Politics of Menopause: The 'Discovery' of a Deficiency Disease." *Social Problems* 31(1): 23.

McKinlay, Sonja, and John McKinlay. 1973. "Selected Studies of the Menopause." *Journal of Biosocial Science* 5: 533–55.

Ravnikar, Veronica. 1990. "Physiology and Treatment of Hot Flushes." *Obstet Gynecol* 75(4) Suppl.: 3S–8S.

Youngs, David. 1990. "Some Misconceptions Concerning the Menopause." *Obstet Gynecol* 75(5): 881–83.

Hormone Replacement Therapy

Seaman, Barbara, and Gideon Seaman. 1977. *Women and the Crisis in Sex Hormones*. Bantam Books, New York.

Greenblatt, Robert (ed.). 1986. *A Modern Approach to the Perimenopausal Years*. De Gruyter, Berlin, New York.

Kaufert, Patricia, and Sonja McKinlay. 1985. "Estrogen-Replacement Therapy: The production of Medical Knowledge and the Emergence of Policy." In *Women, Health and Healing,* ed. Ellen Lewin and Virginia Olesen. Tavistock Press, London.

National Women's Health Network, 1989. *Taking Hormones and Women's Health: Choices, Risks and Benefits*. NWHN, Washington, D.C.

Papers

Corson, Stephen. 1989. "Impact of Estrogen Replacement Therapy on Cardiovascular Risk." *J Repro Med* 34(9) Suppl.: 729–43.

Hulka, Barbara. 1990. "Hormone-Replacement Therapy and the Risk of Breast Cancer." *CA* 40(5): 289–96.

Hunt, Kate, and Martin Vessey. 1987. "Long-term Effects of Postmenopausal Hormone Therapy." *Br Hosp Med* Nov.: 450–60.

Lindsay, Robert. 1987. "Estrogen Therapy in the Prevention and Management of Osteoporosis." *Am Obstet Gynecol* 156(5): 1347–51.

Lobo, Rogerio. 1990. "Cardiovascular Implications of Estrogen Replacement Therapy." *Obstet Gynecol* 75: 18S–25S.

Whitehead, Malcolm, T. Hillard, and D. Crook. 1990. "The Role and Use of Progestogens." *Obstet Gynecol* 75: 59S–75S.

Hysterectomy

Coney, Sandra, and Lyn Potter. 1990. *Hysterectomy.* Heinemann Reed, Auckland.

Breast cancer and Mammography

Australian Health Ministers' Advisory Council and Breast Cancer Screening Evaluation Steering Committee. 1990. *Breast Cancer Screening in Australia: Future Directions.* Australian Institute of Health, Canberra.

Dyson, Linda. 1989. *Breast Cancer.* Heinemann Reed, Auckland.

Love, Susan. 1990. *Dr. Susan Love's Breast Book.* Addison-Wesley, Reading, Mass.

Vessey, Martin, and Muir Gray. 1991. *Breast Cancer Screening 1991: Evidence and Experience since the Forrest Report.* NHS Breast Screening Programme, Sheffield.

Papers

Cancer Society of New Zealand. 1989. "Cancer Society Policy on Breast Self-Examination for Women."

Chamberlain, Jocelyn. 1989. "An Insurance Policy to Reduce the Risk of Dying from Breast Cancer." *Clinical Radiology* 40: 1–3.

Richardson, Ann, Terence Doyle, and Mark Elwood. 1990. "Mammographic Screening for Breast Cancer: Beneficial for Women over 50." *Professional Bulletin,* Cancer Society of New Zealand, No. 3.

Roberts, M. Maureen, 1989. "Breast Screening: Time for a Rethink." *BMJ* 299: 1153–55.

Rodgers, Anthony. 1990. "The UK Breast Cancer Screening Programme: An Expensive Mistake." *Pub Health Med* 12(3/4): 197–204.

Skegg, D., et al. 1988. "Mammographic Screening for Breast Cancer: Prospects for New Zealand." *NZ Med J* 101: 531–33.

Willett, Walter. 1989. "The Search for the Causes of Breast and Colon Cancer." *Nature* 338: 389–94.

Cervical Screening and Cervical Cancer

Expert Group and Department of Health. 1991. *Policy of National Cervical Screening Programme.* Department of Health, Wellington (in press).

Singer, Albert, and Anne Szarewski. 1988. *Cervical Smear Test: What Every Woman Should Know.* MacDonald Optima, London.

Dyson, Linda. 1986. *Cervical Cancer.* Reed Methuen, Auckland.

Hakama, M., A. Miller and N. Day. 1986. *Screening for Cancer of the Uterine Cervix.* International Agency for Research on Cancer, Lyon.

Papers

Bonita, Ruth, and Charlotte Paul. 1991. "The Extent of Cervical Cancer Screening in New Zealand Women 1990." *NZ Med J* (in press).

Cox, Brian, and D. Skegg. 1986. "Trends in Cervical Cancer in New Zealand." *NZ Med J* 99: 795–98.

ARC Working Group on Evaluation of Cervical Cancer Screening Programmes. 1986. "Screening for Squamous Cervical Cancer: Duration of Low Risk after Negative Results of Cervical Cytology and Its Implications for Screening Policies." *BMJ* 293: 659–64.

Mitchell, Heather. 1990. "An Update on Human Papillomavirus Infection of the Cervix." *Aust Fam Phys* 19(6): 887–93.

Paul, Charlotte, et al. 1991. "1991 Cervical Screening Recommendations: A Working Group Report." *NZ Med J* (in press).

Singer, Albert, and David Jenkins. 1991. "Viruses and Cervical Cancer." *BMJ* 302: 251–52.

Index

G

Gall bladder, 5
Genitals, 72, 76, 101–102

H

Hair, 73, 76, 245
Heart disease *see* Coronary heart disease
Hormone replacement therapy, 14,
    23, 27, 32, 61, 75, 76, 77–80,
    98, 127–128, 152, 153, 160,
    182–271
  see also Estrogen therapy *and* Pro-
    gestogen
  after hysterectomy, 225
  after surgical menopause, 225
  and class, 190, 225–226
  and coronary heart disease *see*
    Coronary heart disease
  domino effect of, 228
  effect on: appearance, 200, 236;
    depression, 226, 227; hair, 231,
    233–234; heart *see* Coronary
    heart disease; hot flashes, 200,
    228–229; menopausal symp-
    toms, 220–222; osteoporosis,
    200; psychological symptoms,
    230–232; sexual libido, 229–
    230; vaginal dryness, 200, 229–
    230; well-being, 228, 231–233
  ethics of, 207–109
  forms of therapy: cream, 222–
    223; gel, 223; implants, 221–
    222; oral, 220; transdermal
    (patches), 220–221
  history of, 9, 61, 74–76, 182–211
  long-term use, 228, 242–243,
    265, 270–271
  marketing and promotion, 127–
    128, 182–211
  and osteoporosis, 152, 153, 160,
    201–204, 235–243
  patches—see Hormone replace-
    ment therapy—forms of ther-
    apy—transdermal

premenopausal use, 269–270
  profile of users, 210
  research, 201–204, 212–214, 238–
    239, 240; PEPI study, 212
  placebo effect, 226, 227
  risks, 262–267; breast cancer, 262–
    267; cardiovascular *see* Coro-
    nary heart disease; dilatation
    and curettage, 253; endometrial
    cancer *see* Estrogen therapy *and*
    Progestogen; gall bladder dis-
    ease, 267–268; hysterectomy,
    225, 253; liver, 267–268
  side effects: abnormal bleeding,
    31, 253; bleeding, 218, 249,
    252–253; bloating, 254; nau-
    sea, 254; premenstrual syn-
    drome, 253; sore breasts, 254;
    weight gain, 254
  and smoking, 168, 268, 269
  and stroke, 268
  and thrombosis, 268, 269
  types of therapy: continuous com-
    bined, 214, 217–218; Marvelon
    see Marvelon; estrogen only *see*
    Estrogen; opposed therapy, *see*
    also Progestogen, 214, 216
  unopposed therapy *see* Estrogen
  women's attitudes to, 228, 231–
    233
Hormone tests for menopause, 270
Hormones, function of, 100–102,
    134–135
Hot flashes and night sweats, 34, 64–
    66, 88, 96, 103, 105–108, 200,
    226, 228, 229
Human Papilloma Virus (HPV),
    314–317, 320–321
Hysterectomy, 159, 225, 253
  see also Hormone replacement ther-
    apy—risks—hysterectomy *and*
    Menopause—after hysterec-
    tomy *and* Cervical smears—af-
    ter hysterectomy *and*
    Osteoporosis—risk factors—
    hysterectomy

W

MENOPAUSE WITHOUT MEDICINE
by Linda Ojeda, Ph.D.

This is a book for women of all ages. The revised second edition provides comprehensive guidelines on holistic, natural ways to prepare for menopause and effectively treat major menopausal complaints.

Part One explains the causes of common menopausal symptoms—insomnia, hot flashes, fatigue, osteoporosis—and natural ways to treat them.

Part Two is about aging gracefully and the impact personal appearance, sexuality, and energy level can have on your overall well-being.

Part Three emphasizes good lifestyle habits, which can make the difference between a carefree menopause and a difficult one.

This edition is completely updated with the latest research on nutrition, exercises, and osteoporosis—including good news about the body's ability to rebuild bone late in life. A completely new chapter on breast cancer describes risk factors, possible environmental causes, and the important role that dietary changes can play in beating cancer.

The book debunks many myths, and shows that life—healthy, energetic, and vibrant—can begin again at menopause.

> "Ojeda packs the book with appendixes, charts . . . and suggested resources. These, combined with the accessible, reassuring, and *female* tone of her writing, make this a very useful resource." — *BOOKLIST*

> "Dr. Linda Ojeda has written a book that should be read by any woman concerned with planning for the future . . . . MENOPAUSE WITHOUT MEDICINE could be described as a 'wellness bible.' It really gives women an overall picture of their bodies and how to keep [them] running to optimum proficiency. As menstruation is the beginning of a woman's reproductive cycle; menopause should be seen as the culmination, not the bitter ending." — *WHOLE LIFE TIMES*

Linda Ojeda, Ph.D., is a nutritional consultant and a frequent lecturer at fitness resorts and health clubs. Her first book, *Exclusively Female* (1983), pioneered the nutritional approach to PMS and other menstrual disorders. Her latest book is *Safe Dieting for Teens* (1992).

304 pages ... Paperback ... $12.95 ... Second edition

Prices subject to change . . . to order please see last page

Women's Health & Sexuality

SEXUAL PLEASURE: Reaching New Heights of Sexual Arousal and Intimacy *by* Barbara Keesling, Ph.D.

This book is for all people who are interested in enhancing their sex lives and developing their sensual awareness. A series of graduated exercises reveal the three secrets of sexual pleasure: enjoying touching, enjoying being touched, and merging touching and feeling as an ecstatic experience. Sensual photographs add a note of artistic intimacy and make this book the perfect personal gift for caring partners.

288 pages ... 14 illus ... Paperback $12.95 ... Hardcover $21.95

THE *NEW* A-TO-Z OF WOMEN'S HEALTH *by* Christine Ammer

An up-to-date work that covers all aspects of women's health with over 1000 expert entries. A cross-reference system and subject guide make it easy to use for women and professionals. It discusses timely and important women's health topics, including: drugs, medication, fitness, and vitamins • cholesterol and diet • chronic disease, disabilities, and surgery.

> "The coverage is more extensive than that of *The New Our Bodies, Ourselves* and more current than that of Felicia Stewart's *Understanding Your Body*." — *BOOKLIST*

496 pages ... 10 illus ... Paperback ... $18.95

THE A-TO-Z OF WOMEN'S SEXUALITY *by* Ada P. Kahn and Linda Hughey Holt, M.D.

This sensitively written book presents detailed information on women's sexuality. With over 2000 alphabetically arranged, cross-referenced entries on: sexual fears and disorders • symptoms and complications of STDs, including AIDS, PID, and chlamydia • female and male sexual response cycles • gynecological tests, medications, and contraception methods.

368 pages ... 19 illus ... Paperback ... $14.95

THE A-TO-Z OF PREGNANCY AND CHILDBIRTH *by* Nancy Evans

This book is the perfect gift for expectant parents, answering questions and offering insights into the medical issues and special language surrounding pregnancy and childbirth. Topics include: infertility treatments and reproductive technology • breastfeeding and its effects on mother and baby • the controversy over home vs. hospital births. *Includes a special pull-out illustrated chart that tracks monthly fetal and maternal development.*

416 pages ... 16 illus ... Paperback $16.95 ... Hardcover $29.95

Order all three A-to-Z books for a special price — $34.95
Call toll-free at 1-800-266-5592 to order

ORDER FORM

10% DISCOUNT on orders of $20 or more —
20% DISCOUNT on orders of $50 or more —
30% DISCOUNT on orders of $250 or more —
On cost of books for fully prepaid orders

NAME

ADDRESS

CITY/STATE   ZIP/POSTCODE

PHONE   COUNTRY (outside U.S.)

TITLE	QTY	PRICE	TOTAL
A-to-Z of Pregnancy & Birth *(paperback)*	@	$ 16.95	
A-to-Z of Women's Health *(paperback)*	@	$ 18.95	
A-to-Z of Women's Sexuality *(paperback)*	@	$ 14.95	
Special: **All 3 A-to-Z books** *(paperback)*	@	**$ 34.95**	
Breast Implants	@	$ 7.95	
How Women Can *Finally* Stop Smoking	@	$ 8.95	
The Menopause Industry *(paperback)*	@	$ 14.95	
The Menopause Industry *(hardcover)*	@	$ 24.95	
Menopause Without Medicine	@	$ 12.95	
Running on Empty *(paper/hardcover)*	@	$	
Sexual Pleasure *(paper/hardcover)*	@	$	
Women's Cancers *(paper/hardcover)*	@	$	

Shipping costs:		
First book: $2.50 *($6.00 outside U.S.)*	TOTAL	
	Less discount @_____%	( )
Each additional book: *$.75 ($3.00 outside U.S.)*	TOTAL COST OF BOOKS	
	Calif. residents add sales tax	
For UPS rates and bulk orders call us at (510) 865-5282	Shipping & handling	
	TOTAL ENCLOSED	
	Please pay in U.S. funds only	

☐ Check   ☐ Money Order   ☐ Visa   ☐ M/C

Card # _____ Exp date _____

Signature _____

Complete and mail to:

Hunter House Inc., Publishers

P.O. Box 2914, Alameda CA 94501-0914

Orders: 1-800-266-5592

Phone (510) 865-5282 Fax (510) 865-4295

☐ Check here to receive our FREE book catalog

MPI 06/94